Supporting a Physiologic Approach to Pregnancy and Birth

The optimal role of the attendant—whether physician or midwife—is to be vigilant without being meddlesome.

R. A. Rosenblatt, MD

Supporting a Physiologic Approach to Pregnancy and Birth

A Practical Guide

Edited by

Melissa D. Avery, PhD, CNM, FACNM, FAAN

Professor
Chair, Child and Family Health Co-operative
University of Minnesota, School of Nursing
Minneapolis, Minnesota

WILEY-BLACKWELL

A John Wiley & Sons, Inc., Publication

Editorial Offices
2121 State Avenue, Ames, Iowa 50014-8300, USA
The Atrium, Southern Gate, Chichester, West Sussex, PO19 8SQ, UK
9600 Garsington Road, Oxford, OX4 2DQ, UK

For details of our global editorial offices, for customer services and for information about how to apply for permission to reuse the copyright material in this book please see our website at www.wiley.com/wiley-blackwell.

Library of Congress Cataloging-in-Publication Data is available upon request.

A catalogue record for this book is available from the British Library.

Cover design by Matt Kuhns

Set in 10/12.5pt Times by SPi Publisher Services, Pondicherry, India

1   2013

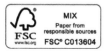

Dedication

To the women—for allowing us the privilege of being present with them during their special time.

And to my husband—Randy Schnoes—who is always there for me.

Contents

Contributors   ix
Foreword by *Holly Powell Kennedy*   xi
Acknowledgments   xiii

Section 1   Understanding a physiologic approach   **1**

1   The case for a physiologic approach to birth: An overview   3
Melissa D. Avery

2   The physiology of pregnancy, labor, and birth   13
Cindy M. Anderson

3   A supportive approach to prenatal care   29
Carrie E. Neerland

4   Supporting a physiologic approach to labor and birth   49
Lisa Kane Low and Rebeca Barroso

Section 2   Interventions and approaches   **77**

5   Promoting comfort: A conceptual approach   79
Kerri D. Schuiling

6   Continuous labor support   91
Carrie E. Neerland

7   Techniques to promote relaxation in labor   105
Kathryn Leggitt

8   Touch therapies in pregnancy and childbirth   119
Deborah Ringdahl

9   Water immersion for labor and birth   157
Michelle R. Collins and Dawn M. Dahlgren-Roemmich

10   Aromatherapy in pregnancy and childbirth   173
Linda L. Halcón

11   Acupressure and acupuncture in pregnancy and childbirth   197
Katie Moriarty and Kennedy Sharp

**Section 3   Organizational approaches to supporting physiologic
pregnancy and birth**   227

12   Rethinking care on the hospital labor unit   229
     Emily Higdon, Rachel Woodard, Kristin Rood and Heidi Jean Bernard

13   Out-of-hospital birth   251
     Marsha E. Jackson and Alice Bailes

14   Educating health professionals for collaborative
     practice in support of normal birth   275
     Melissa D. Avery, John C. Jennings and Michelle L. O'Brien

15   Women's health and maternity care policies: Current
     status and recommendations for change   301
     Heather M. Bradford

Resources for physiologic pregnancy and childbirth   331
Index   335

Contributors

Cindy M. Anderson, PhD, RN, WHNP-BC, FAAN
Associate Professor
Department of Nursing
College of Nursing and Professional Disciplines
University of North Dakota
Grand Forks, North Dakota

Melissa D. Avery, PhD, CNM, FACNM, FAAN
Professor
Chair, Child and Family Health Co-operative Unit
Director, Nurse-Midwifery Program
School of Nursing
University of Minnesota
Minneapolis, Minnesota

Alice Bailes, CNM, MSN, FACNM
Co-Founder
Birth Care and Women's Health
Alexandria, Virginia

Rebeca Barroso, DNP, CNM
Faculty, Frontier Nursing University
Staff Nurse-Midwife
HealthEast Nurse-Midwives
St. Paul, Minnesota

Heidi Jean Bernard, RN, ADN
Staff Nurse
Department of Labor and Delivery
University of Iowa Hospitals and Clinics
Iowa City, Iowa

Heather M. Bradford, MSN, CNM, ARNP, FACNM
Certified Nurse-Midwife
Evergreen Health Midwifery Care
Kirkland, Washington
Affiliate Faculty
Department of Family and Child Nursing
University of Washington
Seattle, Washington

Michelle R. Collins, PhD, CNM
Associate Professor of Nursing
Director, Nurse-Midwifery Program
Vanderbilt University School of Nursing
Nashville, Tennessee

Dawn M. Dahlgren-Roemmich, MS, CNM
Certified Nurse-Midwife
Jordan, Minnesota

Linda L. Halcón, PhD, MPH, RN
Associate Professor
School of Nursing
University of Minnesota
Minneapolis, Minnesota

Emily Higdon, RN, MSN
PhD Student and Jonas Scholar
Staff Nurse
Department of Labor and Delivery
University of Iowa Hospitals and Clinics
Iowa City, Iowa

Marsha E. Jackson, CNM, MSN, FACNM
Director and Co-Founder
Birth Care and Women's Health
Alexandria, Virginia

John C. Jennings, MD
Professor of Obstetrics and Gynecology
Texas Tech University Health Sciences
Odessa, Texas

Kathryn Leggitt, MS, CNM
Certified Nurse-Midwife
Hennepin County Medical Center
Minneapolis, Minnesota

Lisa Kane Low, PhD, CNM, FACNM
Assistant Professor and Director
Nurse-Midwifery Education Program
School of Nursing and Women's Studies
Department
University of Michigan
Ann Arbor, Michigan

Katie Moriarty, PhD, CNM, CAFCI, RN
Clinical Assistant Professor
Associate Director Nurse-Midwifery
Education Program
School of Nursing
University of Michigan
Ann Arbor, Michigan
Certified Acupuncture Foundation of
Canada Institute

Carrie E. Neerland, MS, CNM
Certified Nurse-Midwife
Women's Health Specialists
University of Minnesota Physicians
Adjunct Faculty
University of Minnesota School of
Nursing
University of Minnesota Medical School
Minneapolis, Minnesota

Michelle L. O'Brien, MD, MPH, IBCLC
Adjunct Faculty
Assistant Professor
Department of Family Medicine and
Community Health
University of Minnesota Medical School
Minneapolis, Minnesota

Deborah Ringdahl, DNP, RN, CNM
Reiki Master
Clinical Assistant Professor
School of Nursing
University of Minnesota
Minneapolis, Minnesota

Kristin Rood, RN
Maternal and Infant Staff Nurse
Children and Women's Services Division
University of Iowa Hospitals and Clinics
Iowa City, Iowa

Kennedy Sharp
Licensed Acupuncturist
Masters in Oriental Medicine
NCCAOM Certified
sharpacupuncture.com
Minneapolis, Minnesota

Kerri D. Schuiling, PhD, CNM, FACNM, FAAN
Dean
School of Nursing
Oakland University
Rochester, Michigan

Rachel Woodard, RN, BSN, RNC-OB
Obstetrical Nurse Specialist
Staff Nurse Labor and Delivery
Departments of Pediatrics and Nursing
University of Iowa Hospitals and Clinics
Iowa City, Iowa

Foreword

Birth is an event that carries our universe into the future. Each pregnancy and birth holds the promise of fresh life, renewed faith in our survival, and awe at the magnificence of human reproduction and the power of woman. Every birth is unique and every birth changes the person fortunate enough to witness the emergence of a new life.

Melissa Avery has brought together midwives, nurses, physicians, and other health practitioners in a collective, in-depth discussion of how to support a woman's physiologic capacity to carry and birth her child. This long overdue book is founded on the premise that pregnancy and birth are normal physiologic processes. It takes a direction often missing in traditional texts—that birth is more than simple mechanical, physical processes that can be inherently controlled. Rather, it acknowledges that although there is much we fully understand, there is still much to be learned. Thus, she and her colleagues have expertly woven current scientific evidence and theory with practical clinical expertise for helping women and their families during this life-producing and life-changing event.

The first section grounds the reader in a woman's physiology during pregnancy and birth. Avery starts the section off with a "real-life" scenario that clinicians who attend birth are often faced with each day. This is followed by an exquisite description of the physiologic intricacies of pregnancy and parturition that leaves us breathless in its detail and design and sets the stage for understanding how it all works. Prenatal care is emphasized as the place to work with the woman to establish her confidence in her body and its capabilities. The section closes with a stunning overview of how to keep the woman and her needs central during childbirth. The authors review the evidence on routine maternity care practices that can disrupt normal labor and birth and describe approaches to care that provide step-by-step support of a woman's physiology. Taken together, these four chapters provide the essential elements of the book and lay the underpinning for the following sections, which explore specific techniques and policy.

The second section provides an overview of specific strategies in caring for childbearing women. Different theories and evidence for care strategies are presented, always returning to why and how they support normal physiologic birth. The section begins with an introduction to the theories of "comfort," helping the reader understand how to meet each woman at the intersection of her life and her perception of pain and discomfort. The complexity of labor pain is disentangled through creative descriptions of pain modulation through the release of naturally occurring neuropeptides. The theoretical basis of comfort is extended by presence—the act by which the labor attendant creates a space in which the woman feels safe and thus her body's physiology is supported to do the work of labor. Techniques of relaxation, healing touch, therapeutic use of water, aromatherapy, and acupressure/acupuncture round out the section. Each of the topics is carefully reviewed for current evidence and practical application. The end result of this portion of the book reveals the art and healing science of supporting physiologic birth.

The final section provides a welcome and practical discussion of the realities of change in childbearing care. Since childbirth moved into the hospital it has been regimented to institutional routines not always rooted in evidence. Although these routines were established in good faith and believed to be best for the mother and infant, that was not always the case. Over time routines became so conventional that changing them seemed insurmountable. The section begins by helping us rethink how care is provided in the hospital, where most women in the United States give birth. The challenges of creating a safe environment for the laboring woman within an institutional setting are creatively presented through case studies, principles from major advocacy organizations, and systematically decreasing the use of routine interventions. Complementary to the chapter on hospital birth is a thoughtful presentation on out-of-hospital birth. Both chapters discuss the essential desire of women to be respected for their needs during labor and birth and the right to make decisions about where and how they birth. The authors challenge the idea that medicine is the final word in health care and place the woman at the center of care and as the director. They propose that this change of roles might actually enhance the woman' s physiologic ability to birth. These are hefty sea changes in how we think about the roles of providers and the women for whom they care. Avery, Jennings, and O' Brien emphasize the need for careful nurturing of the professions' young through interdisciplinary education in order to bring these changes about. By exploring issues together during the formative years of their professional identities, nurses, midwives, and physicians can learn together how to best work "with woman" during this profound moment of her life. The book closes by describing the need for policy to undergird the changes needed to best support women—through legislation, regulation, and institutional transformation.

If every clinician and institution that provides care to childbearing women instituted the recommendations in *Supporting a Physiologic Approach to Pregnancy and Birth*, we could truly see change in how women birth in the United States—and I believe improved outcomes. Perhaps the most important message in this book is the blending of our understanding of human birth physiology with human caring. In *Proust Was a Neuroscientist* (Houghton Mifflin, 2007), Jonah Lehrer explored the relationship of artists with concepts in neuroscience, noting, "scientists describe our brain in terms of its physical details . . . what science forgets is that this isn't how we experience the world" (p. x)—artists help us to understand how the world is perceived and lived. Avery and her colleagues help us understand both the science and the art of supporting women' s physiology, how that can actually make birth safer, and how artful presence and caring approaches enhance the woman' s experience and create a powerful mother and healthy child and family in the process. This book is a passage to the future in childbearing care.

Holly Powell Kennedy, PhD, CNM, FACNM, FAAN
Helen Varney Professor of Midwifery
Yale University
January 1, 2013

Acknowledgments

This book would not have been possible without the dedication and hard work of each and every chapter author. Thank you so much for your contributions in providing the background information and practical advice to help maternity care clinicians in their efforts to promote a physiologic approach to pregnancy and childbirth. We have included the physiologic underpinnings, the normal aspects of pregnancy and labor care, multiple integrative therapies, and a focus on the care system including interprofessional education and policy. A special thank you to Deborah Ringdahl, DNP, RN, CNM. In addition to writing a wonderful chapter on touch therapies in pregnancy, her review of multiple chapters and advice on other aspects of the book were immensely helpful. Thank you to Lisa Summers, DrPH, CNM, FACNM, and Joanna King, JD, for their valuable contributions to the policy chapter.

Chapters on acupuncture and acupressure and touch therapies include photographs providing illustrations of the techniques described in the text. We thank Melissa Jackson, Aimee Flood, Beth Kuzma, and Lily Crutchfield for serving as models and helping bring the techniques to life. My research assistant, Colleen Quesnell, reviewed many sections and helped with so many other necessary details that are not evident in the final polished product. A special thanks to Kathe Grooms for expert advice along the way.

For more than three decades as a nurse and midwife, I have had the privilege of working with so many nurses, physicians, midwives, and others that have influenced my day-to-day work as well as broader career trajectory. The faculty and staff at the University of Minnesota, School of Nursing, and the students I have had the pleasure of teaching over the years deserve special thanks for their ongoing support.

Finally, my deepest gratitude to my daughter, Helen Avery Schnoes. Her helpful suggestions as a talented writer and her encouragement were invaluable all along the journey.

Section 1

Understanding a physiologic approach

Chapter 1

The case for a physiologic approach to birth: An overview

Melissa D. Avery

Childbirth is normal until proven otherwise.

Peggy Vincent

Picture yourself at a neighborhood clinic on a typical weekday. You are conducting a health care visit with a woman as her prenatal care provider; she is 32 weeks pregnant. You ask how she has been feeling—she is fine. Her fundal height is 33 cm, the baby feels vertex, fetal heart tones are 134 beats per minute, a 2-pound weight gain since her last visit. No, she has not experienced any bleeding or headaches, no contractions. Yes, she started prenatal classes this week and the instructor reviewed the signs of early labor. Transition to the hospital. You're the nurse admitting a woman in labor to the birthing room with the bed centrally located, the fetal monitor in an attractive wood cabinet next to the bed. You ask when her contractions began, the current frequency and duration, and if her baby has been moving. Her membranes are intact, vital signs are normal, fetal heart rate 148. While you turn down the bedcovers, she changes into a hospital gown and asks if water birth is possible; she read about it on a pregnancy website and thought it might be a nice option.

On the face of it, the daily experiences of many maternity care clinicians and the women we care for seem pretty normal, routine, and positive to a degree. We talk about pregnancy as a normal life process, yet women enter our care system where problems are anticipated rather than emphasizing the normalcy of pregnancy. The number and frequency of technological interventions continue to increase while the outcomes of care have worsened, with some recent abatement. Substantial national resources are spent on what is supposed to be a normal process. From the clinic to the hospital, how do we as nurses, midwives, and physicians provide a safe and high-quality experience for the women we care for during pregnancy and birth? How are we helping women plan for and achieve *their* goals and desires for their birth experiences?

Cesarean section has become the most common operating room procedure in America [1]. The U.S. cesarean section rate is nearly 33%, appearing to at least stabilize in 2010 and 2011 after rising by 60% from 1996 to 2009 [2,3]. The Healthy People 2020 goal is

Supporting a Physiologic Approach to Pregnancy and Birth: A Practical Guide, First Edition.
Edited by Melissa D. Avery.
© 2013 John Wiley & Sons, Inc. Published 2013 by John Wiley & Sons, Inc.

Table 1.1   U.S. maternity care data.

Measure	U.S.	International perspective	Year
Cesarean section	32.8%		2011
Preterm birth	11.72%		2011
Maternal mortality	12.7/100,000	Higher than 49 developed countries	2007
African American women	26.5		2007
White women	10.0		2007
Infant mortality	6.05/1,000	Higher than most OECD countries	2011
African American infants	11.42		2011
White infants	5.11		2011
Portion GDP to healthcare	17.6%	Higher than all OECD countries	2010

a moderate 10% reduction in cesarean births to *low-risk women* (term, singleton, vertex) from a baseline of 26.5% in 2007 to 23.9% by 2020, as well as a 10% increase in vaginal births among women with a previous cesarean [4]. At the same time, infant mortality, a measure used worldwide to reflect care to mothers and families, is 6.05 deaths in the first year of life per 1,000 live births [5]. This is higher than all but three member countries of the Organisation for Economic Co-operation and Development (OECD), an organization of primarily developed countries including Europe, the United States, Canada, and others [6]. Infant mortality in the United States has declined from 6.71 per 1,000 live births in 2006 after remaining stable from 2000 to 2005 [7]. An 8% decline in premature births occurred from 12.80% in 2006 to 11.72% in 2011 [3], along with increased efforts at preventing early elective births such as the March of Dimes and the California Maternal Quality Care Collaborative [8,9]. Maternal mortality was 12.7 per 100,000 live births in 2007 [10], a number that may be increasing [11], with the U.S. rate behind forty-nine other developed nations in 2010 [12]. (See summary data in Table 1.1.)

   Not readily apparent in these statistics are significant racial disparities. For example, infant mortality among African American women was 11.42 per 1,000 live births, 2.2 times greater than the 5.11 for White women [5]. Maternal mortality was approximately 3 times higher for African American women compared to White women [10,11]. These disparities are inexcusable in a country with such vast resources; we must reverse these trends by assuring access to continuous high-quality health care [13]. Returning to a more normal or physiologic approach to maternity care including access to comprehensive continuous care to all women in the United States is one step in that direction.

Spending and doing too much

Nearly 99% of U.S. births occur in hospitals [2], thus "liveborn infant" and "pregnancy and childbirth" are among the most common reasons for hospitalization [1], accounting for nearly a quarter of hospital discharges in 2008, and over $98 billion in hospital charges (amount hospitals bill for a stay). Medicaid payment covers the cost of care for over 40% of pregnancies and births [14]. Of "pregnancy and childbirth" and "liveborn infant" hospitalizations in 2008, $41 billion was paid by Medicaid and $50 billion was paid by private insurers [15]. The United States spent 17.6% of gross domestic product (GDP) on health care in 2010, more than any of the other OECD countries [6]. This phenomenon of doing more in perinatal care without a corresponding improvement in care outcomes was first referred to as the "perinatal paradox" more than 20 years ago [16]. Tremendous resources are allocated to maternal and infant care in the United States and yet our outcomes do not compare well with other developed countries. Although preterm birth has declined in recent years and the cesarean rate may have stabilized, there is much more work to be done.

The passage of the Affordable Care Act (ACA) in 2010 marked the first success in half a century of legislative attempts to change health care in the United States. When fully implemented, millions more Americans will have health care coverage. An important focus of the ACA is on improving health care and reducing costs by enhancing coordination of care for individuals with chronic conditions, reducing medical errors, reducing hospital-acquired infections, and reducing waste in the system. Improving health care, improving care outcomes including client satisfaction, and providing care at lower cost, often referred to as the triple aim, are not only possible but necessary. In addition to improved access to health care, ACA improvements in care options for women include family planning and breast and cervical cancer screening without co-pays, coverage for maternity and newborn care, home-visiting services during pregnancy and early childhood, restricting insurance companies from charging women higher premiums than men, and enhanced support for breastfeeding mothers [17].

Concerns about the increased use of technology and medical intervention overuse in maternity care have been expressed by clinicians, scientists, educators, and others around the world. Multiple health professions and health-related organizations worldwide have issued statements calling for a more normal or physiologic approach to pregnancy and birth. Concerned with the rising rates of interventions in maternity care in the United Kingdom, the Maternity Care Working Party published a normal birth consensus statement in 2007, supported by the Royal College of Obstetricians and Gynecologists and the Royal College of Midwives, defining "normal delivery" as spontaneous labor, labor progression, and birth, without the use of interventions such as labor induction, epidural, cesarean section, and forceps. The statement proposes action steps to increase the proportion of normal births in the four UK countries [18]. Other statements, in some cases endorsed by multiple health professions organizations, have called for support of birth as a normal process, reduced intervention, use of best available evidence, and woman-centered care [19–22]. More recently, in the United States, the American Academy of Family Physicians; American Academy of Pediatrics; American College of Nurse-Midwives; American College of Obstetricians and Gynecologists; American College of Osteopathic Obstetricians and Gynecologists; Association of Women's Health, Obstetric and Neonatal Nurses; and Society for Maternal-Fetal Medicine endorsed a statement on quality patient care in labor and delivery identifying pregnancy and birth as normal processes requiring little if any intervention in most cases [23]. The authors called for effective communication, shared decision making, teamwork, and quality measurement in the provision of maternity care. Three U.S. midwifery organizations partnered in the development of a statement supporting physiologic birth—defining normal physiologic birth, identifying factors that disrupt and factors influencing normal birth, and proposing a set of actions to promote normal birth [24]. Reflecting the growing concern about the U.S. cesarean section rate, authors of a report summarizing a recent workshop held by the American Congress of Obstetricians and Gynecologists, the Society for Maternal-Fetal Medicine, and the Eunice Kennedy Shriver National Institute of Child Health and Human Development, plus a similar commentary, recommended specific practices and actions for clinicians and health systems to prevent the first cesarean section [25,26]. At least on paper, it seems as if we all agree.

Internationally, a series of normal labor and birth conferences have been held beginning in England in 2002 and most recently in China in 2012 [27]. The conferences highlight current research and best practices in promoting normal birth. In the United States, authors of a key report on evidence-based maternity care have identified induction of labor and cesarean section as overused procedures. Additionally, midwives, family physicians, and prenatal vitamins were described as underused interventions [28]. Following that report, Childbirth Connection, a nonprofit organization focused on improving maternity care, held a multistakeholder meeting focused on just how the quality and value of maternity care could be improved in the United States. The resulting "Blueprint for Action: Steps toward a High-Quality, High-Value Maternity Care System" provides clinicians, payers, educators, and care systems with excellent proposals to improve our care to women [29]. Strong Start for Mothers and Newborns, a federally funded program under the Centers for Medicare and Medicaid Services (CMS) Center for Medicare and Medicaid Innovation, has provided funding to reduce early elective births and to test new models of enhanced prenatal care to meet the triple aim. The models include enhanced prenatal care in group prenatal settings, in birth centers, and in maternity care homes [30].

In order to improve quality, health systems need to measure and report on the care provided [29,31,32]. Maternity care measures are available for use to improve quality such as the Joint Commission, the National Quality Forum, and the American Medical Association (AMA). The AMA Physician Consortium for Performance Improvement measure set was developed by an interprofessional work group and includes measures related to overuse of certain care practices as well as a measure for spontaneous labor and birth [33]. These quality measure sets are available to health systems, clinicians, and payers to improve care and achieve better care outcomes. In addition to the national measure sets, a tool to examine the optimal processes and outcomes of normal pregnancies among groups of women has been developed and tested. The Optimality Index-US measures what is "optimal" or best possible care processes and outcomes—within a philosophy of aiming for the best outcome using the least number of interventions [34–36]. Higher Optimality scores in one setting over another may reflect an environment that supports a low intervention and physiologic approach to prenatal and labor care. Available as a research tool, clinicians can also use the index to examine institutional care processes and in peer review and other quality improvement processes [35].

Looking for something different

Women have signaled that they are beginning to look for something different, evidenced by the recent increase in out-of-hospital births [37]. After declining since 1990, home births increased by 29% from 2004 to 2009 [38]. In 2010, the increase in both home and free-standing birth center births was large enough to cross the "99% mark," documenting more than 1% of births occurring outside the hospital [2]. While the absolute number may not seem impressive (47,000 of nearly 4 million), the change is a message that a segment of the U.S. childbearing population is looking for something else. Birth is important to women, often a transformative event that they remember clearly throughout their lives. Many women believe labor and birth should not be interfered with and women understand their right to full information and to accept or refuse specific care processes [39]. Women are asking for specific services in hospitals such as water immersion, aromatherapy, and acupressure as part of the support tools available for labor and birth. Although epidurals remain popular, women are increasingly planning for an unmedicated birth and express a desire to be in control of their birth process [40]. The author of the 2011 consumer book *Natural Birth in the Hospital: The Best of Both Worlds* [41] reaches out to the nearly 99% of women giving birth in hospitals, letting them know that they, too, can have a more normal experience in a hospital and how to get what they want.

Women's partnerships with their care providers are of utmost importance. Return for a moment to your clinic—sit down for a few more minutes with your client. What is it that she and her birth support persons really hope for during her labor and birth? What does the best evidence suggest are the preferred care measures resulting in the least harm? Take a little more time to engage in meaningful discussions with her so she puts aside her fears about labor, forgets the anxiety she's seen in births depicted in the media, and partners with you in understanding options and planning for her labor and birth. When you welcome her to the hospital birthing room, tell her that your goal is to accommodate her and her partner's preferences. Although it sounds easy, and most likely what we are trying to provide, current data support an alternate story.

This book can help you—the clinician "at the bedside"—take a look into the clinic exam rooms and hospital labor units to see what else is possible. The various chapter authors are clinicians and educators just like you. Together we have worked to summarize recent research and other published information and provide some ideas, tools, and solutions to put into the hands of maternity care clinicians including midwives, nurses, physicians, and others. The authors herein argue for supporting and enhancing women's confidence in their ability to give birth. At the same time we aim to increase the confidence of care providers to trust in the normal process and support women expecting a healthy outcome rather than looking for reasons to disrupt the process. It goes without saying that specific conditions warrant medical intervention and higher levels of care such as pre-existing diabetes, hypertension, and multifetal gestation, and yet even women with those conditions can still be supported as mothers, enhancing normal or physiologic processes as much as possible.

A word about language. We have chosen to talk about an approach to physiologic pregnancy and birth with a profound respect for the intricate changes that occur during both pregnancy and labor that result in what is commonly referred to as "the miracle of birth." We use the word "birth" in most cases, to honor the work that women do in giving birth. "Delivery" is retained in some circumstances, primarily to refer to women delivering their newborns. "Normal" is meant to signify the usual process of being pregnant and giving birth without being disturbed by technology or other interventions that are not necessary in supporting the usual processes [42], with no intent to judge any woman's pregnancy or birth experience [43]. Every woman is unique; her process is also unique. Physiologic or normal is not just one variety or type, but each woman's individual experience to be supported, "managing" only when the experience is truly outside the range of normal and thus requiring additional intervention. Even then, aspects of a normal or physiologic approach can be retained, always remembering the unique woman giving birth. Finally, this book is based on a belief that it takes all types of maternity care providers working in partnership to improve maternity care. Thus we refer to providers and clinicians, and the authors represent midwives, nurses, physicians, and others.

A look inside

Section 1 begins with a review of the normal physiologic changes of pregnancy as well as the physiologic uterine phases through pregnancy, labor initiation, continuation, and birth. Although the exact mechanism of the initiation of labor is not completely understood, the known components of pregnancy and labor physiology are fascinating, with increasing understanding through research on the intricacies of the labor process. With the goal of a physiologic approach as the norm, how do we adapt routine prenatal care to enhance women's confidence and understanding of pregnancy as normal and not an illness to be treated? In a woman-centered approach, women are supported to understand the range of tools for comfort in early labor, how to recognize active labor and the best time to transition to the birthing unit (if not the home), and mechanisms to support the process. We work to bring women's knowledge and understanding of the process as close to ours as possible and respect the knowledge and expertise each woman brings to her pregnancy. Originally proposed as a description of exemplary midwifery care, "the art of doing 'nothing' well" [44] is recommended here as an approach for all clinicians providing maternity care unless there is a compelling reason to do something more.

Section 2 begins with a theoretical perspective on promoting comfort for women in labor followed by chapters describing integrative therapies for pregnancy, labor, and birth. Maternity care clinicians may not have sufficient knowledge and understanding about integrative or complementary and alternative medicine (CAM) practices [45]. Midwives appear to have a more positive view of the effectiveness of alternative therapies and are less likely to believe that results of CAM are due to placebo effect than obstetricians [46]. Researchers investigating nurse-midwives' experiences with CAM therapies demonstrated that a majority of certified nurse-midwife respondents reported CAM use. Herbal preparations, pharmacologic/biologic, mind-body interventions, and manual healing/bioelectromagnetic therapies were used most often. Diet and lifestyle therapies were also common [47]. Women have increased their use of CAM therapies during pregnancy, thus maternity care providers need to become knowledgeable about these practices and facilitate communication, cooperation, and respect among alternative and conventional providers [48].

Within the context of promoting comfort, chapters on relaxation, touch therapies, water immersion and water birth, acupuncture and acupressure, and aromatherapy are offered as adjuncts to "doing nothing" in support of women during pregnancy, labor, and birth.

While not an exhaustive representation of possible integrative therapies, reviews of evidence and practical suggestions are offered as tools for maternity care clinicians to assist women in achieving their preferred birth experience. Authors aim to help clinicians understand these therapies better, including specific instructions on how to use certain techniques, as well as information on referring to providers of the therapy and how specific practices, such as acupuncture, are regulated.

Finally, section 3 focuses on the broader care and education systems. Individual clinicians can provide excellent one-on-one care and effect local change. In order to change maternity care in the United States, we must also work within our broader systems to shift to a more physiologic approach. Because nearly 99% of births occur in hospitals, the best opportunity to effect meaningful system change is to adjust the approach to care on labor units. Nurses are key in making that happen, and a group of labor nurses have proposed a possible solution after examining available evidence and related information. The other 1% of births occur outside the hospital; evidence supports the safety of this approach for carefully selected women when out-of-hospital practice is imbedded in a broader system of consultation and referral to more intensive care when needed. Respecting out-of-hospital birth as a safe environment for low-risk women who desire that care is critical. When transfer to the hospital setting is required, the process of transfer and receiving the woman and her family can be more seamless and positive with enhanced understanding and respect among clinicians from both settings.

For the change we desire to be permanent and system-wide, we must promote interprofessional collaborative practices that are built on a foundation of mutual trust and respect, with care decisions made by informed women and their families [23,24,49,50]. Maternity care providers must be educated together so that they will provide the seamless quality care women deserve, with clinical education occurring in environments where students learn with interprofessional care teams. Policy changes to support clinicians practicing together to the full extent of their education and training, in an environment where all women have access to quality health care, is the final critical component to improving maternity care. Legislators and policy-makers need to hear from their constituent clinicians in making those necessary changes.

National attention is focused on maternity care in a way that has not been seen in recent history, providing an opportunity to be transformative [29]. This group of authors, representing committed clinicians, educators, and researchers from multiple professions, invites you to come along on a journey to serve women today to build tomorrow's healthier families. Women and their families deserve the very best that we can collectively provide in an environment that respects pregnancy and birth as normal processes, that respects the women and their families/support networks to lead their care, and where we respect and trust each other as partners in providing excellent care. The change required is larger than any one clinician or profession can accomplish. Indeed, we are encouraged that health professionals are responding to calls for interprofessional practice and education. While we add our voices to the larger discussions in Congress, federal health-related agencies, educational settings, and corporate boardrooms, a more quiet yet powerful change can occur in our care settings through the conversations and plans we make with each other and with our clients every day—clinic by clinic, woman by woman, birth by birth.

References

1. Agency for Healthcare Research and Quality. (2012). Facts and figures 2009—table of contents. Healthcare Cost and Utilization Project (HCUP). www.hcup-us.ahrq.gov/reports/factsandfigures/2009/TOC_2009.jsp. Accessed November 18, 2012.
2. Martin JA, Hamilton BE, Ventura SJ, Osterman MJK, Wilson EC, & Mathews TJ. (2012). Births: Final data for 2010. *National Vital Statistics Reports*, *61*(1). http://www.cdc.gov/nchs/data/nvsr/nvsr61/nvsr61_01.pdf. Accessed November 23, 2012.
3. Hamilton BE, Martin JA, & Ventura SJ. (2012). Births: Preliminary data for 2011. *National Vital Statistics Reports*, *61*(5). Released October 3, 2012. http://www.cdc.gov/nchs/data/nvsr/nvsr61/nvsr61_05.pdf. Accessed November 17, 2012.
4. U.S. Department of Health and Human Services. (2012). Office of Disease Prevention and Health Promotion. Healthy people 2020. Washington, DC. http://www.healthypeople.gov/2020/topicsobjectives2020/objectiveslist.aspx?topicId=26#93911. Accessed November 23, 2012.
5. Hoyert DL & Xu J. (2012). Deaths: Preliminary data for 2011. *National Vital Statistics Reports*, *61*(6). http://www.cdc.gov/nchs/data/nvsr/nvsr61/nvsr61_06.pdf. Accessed November 17, 2012.
6. Organisation for Economic Co-operation and Development. (2012). OECD health data 2012—frequently requested data. http://www.oecd.org/els/healthpoliciesanddata/oecdhealthdata2012-frequentlyrequesteddata.htm. Accessed November 18, 2012.
7. MacDorman MF & Mathews TJ. (2008). Recent trends in infant mortality in the United States. *NCHS Data Brief*, no. 9. Hyattsville, MD: National Center for Health Statistics.
8. March of Dimes. (2012). Healthy babies are worth the wait. http://www.marchofdimes.com/professionals/medicalresources_hbww.html. Accessed November 28, 2012.
9. California Maternal Quality Care Collaborative. (2012). < 39 weeks toolkit. http://www.cmqcc.org/_39_week_toolkit. Accessed November 28, 2012.
10. Xu J, Kochanek KD, Murphy SL, & Tejada-Vera B. (2010). Deaths: Final data for 2007. *National Vital Statistics Reports*, *58*(19). http://www.cdc.gov/nchs/data/nvsr/nvsr58/nvsr58_19.pdf. Accessed November 24, 2012.
11. Singh GK. (2010). Maternal mortality in the United States, 1935–2007: Substantial racial/ethnic, socioeconomic, and geographic disparities persist. Rockville, MD: U.S. Department of Health and Human Services. http://www.hrsa.gov/ourstories/mchb75th/mchb75maternalmortality.pdf. Accessed November 24, 2012.
12. Amnesty International USA. (2011). Deadly delivery: The maternal health care crisis in the USA. One year update spring 2011. http://www.amnestyusa.org/sites/default/files/deadlydeliveryoneyear.pdf. Accessed November 24, 2012.
13. Lu MC. (2008). We can do better: Improving women's healthcare in America. *Current Opinion in Obstetrics and Gynecology*, *20*, 563–565.
14. Agency for Healthcare Research and Quality. (2010). Facts and figures 2008—table of contents. Healthcare Cost and Utilization Project (HCUP). www.hcup-us.ahrq.gov/reports/factsandfigures/2008/TOC_2008.jsp. Accessed November 18, 2012.
15. Wier LM & Andrews RM. (2011). The national hospital bill: The most expensive conditions by payer, 2008. Statistical Brief #107. Agency for Healthcare Research and Quality.
16. Rosenblatt RA. (1989). The perinatal paradox: Doing more and accomplishing less. *Health Affairs*, *8*(3), 158–168. DOI: 10.1377/hlthaff.8.3.158.
17. National Partnership for Women and Families. (2012). http://www.nationalpartnership.org/site/PageServer?pagename=issues_health_reform_anniversary. Accessed November 23, 2012.

18. Maternity Care Working Party. (2007). Making normal birth a reality. Consensus statement from the Maternity Care Working Party. Available from: http://www.nct.org.uk/professional/research/pregnancy-birth-and-postnatal-care/birth/normal-birth. Accessed November 24, 2012.
19. Canadian Association of Midwives. (2010). Midwifery care and normal birth. http://www.aom.on.ca/files/Communications/Position_Statements/CAMNoramalBirth_ENG201001.pdf. Accessed November 24, 2012.
20. International Confederation of Midwives. (2008). Keeping birth normal. http://international midwives.org/assets/uploads/documents/Position%20statements%20-%20English/PS2008_007%20ENG%20Keeping%20Birth%20Normal.pdf. Accessed November 24, 2012.
21. New Zealand College of Midwives. (2006). NZCOM consensus statement normal birth. http://www.midwife.org.nz/index.cfm/3,108,559/normal-birth-ratified-agm-2006-refs-2009.pdf. Accessed November 24, 2012.
22. Society of Obstetricians and Gynaecologists of Canada. (2008). Joint policy statement on normal childbirth. *Journal of Obstetrics and Gynaecology Canada, 30*(12), 1163–1165. http://www.sogc.org/guidelines/documents/gui221PS0812.pdf. Accessed November 24, 2012.
23. American Academy of Family Physicians; American Academy of Pediatrics; American College of Nurse-Midwives; American College of Obstetricians and Gynecologists; American College of Osteopathic Obstetricians & Gynecologists; Association of Women's Health, Obstetric and Neonatal Nurses; & the Society for Maternal-Fetal Medicine. (2012). Quality patient care in labor and delivery: A call to action. *Journal of Midwifery & Women's Health, 57,* 112–113.
24. American College of Nurse-Midwives, Midwives Alliance of North America, & National Association of Certified Professional Midwives. (2012). Supporting healthy and normal physiologic childbirth: A consensus statement by ACNM, MANA, and NACPM. http://www.midwife.org/ACNM/files/ACNMLibraryData/UPLOADFILENAME/000000000272/Physiological%20Birth%20Consensus%20Statement-%20FINAL%20May%2018%202012%20FINAL.pdf. Accessed November 15, 2012.
25. Spong CY, Berghella V, Wenstrom KD, Mercer BM, & Saade GR. (2012). Preventing the first cesarean delivery. Summary of a Joint Eunice Kennedy Shriver National Institute of Child Health and Human Development, Society for Maternal-Fetal Medicine, and American College of Obstetricians and Gynecologists Workshop. *Obstetrics & Gynecology, 120*(5), 1181–1193. DOI: http://10.1097/AOG.0b013e3182704880.
26. Main EK, Morton CH, Melsop K, Hopkins D, Giuliani G, & Gould J. (2012). Creating a public agenda for maternity safety and quality in cesarean delivery. *Obstetrics & Gynecology, 120,* 1194–1198. DOI: http://10.1097/AOG.0b013e31826fc13d.
27. Hanzhou Normal University. (2012). http://www.iresearch4birth.eu/iResearch4Birth/resources/cms/documents/China_English_flyer.pdf. Accessed November 23, 2012.
28. Sakala C & Corry M. (2008). Evidence-based maternity care: What it is and what it can achieve. Co-published by Childbirth Connection, the Reforming States Group, and the Milbank Memorial Fund. Available at: http://www.childbirthconnection.org/pdfs/evidence-based-maternity-care.pdf.
29. Transforming Maternity Care Symposium Steering Committee. (2010). Blueprint for action: Steps toward a high-quality, high-value maternity care system. *Women's Health Issues, 20,* S18–49.
30. Centers for Medicare and Medicaid. (2012). http://www.innovations.cms.gov/initiatives/strong-start/index.html. Accessed November 28, 2012.
31. Joint Commission. (2010). Perinatal care measures. http://manual.jointcommission.org/releases/TJC2011A/PerinatalCare.html. Accessed November 6, 2012.
32. National Quality Forum. (2012). Endorsement summary: Perinatal and reproductive health measures. http://www.qualityforum.org/News_And_Resources/Endorsement_Summaries/Endorsement_Summaries.aspx. Accessed November 6, 2012.

33. American Medical Association and the National Committee for Quality Assurance. (2012). Maternity care performance measurement set. http://www.ama-assn.org/resources/doc/cqi/no-index/maternity-care-measures.pdf. Accessed November 24, 2012.
34. Murphy PA & Fullerton JT. (2001). Measuring outcomes of midwifery care: Development of an instrument to assess optimality. *Journal of Midwifery and Women's Health*, *46*, 274–284.
35. Murphy PA & Fullerton JT. (2006). Development of the Optimality Index as a new approach to evaluating outcomes of maternity care. *JOGNN*, *35*, 770–778.
36. Kennedy HP. (2006). A concept analysis of "optimality" in perinatal health. *JOGNN*, *35*, 763–769.
37. MacDorman M, Menacker F, & Declercq E. (2010). Trends and characteristics of home and other out-of-hospital births in the United States, 1990–2006. *National Vital Statistics Reports*, *58*(11).
38. MacDorman MF, Mathews TJ, & Declercq E. (2012). Home births in the United States, 1990–2009. *NCHS Data Brief*, no. 84.
39. Declercq ER, Sakala C, Corry MP, & Applebaum S. (2006). Listening to Mothers II: Report of the Second National U.S. Survey of Women's Childbearing Experiences. Retrieved from: http://www.childbirthconnection.org/article.asp?ck=10396. Accessed November 24, 2012.
40. Stewart NR. (2012). What women want in the delivery room. *Boston Globe*, June 18, 2012. http://www.bostonglobe.com/lifestyle/health-wellness/2012/06/17/hospitals-are-offering-spa-like-services-maternity-ward/itm5E5y5fM8bq1b7LDLaeL/story.html. Accessed November 24, 2012.
41. Gabriel. Cynthia. (2011). Natural Hospital Birth: The Best of Both Worlds. Boston, MA: The Harvard Common Press.
42. Kennedy HP. (2010). The problem of normal birth. *Journal of Midwifery & Women's Health*, *55*, 199–201.
43. Zeldes K & Norsigian J. (2008). Encouraging women to consider a less medicalized approach to childbirth without turning them off: Challenges to producing *Our Bodies Ourselves: Pregnancy and Birth*. *Birth*, *35*, 245–249.
44. Kennedy HP. (2000). A model of exemplary midwifery practice: Results of a Delphi study. *Journal of Midwifery & Women's Health*, *45*, 4–19. DOI: 10.1016/S1526-9523(99)00018-5.
45. Tiran D. (2006). Complementary therapies and risk: Midwives' and obstetricians' appreciation of risk. *Complementary Therapies in Clinical Practice*, *12*, 126–131.
46. Gaffney L & Smith CA. (2004). Use of complementary therapies in pregnancy: The perceptions of obstetricians and midwives in South Australia. *Australian and New Zealand Journal of Obstetrics and Gynaecology*, *44*, 24–29.
47. Hastings-Tolsma M & Terada M. (2009). Complementary medicine use by nurse midwives in the U.S. *Complementary Therapies in Clinical Practice*, *15*, 212–219.
48. Adams J, Lui CW, Sibbritt D, Broom A, Wardle J, & Homer C. (2010). Attitudes and referral practices of maternity care professionals with regard to complementary and alternative medicine: An integrative review. *Journal of Advanced Nursing*, *67*(3), 472–483.
49. Waldman RN & Kennedy HP. (2011). Collaborative practice between obstetricians and midwives. *Obstetrics & Gynecology*, *118*, 503–504.
50. Avery MD, Montgomery O, & Brandl-Salutz E. (2012). Essential components of successful collaborative maternity care models: The ACOG-ACNM Project. *Obstetrics and Gynecology Clinics of North America*, *39*, 423–434. DOI: 10.1016/j.ogc.2012.05.010.

Chapter 2

The physiology of pregnancy, labor, and birth

Cindy M. Anderson

Key points

- The placenta is the interface between the mother and fetus supporting perfusion to meet fetal growth and development needs; transport is influenced by placental area, diffusing distance, permeability of placental barrier, and maternal-fetal blood flow in the intervillous spaces.
- The placenta assumes the neuroendocrine functions that are regulated in the nonpregnant state by the typical hypothalamus-pituitary-end organ feedback mechanisms.
- Progesterone is the dominant hormone during pregnancy, its inhibitory effects largely responsible for the uterine quiescent phase during pregnancy.
- To meet the increased demand for maternal and fetal oxygen and oxygen transport during pregnancy, cardiac output, oxygen consumption, and left ventricular stroke volume increase, along with a 40% increase in blood volume primarily comprised of the plasma component. Maternal pulmonary tidal volume and inspiratory capacity increase while residual volume, expiratory reserve volume and functional residual capacity decline.
- Changes in the firm cervical structure to more pliable and distensible occur in later pregnancy as water concentration increases relative to collagen, resulting from an increase in highly hydrophilic glycoaminoglycans such as chondroitin sulfate and hyaluronan.
- The complex signaling between mother, placenta, and fetus that triggers labor initiation and progression are not completely understood, however likely involve the interplay among hormonal, mechanical, and immune factors.
- The transition from progesterone dominance in the uterine quiescent phase to the estrogen dominance in the activation phase stimulates coordinated, synchronous contractions in myometrial cells in the contractile fundus. Uterine contractions are promoted by increased myometrial oxytocin receptors and increased prostaglandin production in the fetal membranes.
- Stress and anxiety during labor can be exacerbated by fear, thus triggering cognitive pain perception and increasing sensitivity to pain.

[I]t is time that professionals regain their trust in the physiology which enables healthy women to labour and deliver, mostly without interference.

Marianne Mead

Supporting a Physiologic Approach to Pregnancy and Birth: A Practical Guide, First Edition.
Edited by Melissa D. Avery.
© 2013 John Wiley & Sons, Inc. Published 2013 by John Wiley & Sons, Inc.

Introduction

The processes of the initiation and progression events characteristic of the intrapartum period are critically important for optimal care of pregnant women, yet the underlying mechanisms of labor physiology are poorly understood. The physiologic changes of pregnancy are necessary to prepare women for the unique challenges brought on by the significant demands placed on multiple maternal body systems, required to support ideal function of the maternal-placental-fetal unit. The intrapartum period presents new challenges associated with unique adaptations associated with initiation and progression of labor, culminating in birth of a newborn and the return to maternal prepregnant physiologic function. Theories surrounding the relatively mysterious biochemical events that prompt intrapartum events abound, though a single explanation for the processes of labor and birth is elusive. The complex signaling between mother, placenta, and fetus that triggers labor initiation and progression is unclear but likely involves interplay between hormonal, mechanical, and immune factors. This chapter presents a detailed discussion of maternal physiologic adaptations in pregnancy as well as labor and birth and the known and postulated mechanisms surrounding the intrapartum events of labor and delivery.

Physiologic adaptive changes in pregnancy

Adaptations of maternal physiology during pregnancy involve the accommodations in multiple systems to support the increasing demands with progressive gestation. Pregnancy adaptations are essential foundations for the unique adjustments required to support the processes of labor and to support the increased demands placed on the maternal-placental-fetal unit during the intrapartum period. Pregnancy can be considered in four separate phases: quiescence, activation, stimulation, and involution [1]. The antepartum period prior to the onset of labor is characterized by quiescence, suppression of uterine activity, reflecting the exquisite balance between the hormonal mileu and responsiveness of the uterus and cervix. Quiescence is mediated by inhibitor hormones, including progesterone, prostacyclin, relaxin, nitric oxide (NO), corticotropin-releasing hormone (CRH), and human placental lactogen (hPL).

Placenta

The placenta, formed by the union of the maternal decidua basalis and the fetal trophoblast, develops in the early days of pregnancy with implantation of the blastocyst. Placental growth continues throughout gestation until term, when the average surface area reaches $12.6 \, m^2$, increasing to a functional surface area of $90 \, m^2$ when microvilli surface is considered. Placental weight at term equals approximately $500 \, g$, with dimensions of a diameter of 15–20 cm and thickness of 3 cm [2, p. 3].

The placenta serves as the interface between mother and fetus, supporting perfusion to meet fetal needs in the intrauterine environment. Progressive placental vascular development is stimulated by the hypoxic intrauterine environment characteristic of early pregnancy. Fetal deoxygenated blood passes from the dual umbilical arteries to the placenta.

Maternal blood supply is delivered to the placenta by the remodeled spiral arteries, bathing the spaces between chorionic villi (intervillous) with arterial blood at approximately 8–9 weeks of gestation [3]. The chorionic villi contain fetal blood vessels, tightly packed with extensive branching. Maternal-fetal circulatory separation is achieved by several layers of tissue known as the placental barrier or membrane, providing structural separation between fetal vessels within the chorionic villi and maternal blood. Chorionic villi represent the anatomic structure across which essential substrates including gases, nutrients, drugs, and wastes must be transported bidirectionally between the maternal and fetal circulations. Transport processes include simple diffusion as the primary mechanism, followed by facilitated diffusion and active transport of select nutritionally essential molecules. Efficiency of placental transport is influenced by placental area, diffusing distance, permeability of placental barrier and maternal-fetal blood flow in the intervillous spaces. Additionally, the characteristics of the transported substance that influence transport include concentration and electrical potential gradients, molecule size, binding affinity of substance to carrier protein (e.g., hemoglobin), and solubility (e.g., water, lipid). Factors impacting fetal blood flow include fetal heart activity, influenced by fetal blood pressure, right to left shunts, and vascular resistance, both pulmonary and systemic. Maternal blood flow is determined by perfusion to the uterine and spiral (uteroplacental) arteries, influenced by cardiac output, systemic, peripheral, and uteroplacental resistance.

Endocrine adaptations

Placental endocrine functions are central to the establishment and maintenance of pregnancy. Optimal placental endocrine function requires the involvement of the maternal-placental-fetal unit, reflecting the adaptive transition from independent maternal production [4]. The array of endocrine substances produced by the placenta includes, but is not limited to, polypeptide hormones adrenocorticotropic hormone (ACTH), human chorionic gonadotropin hormone (hCG) and hPL, steroid hormones estrogen and progesterone, neurohormones oxytocin and releasing hormones (gonadotropin, thyroid, growth, corticotropin), growth factors (placental, PlGF; transforming, TGF; insulin-like, IGF), and cytokines (interleukins, IL; tumor necrosis factor, TNF). The placenta assumes neuroendocrine functions during pregnancy, typically regulated by the hypothalamus-pituitary-end organ feedback mechanisms in the nonpregnant state [4].

Progesterone is often referred to as the hormone of pregnancy, reflecting the dominance of this steroid hormone during gestation. The quiescent phase of pregnancy is largely attributed to the inhibitory effects of progesterone. Progesterone inhibits formation of estrogen receptor alpha (ER-α), limiting estrogen sensitivity [5]. The effects of estrogen are opposed by progesterone, resulting in inhibition of gap junction formation and uterine activity. A progesterone-induced increase in NO synthase activity, decreased prostaglandin (PG) production, and reduced development of oxytocin receptors and calcium ion channels combine to enhance uterine quiescence. Cervical integrity is also promoted by progesterone through the inhibition of collagen breakdown.

The ovarian corpus luteum is the primary source of progesterone in early pregnancy, transitioning to primary production from acetate and cholesterol by the placenta with advancing gestation. Progesterone binds to two primary receptor isoforms: progesterone receptor (PR)-A and PR-B. Binding of progesterone to PR-B enhances progesterone function compared to progesterone binding to the truncated PR-A, which antagonizes the effects of progesterone–PR-B binding [6]. During pregnancy, the progesterone binding to PR-B exceeds that of PR-A, promoting the characteristic effects of progesterone. During labor, the PR-A to PR-B ratio changes, promoting the dominant proinflammatory effects of progesterone–PR-A binding [7].

During pregnancy, the delicate balance between estrogen and progesterone is critical to suppression of uterine activity. Progesterone dominance over estrogen during the quiescent period of pregnancy overcomes the influence of estrogen-associated effects prior to labor initiation. The placenta is a major source of estriol, the major circulating estrogen in pregnancy. Placental production of estriol is primarily dependent on fetal adrenal production of dehydroepiandrosterone sulfate (DHEAS), hydroxylation of DHEAS by the liver, and aromatization by the placenta [8]. Placenta estriol leads to an increase in the release of maternal prostaglandins, prostaglandin receptors, and oxytocin receptors. An increase in gap junctions, necessary for the rapid transmission of contractile signals, is also due to the influence of estrogen [9]. During the last few weeks of pregnancy, cervical ripening is enhanced by estrogens, promoted by remodeling of collagen and elastin that soften the cervix. Estrogen binding to the ER-α promotes cellular signaling with outcomes associated with the actions of estrogen.

Oxytocin is a peptide hormone that has a important role in the labor process. Its relatively short half-life of 3–4 minutes is reduced further when exogenous high doses of oxytocin are infused [10]. Synthesized in the hypothalamus, oxytocin is released from the posterior pituitary and binds to oxytocin receptors for the primary action of uterine contraction stimulation.

Uterine adaptation

The adaptations of the uterus accommodate the increasing intrauterine contents as gestation advances. Enlargement of the uterus is due to progressive elasticity and proliferation of smooth muscle contractile units, the myocytes [11]. Early uterine growth is due to myocyte hyperplasia, increase in cell number. Progressive growth with continued gestation is the result of the combined effect of both hyperplasia and hypertrophy, enlargement of existing cells, increasing uterine capacity from 10 ml to 5000 ml at term. The longitudinal and circular muscles of the uterus gain equilibrium in contractile ability by term. Contractile ability is influenced by electrical events in myocyte cellular membranes leading to action potential, the propagation of the action potential to nearby cells via gap junctions, and intracellular calcium availability. The organization of uterine smooth muscle cells promotes a great deal of force along a short distance at low velocity [12].

The coordinated, synchronous contraction of myometrial cells in the contractile fundus is the hallmark of labor onset and progression. Of critical importance is the regulation of uterine contractile function during gestation, delayed until the onset of parturition. The quiescent period prior to labor initiation is characterized by uterine relaxation, with intermittent dyssynchronous uterine activity [8]. The suppression of uterine contractile activity is the combined effect of inhibitors of myometrial activity, which include progesterone, prostacyclin (PG I_2), relaxin, NO, and CRH.

Cervical remodeling

During pregnancy, the cervix changes from a firm, rigid structure to one that is pliable and distensible. The cervix is primarily comprised of collagen-producing fibroblasts and smooth muscle cells comprised of cross-linked collagen fibers, elastin, and proteoglycans (glycoaminoglycans attached to a protein). As pregnancy advances, water concentration increases relative to collagen as a result of an increase in highly hydrophilic glycoamino-glycans such as chondroitin sulfate and hyaluronan. The tight collagen bundles relax as a result of remodeling of collagen linkages, maximized by collagen degradation during the process of mechanical stretch during labor. Cervical vascular permeability is promoted by the presence of fibroblasts, leukocytes, macrophages, and eosinophil infiltration.

PGs, a group of hormones resulting from metabolism of arachidonic acid, are produced by the placental and fetal amnion/chorion and are involved in the regulation of uterine activity. Inhibitory PGs (PG I_2) reduce uterine activity while stimulatory PGs (PG $F_2\alpha$ and E_2) promote myometrial contraction [8]. PG production is increased under the influence of estrogens, CRH, and inflammatory cytokines and decreased by progesterone.

CRH is a hypothalamic-releasing hormone regulating ACTH and adrenal cortisol via a negative feedback loop. Beginning in the second trimester, the major source of CRH production transitions from the hypothalamus to the placenta along with a change from negative to positive feedback, with cortisol serving to increase placental CRH production [8]. Stimulants of placental CRH production include PGs, inflammatory cytokines, and neuropeptides. Progesterone and NO inhibit CRH production [11]. The shift to estrogen dominance may be influenced by CRH through stimulation of fetal adrenal activity, promoting release of DHEAS, the precursor of estriol [8]. CRH increases dilation of uterine, fetal, and placental blood vessels and promotes uterine contraction, possibly through the effect on increased fetal membrane production of stimulatory PGs $F_2\alpha$ and E_2.

Hematologic and cardiac adaptations

Hematologic and cardiac adaptations in pregnancy are essential to promote fetal tolerance for the challenges during labor and blood loss in the third stage of labor. Cardiac output, oxygen consumption, and left ventricular stroke volume are increased with progressive increases in blood volume [13]. Increased maternal blood volume of approximately 40%, composed primarily of increased plasma component due to retention of sodium and body water, peaks in the early third trimester. Red blood cells (RBCs) increase approximately 33%, maximizing oxygen-carrying capacity and provision of oxygen to the fetus. Increased RBC production is promoted by hormone stimulated release of erythropoietin but occurs more slowly than plasma volume adaptations. Plasma proteins are reduced by approximately 10–14%, with implications for drug binding, calcium binding, and metabolism of anesthetic agents during the intrapartum period. Increased production of coagulation factors contributes to a hypercoagulable state, characterized by increased clot formation and inhibition of clot breakdown. Thrombin, the clotting cascade enzyme responsible for the irreversible conversion of soluble fibrinogen to an insoluble fibrin clot, is increased during pregnancy. Thrombin also potentiates clotting through activation of clotting factors V, VII, XI, and XII. During labor and delivery, further increases in factor V and VII provide protection against hemorrhage after placental separation. Fibrinolytic activity is reduced during labor due primarily to plasminogen-activating inhibitor and fibrin-degradation products that peak at placental separation.

The hypertrophy of the maternal vascular system, promoted by NO-mediated vasodilation and progesterone-mediated reduction in vascular tone and resistance, accommodates the increased blood volume and perfusion requirements of the maternal-placental-fetal unit. Increased plasma volume is accompanied by decreased viscosity, reducing resistance to flow. The decreased resistance in the uteroplacental circulation is in part the result of a physiologic arteriovenous shunt that promotes accommodation of increased blood volume and cardiac output.

Respiratory adaptations

In concert with hematologic changes, respiratory adaptations in pregnancy serve to maximize oxygen delivery to meet maternal and fetal needs. Pulmonary functional adaptations include increase in tidal volume (30–40%) and inspiratory capacity (5–10%). Decreases in residual volume, expiratory reserve volume and functional residual capacity of approximately 20% occur during pregnancy in the absence of changes in respiratory pressures [14]. Pregnancy-induced respiratory adaptations combine to promote oxygenation and reduce carbon dioxide retention, maximizing efficiency of respiration [15]. Relaxation of smooth muscle in the ventilator and respiratory airways due to the influence of progesterone increases the airway lumen radius, promoting the ability to move more air in and out of the respiratory system. A state of chronic mild hyperventilation and compensated respiratory alkalosis in pregnancy is maintained, associated with increased renal secretion of bicarbonate to achieve a maternal pH of 7.4. The result of these changes includes reduced affinity of oxygen binding to maternal hemoglobin, releasing oxygen more readily to the fetus in the low oxygen in-utero environment. The increased oxygen consumption of 20–40% during pregnancy is further enhanced during labor to meet the demands of the fetus, placenta, and maternal system. Of particular significance is the influence of contractions on oxygen consumption during labor, as maternal oxygen reserve is lowered as a result of reduced functional residual capacity.

The combined effects of estrogen and progesterone contribute to rhinitis, the most common respiratory complaint in pregnancy. Increased blood flow and nasal mucus due to estrogen combined with progesterone-induced relaxation of vascular smooth muscle in the nasal turbinates induce feelings of stuffiness and runny nose similar to allergies or the common cold. Dyspnea is also a common complaint during pregnancy [16], with worsening of symptoms associated with increasing gestation.

Pregnancy adaptations and nutritional requirements

The nutritional needs of both mother and fetus are significant in the period of growth, development, and physiologic change characteristic of pregnancy. Maternal weight gain is typically greater in the second and third trimesters and is associated with fetal weight, both fat mass and fat-free mass [17]. Maternal intake of energy, protein and essential fatty acids, iron, folate [18], vitamin D [19], and calcium [20] is among the essential dietary factors central to promoting achievement of optimal nutrition in pregnancy for both mothers and their fetuses. Beyond the acute concerns of assuring adequate fetal growth and maternal function, maternal dietary intake in pregnancy can have long-lasting consequences on future health [21]. Nutrient-sensing mechanisms in the placenta are central to transfer of nutrients to the fetus, further necessitating the adequate intake of maternal macro- and micronutrients [22]. Fatty acid, amino acid, and glucose sensing promote transfer of essential nutrients to the fetus in competition with maternal demands [23,24]. Optimizing the nutritional status of both the mother and fetus during pregnancy supports their abilities to meet the additional physiologic challenges during labor.

Physiology of labor

The processes of labor initiation are complex, integrating biochemical, hormonal, and mechanical events that culminate with delivery of the fetus. The interplay between estrogen, progesterone, oxytocin, prostaglandins, and immune mediators results in the initiation and progression of labor. Endocrine, autocrine, and paracrine interactions involve the mother, fetus, placenta, and membranes and are critical to generation of uterine contractions and fetal expulsion.

The intrapartum period of labor includes the activation and stimulation phases, characterized by progressive uterine activity required for expulsion of the fetus. Activation is mediated by uterotropin hormones, including estrogen, to facilitate effective contractions. The activation phase also prepares the uterus for the stimulation phase, at which time the uterotonics PG and oxytocin stimulate regular contractions required for delivery.

The onset of contractions with a regular pattern and increasing duration and intensity indicates the onset of labor [25]. Triggers of the calcium-dependent contractile pathway (oxytocin, stimulatory PGs) stimulate phosphoinositol cell signaling, promoting the influx of extracellular calcium via ion channels and intracellular calcium release from the sarcoplasmic reticulum, providing calcium availability to support the contractile response. Calcium binding to calmodulin prompts the phosphorylation of myosin light chain kinase (MLCK), initiating the interaction of actin and myosin and uterine smooth muscle contraction. The inhibition of myosin phosphatase, the enzyme that catalyzes dephosphorylation ending the contraction, combined with increased MLCK phosphorylation is the outcome of activation of the calcium-independent pathway leading to uterine muscle contraction. Action potentials are propagated to adjacent myocytes via gap junctions, facilitating coordinated contractile activity [25]. Factors inhibitory to this process include progesterone and drugs that stimulate the β-adrenergic signaling pathway (e.g., terbutaline), inhibit inflammatory pathways (e.g., indomethacin), block calcium channels (e.g., nifedipine), and inhibit myosin light chain (e.g., magnesium sulfate), reducing myometrial contraction.

The transition from progesterone dominance in the quiescent phase to the estrogen dominance in the activation phase provides the primary stimulus for initiation and progression of labor, with onset of uterine contractions resulting from coordinated changes in hormone balance (Figure 2.1). The previous dominance of progesterone gives way to estrogen dominance, in large part due to reduced progesterone sensitivity, increased

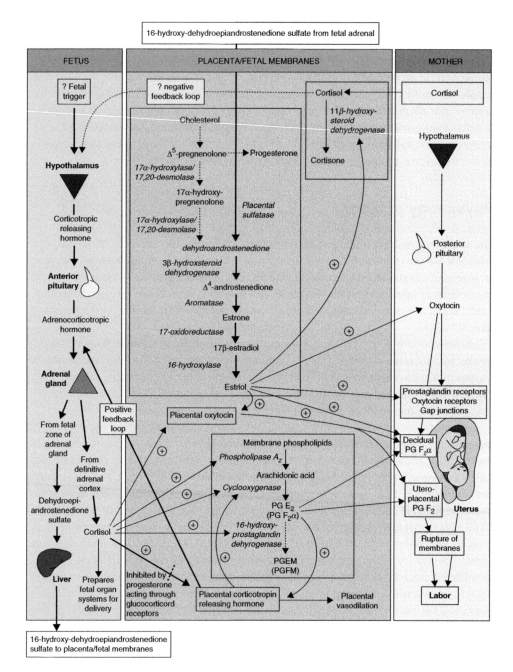

Figure 2.1   Maternal, fetal, and placental influences combine to regulate the onset and progression of labor through hormonal interactions. From Gabbe SG, *Obstetrics: Normal and Problem Pregnancies*, 5th ed. Copyright 2007 Churchill Livingstone, An Imprint of Elsevier. Modified from Norwitz ER, Robinson JN, Repke JT. (1999). The initiation of parturition: A comparative analysis across the species. *Current Problems in Obstetrics, Gynecology, and Fertility,* 22(41).

oxytocin sensitivity, and increased prostaglandin $F_2\alpha$ and E_2 activity in the activation phase of labor. The decreased gene transcription of progesterone receptor may lead to reduced availability of receptor and progesterone receptor binding, reducing receptor responsiveness and altering the ratio of progesterone receptor subtypes. The ratio of progesterone receptor subtypes transitions to that favoring increased progesterone receptor-A (PR-A) compared to progesterone receptor-B (PR-B), promoting reduced receptor sensitivity to progesterone. PR-A suppresses progesterone responsiveness, while PR-B promotes progesterone responsiveness. PR-A is found in increasing concentrations in the laboring myometrium, thus enhancing progesterone antagonism. The outcome of progesterone receptor antagonism is functional progesterone withdrawal, which occurs despite the stable levels of circulating progesterone [5]. In the absence of the influence of progesterone, estrogen suppression is removed. Estrogen increases ion channel activation, enhancing extracellular calcium entry into the myometrial cells. The PR ratio favoring increased PR-A also increases estrogen-responsive genes, including those that promote formation of gap junctions, cyclooxygenase (COX)-2, and oxytocin receptor production. An increased formation of gap junctions promotes transmission of contractile signals, leading to a coordinated, synchronous contractile pattern [8].

Oxytocin sensitivity increases in early labor, enhanced by the shift to estrogen dominance and increased production of PGs. It is the change in oxytocin receptor number and sensitivity, rather than the production and release of oxytocin itself, that appears to hold the greatest influence for the initiation of labor [8]. The high affinity of the oxytocin receptor increases sensitivity to oxytocin, further enhancing oxytocin receptor binding. The oxytocin receptor number increases 100- to 200-fold during pregnancy, reaching maximal concentrations in early labor. The number of oxytocin receptors in the contractile segment of the uterine fundus far exceeds the number located in the more passive lower uterine segment and cervix. The level of oxytocin peaks in the second stage of labor, possibly enhanced by fetal oxytocin release and transport to the maternal side of the placenta. Oxytocin receptor binding induces the phosphoinositide cycle and activation of phospholipase C (PLC), initiating a complex cell signaling cascade involving both calcium dependent and independent pathways leading to myometrial contraction.

The role of oxytocin receptor binding in the noncontractile amnion is less clear. The amnion increases prostaglandin synthesis prior to labor onset through oxytocin receptor binding, resulting in increased COX-2 production, the enzyme responsible for catalyzing the production of PGs [26]. The production of PGs in the amnion and decidua is an indirect consequence of phosphoinositide cycle activation, the result of arachidonic acid generation [9]. Activation of PLC promotes release of PG $F_2\alpha$ and E_2 from the fetal membranes; however, the effect of this action is not well described. Similarly, the effect of oxytocin on cervical ripening is unclear, despite the frequent use of exogenous low-dose oxytocin for this purpose in the clinical setting [8].

The neurohormone prolactin has been shown to increase the secretion of oxytocin, facilitating parturition [27]. Estrogen-mediated increase in oxytocin receptors contributes to the significantly increased receptor concentration in the uterine fundus, promoting sensitivity to circulating oxytocin. Labor and mechanical stretch significantly increases oxytocin receptor expression in uterine myocytes, further enhancing the potential for oxytocin receptor binding [26,28]. Oxytocin receptor binding stimulates the amnion and decidua to increase PG production and promotes myometrial contraction through the calcium-dependent and -independent pathways. Oxytocin works to promote uterine contractions by increasing the release of PG $F_2\alpha$ and E_2 in the fetal membranes and by increasing the activity of PLC.

Uterine increases in PGs thromboxane, $F_2\alpha$, and E_2 prime the myometrium for the onset of parturition, promoted by increased COX-2 activity on arachidonic acid [29]. Through a paracrine effect, relaxin inhibits production of PG E_2 by the fetal membranes during pregnancy. However, the increased production of CRH in late gestation stimulates the production of estriol and stimulatory PGs, perhaps overcoming the effect of relaxin on PG production. Further, the influence of CRH on uterine activity and blood vessel tone supports the transition to the activation phase of parturition [4]. Inflammatory cytokines may also play a role in initiation of labor through the increased CRH receptor and COX-2 activity.

PG activity increases during parturition, stimulated by the inhibition of progesterone, the stimulation of estrogen, inflammatory cytokines, and the oxytocin receptor binding [30]. PG F_2 is also thought to induce increases in PR-A, contributing to estrogen dominance. The increased PG sensitivity common in parturition may result from the differential regulation of PG receptor formation. Receptors with high affinity for stimulatory PGs promote myometrial contraction through increase in intracellular calcium and decrease in cyclic adenosinemonophosphate (cAMP). Further, the enzyme that catabolizes PG (15-hydroprostaglandin dehydrogenase [PGDH]) is decreased in the chorion and lower uterine segment during labor, promoting increased PG availability.

The cervix responds to mechanical pressure and stretch during labor by dilating and effacing in preparation for fetal expulsion. The loss of progesterone influence in late gestation is associated with removal of inhibition of collagen breakdown. A peptide hormone product of the ovarian corpus luteum, relaxin, is also produced by the placenta and decidua exerting local actions. Binding of relaxin to cervical receptors results in cervical softening via stimulation of collagen remodeling.

Cervical adaptations in pregnancy culminate with degradation of the collagen matrix, triggered by increased activity of matrix-degrading enzymes collagenase, protease, elastase, and matrix metaloproteinases (MMPs) and reduced activity of tissue inhibitors of MMPs (TIMMPs). The cervical tissue becomes soft due to the relaxed collagen bundles and high water content progressively developed during gestation. The influence of inflammatory mediators in cervical ripening is evidenced by cervical leukocyte invasion, inflammatory cytokine expression, and decreased production of suppressors of cytokine signaling, promoting progressive remodeling that includes changes in collagen, elastin, proteoglycans, and smooth muscle. Cervical stretching contributes to PG F_2 and oxytocin-stimulated uterine activity. Increased perfusion to the cervix is due in part to increased NO and PG E_2, promoting cervical vasodilation.

The outcome of uterine activity generated by utertonics in the stimulation phase is the generation of force in the uterine musculature, also known as the power [25]. Electrical activity initiated by action potentials and propagated by gap junctions translates into the frequency of contractions determined by speed of impulse and strength of contractions determined by number of myocytes recruited for action. The traction of the contractile uterus on the cervix likely contributes to dilation and effacement, facilitated by the preparatory connective tissue remodeling of late pregnancy. The pressure of the descending fetal head may also contribute to cervical effacement and dilation.

Hemodynamic adaptations to active labor are intensified beyond those in the quiescent phase. During each contraction in the second stage of labor, cardiac output increases by 50% along with an increase of up to 500 ml in blood volume, systemic vascular resistance, and oxygen consumption [13].

The last phase of labor is involution, characterized by oxytocin-mediated contraction of the uterus after fetal and placental delivery. An additional increase in the cardiac output of 60–80% in the immediate fourth stage of labor is accompanied by adaptations that promote return to baseline for blood volume, heart rate, and blood pressure [13]. Blood vessels that previously provided perfusion for the uteroplacental unit are compressed with uterine contractions, initiated immediately after the birth of the infant. Thrombin is active during involution to promote clotting, further contributing to control of blood loss. Contractile and hemostatic events promote separation and then delivery of the placenta. Uterine contractions cause a mechanical reduction in the placental site, limiting blood loss after delivery [12].

Involution involves physiologic mechanisms that eliminate altered uteroplacental vessels involving occlusive fibrointimal thickening, thrombosis, regeneration of vascular connective tissue, endothelial cell, and smooth muscle morphology [3]. The absence of the influence of placental estrogen promotes reduction in contractile proteins actin and myosin and cellular cytoplasm, leading to a decrease in cell size. Autolysis of myometrial cells also contributes to reduction in the size of the uterus. Epithelial regeneration promotes restoration of the postpartum endometrium as early as 2 days after delivery [12].

The removal of the placenta alters the endocrine environment, discontinuing placental production of pregnancy hormones [12]. A return to prepregnancy hormone production via negative feedback regulation resumes and returns prepregnant levels by 6 weeks postpartum. Estrogen levels drop rapidly, followed by progesterone. Production of these steroid hormones resumes with the resumption of hypothalamic-pituitary-ovarian feedback regulation. The sensitivity of the myometrium to oxytocin that progressively increased throughout pregnancy and labor promotes contraction of the myometrium, particularly when released during periods of infant suckling. The influence of oxytocin on myometrial contraction contributes to the progressive involution in the size of the uterus and subsequent return to pelvic location. An overview of uterine physiologic changes is presented in Box 2.1.

Psychobiological responses to labor

The physiology of labor induces responses among women that reflect the physical, psychological, social, and environmental context of the birth experience. The responses can be predicted but are as widely variable as the women themselves. Pain during labor is due predominantly to the characteristic uterine and cervical changes. Sensations of contractile pain are conducted from pain receptors (nociceptors) to afferent type A delta and C neurons extending from the uterus to the dorsal spinal cord, entering through

---

Box 2.1   Summary of uterine physiologic changes by phase

Quiescence: suppression of uterine activity
• Progesterone dominance.
• Estrogen sensitivity reduced.
• Decreased prostaglandin production.
• Reduced oxytocin receptors.

Activation: cervical ripening and initiation of uterine activity
• Estrogen dominance.
• Decreased progesterone sensitivity.
• Increased oxytocin sensitivity.
• Increased stimulatory prostaglandin activity.
• Relaxin binding to cervical receptors.

Stimulation: cervical dilation and effacement, increased frequency and intensity of uterine activity
• Estrogen dominance.
• Increased oxytocin and receptors.
• Increased stimulatory prostaglandins and receptors.

Involution: uterine return to prepregnancy state
• Oxytocin-mediated contraction.
• Thrombin activation.
• Removal of placental endocrine production.

---

segments of the thoracic spinal nerves (10–12) [31]. Mechanical pressure on the pelvic floor, vagina, and perineum due to fetal descent during the second stage of labor triggers sensory pain impulses to the sacral spinal nerves (2–4) along the pudendal nerve. The pain impulse travels up the spinal cord to higher cortical brain centers where interpretation of the sensation occurs. Interruption of the pain pathway at any point (entry into the spinal cord, spinal neurons, and higher brain centers) can modulate the pain sensation, promoting the effective strategies for pain relief that are at the heart of pain management in labor [32]. Stimulation of inhibitory afferent type A beta fibers through interventions such as massage can decrease the transmittal of the pain sensation at the entry to the spinal cord. Endogenous responses via enkephalinergic or other inhibitory neurons can decrease pain perception via the descending spinal nerves. Strategies including cognitive manipulation (e.g., distraction) target higher cortical brain centers, reducing the interpretation of the pain stimulus.

Stress and anxiety during labor are exacerbated by fear, past traumatic birth experiences, and hormonal responses associated with physiologic events during labor [33]. Anxiety in women is a particularly important trigger for cognitive pain perception, increasing sensitivity to pain [34]. Cortisol, a biomarker for anxiety and stress, is a likely target to explain variations in psychological responses to labor, though there is inadequate evidence to support this link [35]. The potential advantages for strategies aimed at reducing fear, stress, and anxiety in women during labor include improved birth outcomes and experiences [36]. Factors contributing to the psychobiological response to labor include opportunities for decision making, access to information, emotional well-being and satisfaction with the birth experience [37], serving as natural targets for interventions to reduce fear, stress, and anxiety during the process.

Pain during labor is anticipated with varying degrees of concern among pregnant women. Pre-existing fears, ineffective coping skills, and high levels of anxiety can potentiate the subjective interpretation of pain. Characteristics of the birth experience such as knowledge, attention to goals, companionship, feelings of reassurance, and safety and can positively modulate pain, distinguishing it from trauma and suffering [38]. Implementation of nonpharmacologic strategies (e.g., relaxation, water immersion, acupuncture) and activities such as yoga during labor have the potential to reduce the sensation of pain intensity, promoting control and achievement of a positive birth experience [39,40].

Summary

Pregnancy adaptations prime the maternal-placental-fetal systems for labor and birth, prompted in large part by placenta-induced changes in endocrine regulation. While direct actions on reproductive organs provided the primary focus of this chapter review, the endocrine milieu of pregnancy impacts responsive cells throughout the system. A clear understanding of the physiologic basis for pregnancy, labor, birth, and recovery provides the rationale basis for therapeutic management.

A philosophical appreciation of pregnancy as a normal physiologic event in women's lives, in addition to current knowledge about labor initiation and progression, is foundational to an approach to clinical care during pregnancy that, in fact, supports and encourages women's confidence in these normal processes. The combination of basic science and philosophy, grounded in the best research evidence, with a healthy respect for individual normal variation, prepares clinicians to partner with women and their families during this critical developmental and indeed magical time in their lives.

References

1. Norwitz ER, Robinson JN, & Challis JR. (1999). The control of labor. *New England Journal of Medicine, 341*(9), 660–666. DOI: 10.1056/NEJM199908263410906.
2. Burton GJ, Sibley CP, & Jauniaux ERM. (2012). Placental anatomy and physiology. In SG Gabbe, JR Niebyl, JL Simpson, MB Landon, HL Galan, ER Jauniaux, & DA Driscoll, eds., *Obstetrics: Normal and problem pregnancies*, 6th ed., pp. 3–19. Philadelphia: Elsevier.
3. Weydert JA & Benda JA. (2006). Subinvolution of the placental site as an anatomic cause of postpartum uterine bleeding: A review. *Archives of Pathology & Laboratory Medicine, 130*(10), 1538–1542.
4. Petraglia F, Imperatore A, & Challis JR. (2010). Neuroendocrine mechanisms in pregnancy and parturition. *Endocrine Reviews, 31*(6), 783–816. DOI: 10.1210/er.2009-0019.
5. Kamel RM. (2010). The onset of human parturition. *Archives of Gynecology and Obstetrics, 281*(6), 975–982. DOI: 10.1007/s00404-010-1365-9.
6. Lei K, Chen L, Cryar BJ, Hua R, Sooranna SR, Brosens JJ, & Johnson MR. (2011). Uterine stretch and progesterone action. *Journal of Clinical Endocrinology and Metabolism, 96*(6), E1013–1024. DOI: 10.1210/jc.2010-2310.

7. Tan H, Yi L, Rote NS, Hurd WW, & Mesiano S. (2012). Progesterone receptor-A and -B have opposite effects on proinflammatory gene expression in human myometrial cells: Implications for progesterone actions in human pregnancy and parturition. *Journal of Clinical Endocrinology and Metabolism, 97*(5), E719–730. DOI: 10.1210/jc.2011-3251.

8. Weiss G. (2000). Endocrinology of parturition. *Journal of Clinical Endocrinology and Metabolism, 85*(12), 4421–4425.

9. Vidaeff AC & Ramin SM. (2008). Potential biochemical events associated with initiation of labor. *Current Medicinal Chemistry, 15*(6), 614–619.

10. Kilpatrick S & Garrison E. (2012). In SG Gabbe, JR Niebyl, JL Simpson, MB Landon, HL Galan, ER Jauniaux, & DA Driscoll, eds., *Obstetrics: Normal and problem pregnancies,* 6th ed. Philadelphia: Elsevier.

11. Shynlova O, Tsui P, Jaffer S, & Lye SJ. (2009). Integration of endocrine and mechanical signals in the regulation of myometrial functions during pregnancy and labour. *European Journal of Obstetrics, Gynecology, and Reproductive Biology, 144* (Suppl 1), S2–10. DOI: 10.1016/j.ejogrb.2009. 02. 044.

12. Blackburn ST. (2007). *Maternal, fetal, & neonatal physiology: A clinical perspective.* St. Louis: Elsevier.

13. Fujitani S & Baldisseri MR. (2005). Hemodynamic assessment in a pregnant and peripartum patient. *Critical Care Medicine, 33* (10 Suppl), S354–361.

14. Gordon MC. (2012). Maternal physiology. In SG Gabbe, JR Niebyl, JL Simpson, MB Landon, HL Galan, ER Jauniaux, & DA Driscoll, eds., *Obstetrics: Normal and problem pregnancies,* 6th ed., pp. 49–51. Philadelphia: Elsevier.

15. Curran CA. (2006). The effects of rhinitis, asthma, and acute respiratory distress syndrome as acute or chronic pulmonary conditions during pregnancy. *Journal of Perinatal & Neonatal Nursing, 20* (2), 147–154, quiz 155–156.

16. Sroczynski T, Gawlikowska-Sroka A, Dzieciolowska-Baran E, & Poziomkowska-Gesicka I. (2010). Causes of respiratory ailments in pregnancy. *European Journal of Medical Research, 15*(Suppl 2), 189–192.

17. Institute of Medicine (U.S.) and National Research Council (U.S.) Committee to Reexamine IOM Pregnancy Weight Guidelines. (2009).

18. Abu-Saad K & Fraser D. (2010). Maternal nutrition and birth outcomes. *Epidemiologic Reviews, 32*(1), 5–25. DOI: 10.1093/epirev/mxq001.

19. Hollis BW & Wagner CL. (2012). Vitamin D and pregnancy: Skeletal effects, nonskeletal effects, and birth outcomes. *Calcified Tissue International,* DOI: 10.1007/s00223-012-9607-4.

20. Buppasiri P, Lumbiganon P, Thinkhamrop J, Ngamjarus C, & Laopaiboon M. (2011). Calcium supplementation (other than for preventing or treating hypertension) for improving pregnancy and infant outcomes. *Cochrane Database of Systematic Reviews, 10* (10), CD007079. DOI: 10.1002/14651858.CD007079.pub2.

21. Barger MK. (2010). Maternal nutrition and perinatal outcomes. *Journal of Midwifery & Women's Health, 55*(6), 502–511. DOI: 10.1016/j.jmwh.2010.02.017.

22. Sandovici I, Hoelle K, Angiolini E, & Constancia M. (2012). Placental adaptations to the maternal-fetal environment: Implications for fetal growth and developmental programming. *Reproductive Biomedicine Online.* DOI: 10.1016/j.rbmo.2012.03.017

23. Gil-Sanchez A, Koletzko B, & Larque E. (2012). Current understanding of placental fatty acid transport. *Current Opinion in Clinical Nutrition and Metabolic Care, 15*(3), 265–272. DOI: 10.1097/MCO.0b013e3283523b6e .

24. Jansson T, Aye IL, & Goberdhan DC. (2012). The emerging role of mTORC1 signaling in placental nutrient-sensing. *Placenta,* DOI: 10.1016/j.placenta.2012.05.010.

25. Liao JB, Buhimschi CS, & Norwitz ER. (2005). Normal labor: Mechanism and duration. *Obstetrics and Gynecology Clinics of North America, 32*(2), 145–164, vii. DOI: 10.1016/j. ogc.2005.01.001.
26. Terzidou V, Blanks AM, Kim SH, Thornton S, & Bennett PR. (2011). Labor and inflammation increase the expression of oxytocin receptor in human amnion. *Biology of Reproduction, 84*(3), 546–552. DOI: 10.1095/biolreprod.110.086785.
27. Vega C, Moreno-Carranza B, Zamorano M, Quintanar-Stephano A, Mendez I, Thebault S, & Clapp C. (2010). Prolactin promotes oxytocin and vasopressin release by activating neuronal nitric oxide synthase in the supraoptic and paraventricular nuclei. *American Journal of Physiology—Regulatory, Integrative and Comparative Physiology, 299*(6), R1701–1708. DOI: 10.1152/ajpregu.00575.2010.
28. Terzidou V, Sooranna SR, Kim LU, Thornton S, Bennett PR, & Johnson MR. (2005). Mechanical stretch up-regulates the human oxytocin receptor in primary human uterine myocytes. *Journal of Clinical Endocrinology and Metabolism, 90*(1), 237–246. DOI: 10.1210/jc.2004-0277.
29. Makino S, Zaragoza DB, Mitchell BF, Robertson S, & Olson DM. (2007). Prostaglandin F2alpha and its receptor as activators of human decidua. *Seminars in Reproductive Medicine, 25*(1), 60–68. DOI: 10.1055/s-2006-956776.
30. Olson DM. (2003). The role of prostaglandins in the initiation of parturition. *Best Practice & Research: Clinical Obstetrics & Gynaecology, 17*(5), 717–730.
31. Hawkins JL & Bucklin BA. (2012). Obstetrical anesthesia. In SG Gabbe, JR Niebyl, JL Simpson, MB Landon, HL Galan, ER Jauniaux, & DA Driscoll, eds., *Obstetrics: Normal and problem pregnancies*, 6th ed., pp. 362–365. Philadelphia: Elsevier.
32. Marchand S. (2008). The physiology of pain mechanisms: From the periphery to the brain. *Rheumatology Disease Clinics of North America, 34*(2), 285–309. DOI: 10.1016/j.rdc.2008.04.003.
33. Alder J, Breitinger G, Granado C, Fornaro I, Bitzer J, Hosli I, & Urech C. (2011). Antenatal psychobiological predictors of psychological response to childbirth. *Journal of the American Psychiatric Nurses Association, 17*(6), 417–425. DOI: 10.1177/1078390311426454.
34. Goffaux P, Michaud K, Gaudreau J, Chalaye P, Rainville P, & Marchand S. (2011). Sex differences in perceived pain are affected by an anxious brain. *Pain, 152*(9), 2065–2073. DOI: 10.1016/j.pain.2011.05.002.
35. Giurgescu C. (2011). A clinical translation of the research article titled "Antenatal psychobiological predictors of psychological response to childbirth." *Journal of the American Psychiatric Nurses Association, 17*(6), 426–430. DOI: 10.1177/1078390311424908.
36. Haines HM, Rubertsson C, Pallant JF, & Hildingsson I. (2012). The influence of women's fear, attitudes and beliefs of childbirth on mode and experience of birth. *BMC Pregnancy and Childbirth, 12*(1), 55. DOI: 10.1186/1471-2393-12-55.
37. Meyer S. (2012). Control in childbirth: A concept analysis and synthesis. Journal of Advanced Nursing. DOI: 10.1111/j.1365-2648.2012.06051.x; 10.1111/j.1365-2648.2012.06051.x.
38. Simkin P. (2011). Pain, suffering, and trauma in labor and prevention of subsequent posttraumatic stress disorder. *Journal of Perinatal Education, 20*(3), 166–176. DOI: 10.1891/1058-1243.20.3.166.
39. Jones L, Othman M, Dowswell T, Alfirevic Z, Gates S, Newburn M, & Neilson JP. (2012). Pain management for women in labour: An overview of systematic reviews. *Cochrane Database of Systematic Reviews, 3*, CD009234. DOI: 10.1002/14651858.CD009234.pub2.
40. Smith CA, Levett KM, Collins CT, & Crowther CA. (2011). Relaxation techniques for pain management in labour. *Cochrane Database of Systematic Reviews, (12)*(12), CD009514. DOI: 10.1002/14651858.CD009514.

Chapter 3

A supportive approach to prenatal care

Carrie E. Neerland

Key points

- Prenatal care in the United States continues to be focused on risk assessment.
- A supportive approach to prenatal care emphasizing normal pregnancy ideally begins preconceptionally or interconceptionally.
- Supportive prenatal care means a woman-centered approach where care is focused on the woman's concerns and emphasizes the normalcy of pregnancy.
- Components of prenatal care include anticipatory guidance, listening to women, active participation, women-/family-centered care, and an "optimized" prenatal care setting.
- Group prenatal care is an alternative care model that is woman-centered and provider-facilitated.
- Prenatal strategies to help a woman achieve her preferred labor and birth experience include shared decision making, evidence-based information, and development of the birth plan or birth preferences.

[A] climate of confidence focuses on our bodies' capacity to give birth. Such a climate reinforces women's strengths and abilities and minimizes fear.
The Boston Women's Health Book Collective

Introduction

The current model of prenatal care in the United States has been in place for more than a century and is based on risk assessment and recognizing complications of pregnancy such as preeclampsia [1,2]. Not much has changed in the way prenatal care is provided in the United States aside from the addition of newer technologies and increased testing to detect problems and high-risk factors. There is little evidence, however, to suggest that this model of prenatal care is effective with approximately one-third (32.8% in 2010) of all births being cesarean sections, 11.99% preterm (although down for the fourth year in a row), and 8.15% of infants born low birth weight [3]. Black infants are more than

---

Supporting a Physiologic Approach to Pregnancy and Birth: A Practical Guide, First Edition.
Edited by Melissa D. Avery.

2 times as likely as white or Hispanic infants to be low birth weight and/or preterm [4,5], and their infant mortality rate is higher than most other developed countries [5].

In this chapter, suggestions for emphasizing the normalcy of pregnancy for low-risk women to encourage a physiologic approach to prenatal care and preparation for labor and birth are presented. It is assumed that clinicians reading this chapter are already familiar with the basics of providing prenatal care including providing or referring for higher levels of care where a woman's condition warrants such care. Building women's confidence in the normalcy of pregnancy and birth and their capability to grow and give birth to a healthy newborn are emphasized.

Typical approach to prenatal care

The prenatal care schedule typically consists of an initial visit with a complete history and physical examination and is followed by twelve to sixteen short one-on-one visits (monthly earlier in pregnancy, weekly by the final month) with a provider (obstetrician-gynecologist, family medicine physician, midwife, or nurse practitioner) that consist of physical assessment, risk assessment, and counseling on specific pregnancy issues based on gestational weeks. In 1989, the U.S. Public Health Service's Expert Panel on the Content of Prenatal Care established guidelines on the timing and the content of prenatal care, including a reduced visit schedule for those women considered at lower risk for adverse outcomes [6]. A preconception visit followed by seven to nine prenatal visits, depending on parity, was recommended for low-risk women. Since the report was published, several randomized clinical trials have been conducted validating the safety and efficacy of reduced visits and finding this approach to be equivalent in outcomes for preterm delivery, preeclampsia, cesarean section, and low birth weight infants [7]. Fewer visits, however, have been associated with decreased satisfaction with care among low-risk women [8]. Therefore, with ongoing assessment of women's individual health needs, visit frequency can be adjusted or modified for each woman according to her preferences in partnership with the care provider.

With the typical schedule, or even with a reduced schedule of prenatal visits, the emphasis continues to be placed on risk even though the majority of pregnancies progress normally. This risk-based approach can result in more visits than necessary, increased use of ultrasonography, increased prenatal testing, and continued use of tests and assessments that are not based on evidence (e.g., routine urine dipstick testing for protein and glucose). A culture where pregnancy is automatically considered risky results in normalizing the unnecessary testing and resulting interventions. This pattern also has the potential to lead to a culture of fear surrounding pregnancy and birth, with negative psychological effects on women and undermining women's own knowledge of pregnancy and birth [9].

Midwifery care is based on a philosophy of pregnancy and birth as normal events in women's lives. Care provided during pregnancy is focused on the woman and includes education and counseling as well as specific care components, referring to or collaborating with physicians and others when higher care levels are needed. A Cochrane review and meta-analysis of midwife-led care compared to other models of care was published in 2009. Eleven trials with over twelve thousand women randomized were included in the meta-analysis. Midwife-led care meant that a midwife was the "lead professional" for maternity care, although there may have been visits with other care providers. Midwife-led care resulted in fewer antenatal hospitalizations, instrumental births, regional anesthesia use, and episiotomies, as well as more spontaneous vaginal births, breastfeeding initiation, and women's perception of control in labor was improved. There was no difference in the cesarean section rate. Maternal satisfaction was difficult to analyze statistically because of significant heterogeneity in concept and measurement, although it appeared to be higher among women randomized to midwife-led care [10]. Evidence supports more frequent use of this care model for low-risk women in the United States [11].

Preconception and interconceptional care: Begin a supportive approach early

A supportive approach to normal pregnancy commonly begins following the diagnosis of pregnancy. However, this approach can be initiated prior to conception and/or continued between pregnancies. Pregnancy, viewed as a normal life event along the continuum of women's health, allows for a discussion of reproductive planning at each health care visit for all women of reproductive age. Referred to as the reproductive life plan [12,13], asking about if and when a woman might wish to conceive her first (or next) child will help to frame her goals in terms of overall health and childbearing. In addition, sexual history, current sexual activity, contraceptive use, and health status all warrant inquiry. Assisting women to optimize their health prior to a pregnancy or between pregnancies can help them develop lifelong healthy habits. Additionally, when providing care to women with previous adverse outcomes, the objectives are to optimize health prior to conception, initiate early prenatal care, and detect and prevent obstetrical complications early. The reproductive life plan may be addressed as part of an annual physical exam, contraception counseling visit, or exam for sexually transmitted infections, as well as a formal preconception visit.

Helpful questions to ask when discussing a woman's reproductive life plan include:

- Do you hope to have any (more) children?
- How many children to do you hope to have?
- How long do you plan to wait until you (next) become pregnant?
- How much space do you plan to have between pregnancies?
- What do you plan to do until you are ready to become pregnant?
- What can I do today to help you achieve your plan? [14]

Interventions recommended for all women planning a pregnancy include folic acid supplementation; immunizations as needed such as MMR, varicella, influenza; diet and exercise advice; and screening for other specific risk factors that may warrant intervention prior to pregnancy such as substance use, obesity, specific medical conditions, and any social issues that should be addressed [15]. Preconception and interconception periods are important opportunities to emphasize pregnancy as a normal process in women's lives.

1   Folic acid: Folic acid is an essential B vitamin important in the development of the fetal neural tube. The CDC and the U.S. Public Health Service recommend that all women of childbearing age consume 0.4 mg (400 mcg) of folic acid daily in order to prevent spina bifida and other neural tube defects [16]. All women between 15 and 45 years of age are recommended to consume folic acid daily because half of U.S. pregnancies are unplanned or unintended and because neural tube defects occur very early in pregnancy (3–4 weeks after conception), before most women know they are pregnant [16]. The CDC estimates that 50–70% of neural tube birth defects could be prevented if this recommendation were followed before and during early pregnancy [16].

2   Healthy weight: Being overweight or underweight can make conception more difficult, and while being underweight can lead to low birth weight babies, being overweight can also contribute to pregnancy and birth complications such as diabetes, hypertension, and increased risk of cesarean section [17]. A healthy body mass index (BMI) is 18.5 to 24.9; 25.0 to 29.9 is considered overweight and a BMI greater than 30 is defined as obese. Helping women to achieve a healthy weight should be a public health priority. Convenient BMI calculators easily found online can be shared with women (see http://nhlbisupport.com/bmi/).

3   Nutrition: Achieving good nutritional status before becoming pregnant or between pregnancies is an important topic, particularly in relation to folic acid. Attaining a healthy weight, addressing any eating disorders, and developing nutritionally balanced eating habits are essential for growing healthy newborns and extend beyond pregnancy to choosing and preparing healthy food for children. Recognition of nutritional deficits may lead to nutritional counseling, while more significant issues such as obesity or an eating disorder may require referral to a nutritionist or a psychological evaluation [18].

4   Exercise: Exercise is an important way for women to stay healthy during and between pregnancies. If a woman does not exercise prior to pregnancy, she should be encouraged to initiate a regular physical activity program. Good options for exercise include walking, swimming, biking, or low-impact aerobics. When beginning a program, a woman should be encouraged to start slowly with 10–20 minutes of an activity initially, increasing to 60 minutes over time. If already exercising, she should be encouraged to continue her current exercise regimen [19]. Yoga is also an excellent option, as it helps to build strength and flexibility and includes a focus on breathing and concentration that may aid relaxation during labor.

5   Cessation of any unhealthy practices—tobacco, alcohol, drugs: During the preconception/interconception period, women can be assisted and supported in cessation of unhealthy practices such as tobacco, alcohol, and nonprescription drug use [20]. A careful history should be obtained to identify use of these substances. Screening guidelines and suggested tools are widely available [21–24] and can be used in combination with local resources and referrals.

   It is well established that tobacco use (smoking) in pregnancy is associated with preterm birth, low birth weight, and small for gestational age babies [25]. Counseling should be offered to women describing the effects of smoking prior to, during, and after pregnancy as well as a discussion of treatment options including medications and counseling options such as individual, group, and telephone.

All women of childbearing age should be screened for alcohol use during the preconception or interconceptional period. Interventions include providing information about the effects of alcohol during pregnancy and that no safe level of consumption has been established. Women with alcohol dependence should be offered education about the risks of alcohol consumption and efforts should be made to find programs to help them achieve cessation. Contraception counseling should be offered and pregnancy postponed until an alcohol-free pregnancy is possible.

Similarly, women of childbearing age should be asked about illicit drug use and counseled on the risks of drug use before and during pregnancy. Information should then be offered on treatment programs and contraceptive options offered so that pregnancy may be delayed until the woman is no longer using these substances.

Tobacco, alcohol, and drug use can cause health risks both for women of childbearing age and their children. Screening during the preconception or interconception period creates an opportunity to identify these issues and help women reduce their health risks.

6 Previous risks/adverse outcomes: Obstetric history should be included during any interconceptional visit. Having had a previous preterm birth, a low birth weight or small for gestational age infant, or a fetal demise are risk factors for having a subsequent poor birth outcome.

Women who have experienced gestational diabetes in a previous pregnancy should be tested postpartum, triennially, or prepregnancy with a 75 g 2-hour OGTT [26]. Additionally, first trimester testing is recommended in subsequent pregnancies.

Women with a history of preeclampsia are at increased risk for preeclampsia and other adverse outcomes. Preconception counseling regarding recurrence is important as well as identification and treatment of underlying disorders. Once pregnant, antenatal care may include more frequent visits, baseline laboratory work, and home blood pressure monitoring [27].

Supportive physiologic prenatal care: What is it?

Supportive prenatal care is care that supports normal physiologic changes of pregnancy and where the provider recognizes that pregnancy, labor, and birth are normal, healthy processes that result in healthy outcomes for the vast majority of mothers and newborns. The focus on pregnancy as normal is communicated clearly to women as part of their prenatal care. Care is woman-centered and includes education and support based on her individual needs, questions and concerns, and sociocultural preferences rather than a checklist of questions and measurements provided to all women. However, pregnancy is also a time of great change for a woman and her family. As a woman experiences the physiologic changes of pregnancy she may be anxious, uncomfortable, overwhelmed, or blissfully unaware. It is the role of the health care clinician to integrate the best evidence available into a model of shared decision making in order to meet the woman "where she is" and to offer support in managing common pregnancy changes. The components of supportive prenatal care include anticipatory guidance, individualized and comprehensive care, and engaging the woman in active participation in decision making.

Components of supportive prenatal care

Anticipatory guidance

Anticipatory guidance is the "psychological preparation of a person or group of people to help relieve fear and anxiety regarding an anticipated development or event expected to be stressful" [28]. Along with psychological preparation, anticipatory guidance can also assist in achieving health promotion and disease prevention. Using anticipatory guidance, providers can help expectant mothers understand the changes they are experiencing in pregnancy and how to have the most healthy pregnancy possible. Providers also help women and families prepare both physically and psychologically for a normal pregnancy and birth. This process includes information gathering, establishing a therapeutic alliance, and finally providing education and guidance.

Gathering information and individualizing care: Really listening to women

In order to meet the needs of a pregnant woman during her prenatal visits, it is important to first gather information. The plan of care not only involves her historical and physical data but addressing any concerns that the woman and her family may have at each visit. The needs of the woman are primary over the needs of the clinician and/or educator. Individualizing care is an important feature described in the philosophy of the American College of Nurse-Midwives: "the best model of care for a woman and her family includes individualized methods of care and healing guided by the best evidence available." Utilizing this standard of care, a clinician collects and assesses client care data, develops and implements an individualized plan of care, and evaluates care outcomes. In studies, women consistently report higher satisfaction with care when it is individualized to meet their needs [29].

Reminding women about the normalcy of their pregnancy and asking how they perceive their progress and change since the previous visit and how they would like to focus the current visit is a good place to begin. Ask open-ended questions: "What would you most like to talk about today?" or "What questions or concerns do you have today?" These questions offer a starting point at which the clinician can address the woman's needs and then adapt care accordingly. It is equally important to take the time to listen to women's concerns. A study in the *Journal of the American Medical Association* demonstrated that physicians interrupt patients, on average, only 23 seconds into the interview [30]. Often, if patients are interrupted, they may not return to talking about their own needs or they may feel they were not listened to, thus damaging trust and ultimately the provider-patient relationship. Truly, providers must listen to women. In a recent online survey of more than 1,200 women conducted by the American College of Nurse-Midwives, 62% of women reported that their care provider did not discuss how to stay healthy in pregnancy [31].

Creating therapeutic alliance/engaging in active participation

Engaging a woman in active participation increases her sense of control in the care process and enables the woman and her family to make informed choices. Participation in health care decision making is correlated with improvement in provider-patient relationships and trust in the provider, thus contributing to positive patient satisfaction and greater adherence to the plan of care [32]. The physiologic benefits associated with patient involvement in decision making include increased adherence to treatment plan, improved clinical outcomes, increased sense of responsibility for health of self and baby, and shorter recovery periods [32]. The psychological benefits associated with patient involvement in decision making include increased patient satisfaction and perception of experience, enhanced emotional well-being, and increased sense of patient empowerment and self-esteem. Benefits specifically related to women's involvement in childbirth decision making and patient control include lower levels of fear and less depressive and posttraumatic stress symptoms after birth [32].

Although this is information familiar to health care clinicians, today's health care environment can make the provision of care that is truly woman-centered difficult and thus is a topic worth revisiting. To actively engage women and to create a therapeutic alliance, providers ask open-ended questions and take the time to listen, encourage women to write down their questions and bring them to their prenatal visits, encourage involvement in the care process, and discuss care options and jointly make decisions with women and their families.

Partners involved in decision making, family centered care

Pregnancy is a time of change for families as well as pregnant women. Involving a woman's support person(s) and an approach to care that is family centered facilitates individualized care and active participation. Recognizing that each woman and her family or support person(s) are unique will help the clinician to provide the best care for the woman. Women desire to have their partners involved in discussions, often look for information as to how their partners can be involved in pregnancy and childbirth, and may have increased adherence and satisfaction when partners are involved [29].

Further, the family friendliness of the clinic culture including adequate space for the woman's partner and providing family friendly waiting areas supports the philosophy of family centered care. Ensuring that women feel comfortable bringing children to the clinic if they need to or so desire, offering children toys to play with while they wait, and keeping women informed of wait times are important details and impact satisfaction as well as how a woman feels supported within the clinic culture [29]. Care is culturally competent and family centered when a broad definition of family, including all significant others important to the pregnant woman, is incorporated in providing prenatal care.

Comprehensive care/psychosocial care

In addition to the physical changes of pregnancy, pregnancy is a time of significant emotional changes as well as changes in roles and relationship dynamics. Comprehensive health care that includes mental health assessment and psychological support services is essential. Women value and benefit from counseling services, psychosocial assessments, or even just the opportunity to talk informally about concerns [29]. Counseling services, social services, and nurse support and coordination can impact outcomes as well as women's satisfaction with prenatal care [29]. Support groups can also offer peer-to-peer support during pregnancy and often continue through the postpartum period. Peer support can aid in normalizing pregnancy and parenting concerns and enhance self-esteem. If psychological care, counseling services, or social services are not immediately part of the prenatal care setting, information regarding how women can access these services should be made available.

Optimizing the prenatal care setting

The clinical care setting can be optimized for education and support of normal pregnancy and birth. Having reading materials and handouts about important pregnancy topics can help to answer common questions for women. If possible, provide reading materials in multiple languages if serving a diverse population. Posters of pregnancy changes as well as diagrams of the labor process, including pictures of labor positions, can be helpful when answering women's questions about labor and birth. Portable DVD players also offer an opportunity to watch videos about childbirth or breastfeeding, for example, while the woman is waiting for her appointment or for laboratory or other tests.

Lending libraries in clinics give women an opportunity to read about pregnancy topics while they wait, or materials can be made available to take home and return on a subsequent visit. Providing a list of reliable websites and Internet resources that support physiologic birth is helpful in our current technology-rich environment. Providing web resources on individual clinic websites, including a list of evidence-based and reliable resources for women, is a plus. Taking it a step further, Facebook and Twitter accounts can be created and managed to provide information on evidence-based care during normal pregnancy, including local resources for childbirth education, doulas, birth plans, and individual hospital or birth center statistics. The bottom line is this: the message that pregnancy is normal and that physiologic birth is supported and achievable should be *everywhere*.

"The Rights of Childbearing Women" [33] was developed in 2006 to help assure that childbearing women have access to the best evidence about maternity care and are able to participate meaningfully in their care. Providing a copy of the rights to each woman as part of her prenatal care gives the message that it is her pregnancy and she is at the center of the care team.

Group prenatal care as an alternative to individual care

Group prenatal care has been suggested as an alternative to the traditional individual prenatal care visit structure. Group prenatal care, or more specifically the Centering Pregnancy model, is based on assessment, education and skill-building, and support. After an individual initial prenatal visit and examination with a provider, eight to twelve women with similar expected due dates meet beginning at approximately 12–16 weeks of pregnancy. The women and provider group facilitators then meet ten times for 2-hour sessions through the rest of their pregnancies—first monthly and then biweekly.

Each group session has a similar format. During an initial self-assessment period, women each take their own blood pressure and weight, determine their gestational age, and review self-assessment materials. Next, a health care provider completes individual physical assessments with each woman including measuring her fundal height, listening to fetal heart tones, reviewing vital signs and any new lab findings, and identifying any concerns a woman might have. Women are encouraged to bring their general concerns to the group, as it is likely these issues will be pertinent to the other women and all will benefit from the discussion. While the physical assessments are being performed, women complete self-assessment worksheets, which help to stimulate discussion regarding common pregnancy topics such as discomforts in pregnancy, nutrition, exercise, preparation for labor and birth, contraception, stress reduction, and parenting issues. The group then comes together for introductions, reminders of guidelines (e.g., confidentiality), and facilitated discussion.

The benefits of group prenatal care include more provider time spent with women, improved satisfaction with care, increased feeling of preparedness for labor and birth, increased knowledge, reduced rates of cesarean section, increased breastfeeding rates, and reduced rates of preterm birth [34–36]. The mutual support and community building are also a great benefit to women, with many exchanging contact information and continuing to meet after the birth of their babies to offer each other support regarding postpartum, breastfeeding, and parenting issues. This group model of prenatal care by definition is woman-centered and utilizes an approach supporting normal pregnancy where the provider is a facilitator rather than the director of the care process. Women choose the focus for the group visits, resulting in an approach to pregnancy care that is shaped by the women.

Common discomforts of pregnancy

Addressing the common discomforts of pregnancy, reassuring women of their normalcy, explaining normal physiologic pregnancy changes, and providing constructive and practical advice to meet women's needs are essential components of prenatal care. Although common to clinicians, who may discuss similar topics multiple times throughout a clinic day, these topics should not be trivialized or downplayed. Women may need to express their emotions about a particular discomfort or may be seeking information about the cause of the problem, whether or not it is normal, and want help identifying a solution or therapy for the issue. Women can be reminded that most symptoms are good news and are the result of a growing fetus and the subsequent hormonal changes or the result of the growing uterus. Provide specific suggestions to help the woman's significant other provide emotional and physical support during the changes of pregnancy. This is especially important early in pregnancy when she may be experiencing symptoms but the pregnancy is not yet physically apparent, and in late pregnancy when physical discomforts can be numerous. Nonpharmacologic remedies that are evidence based can be recommended as a way to promote the normalcy of common pregnancy symptoms.

When women present with common pregnancy discomforts such as nausea and vomiting, low back pain, or constipation (to highlight a few), providers have an opportunity to offer a supportive physiologic approach, including education and nonpharmacologic relief measures, instead of immediately pulling out the prescription pad. Offering reassurance that many of these discomforts are normal helps women to feel more at ease and oftentimes less anxious about the physical changes they are experiencing. Although not an exhaustive list of nonpharmacologic comfort measures in pregnancy, a few are worth mentioning here.

Nausea and vomiting in pregnancy: There is some evidence that acupressure (of the P6 point) may be helpful in relieving some of the nausea and vomiting of pregnancy. Wrist acupressure of the P6 either manually or with the use of acupressure bands is an inexpensive method with no known negative side effects or harm. Ginger-containing foods such as ginger tea, ginger ale, or ginger pops may offer some relief as well. Women can also be reminded to eat small, frequent meals, to avoid triggers of nausea and vomiting, and may take their prenatal vitamins at bedtime instead of morning. Definitive safety and efficacy of these measures are not supported in systematic reviews of research and further high-quality research is needed [37].

Low back pain in pregnancy: Women can benefit from education regarding posture, ergonomics, pain management strategies, and relaxation techniques. Additionally, maternity support belts, tailored exercise, and acupuncture have been shown to be beneficial. Massage and the use of heat or cold also offer relief from low back pain and offer no risk to women [38].

Constipation: Many women suffer from constipation in pregnancy and it is thought to be a result of the increase in progesterone and resulting decrease in gastrointestinal motility. Education, lifestyle and diet modifications, and reassurance are the first line in treating constipation in pregnancy. Along with education regarding the physiology, women with constipation should be encouraged to increase their fluid intake along with increasing fiber in their diet and to participate in regular physical activity [39].

Preparation during pregnancy for a physiologic approach to labor and birth

Preparation for physiologic birth includes woman-centered prenatal care (either group or individual), childbirth education that focuses on preparation for labor and birth rather than common hospital routines, continuity in care, and creating a climate of confidence.

Prenatal care

Preparation during pregnancy for a physiologic approach can begin at the very first prenatal appointment and, as already discussed, can even begin during the preconception or interconception period. Offer reassurance to the pregnant woman that pregnancy is a normal, healthy process and that most women proceed through their pregnancy without complications. Breastfeeding is supported as the preferred infant feeding method when possible. It is important to help manage normal fears and help women develop confidence in self and the process of pregnancy and birth.

Childbirth education

Although some controversy exists regarding the effectiveness of childbirth education [40], many clinicians and educators continue to encourage childbirth education with the view that with increased knowledge there is decreased fear and stress (fear-tension-pain cycle) and that there is no known harm that comes from formal preparation for labor and birth.

The goals of childbirth education are to provide women and their support person(s) an opportunity to explore beliefs about pregnancy and birth, to help women feel confident in their own ability to give birth, to provide coping skills women can use as labor progresses in order to have a sense of control and to minimize discomfort, and to provide information to enhance the knowledge and skills of support persons [41].

The benefits of childbirth education include building a woman's confidence in her body's ability to give birth; opportunity to discuss fears about labor and birth with the educator and others who may have similar concerns; partners learn methods of offering support in labor; increased bonding with partner; overview of pain relief options and comfort measures including hydrotherapy, massage, relaxation, breathing, and medications; tour of birthing facility; and creating a social support network.

Continuity in care

Women often state that they desire to receive care during pregnancy from one provider or from a small group of providers. Novick found that women were more satisfied with prenatal care provided by a designated health care provider. Additionally, women were more accepting if they understood in advance that they would be seeing multiple providers within a group [29]. Women receiving care from a small group of midwives with whom they established a trusting relationship developed confidence during pregnancy and appreciated being supported to labor without pharmacologic methods [42]. Many different models of care can be utilized, and women appreciate a description of the type of care they will receive as well as being informed throughout the pregnancy.

Building the climate of confidence

As the climate around birth has evolved into one of fear, risk, and interventions, many women have lost the confidence to give birth in a normal, physiologic manner. Media depictions of birth have also contributed to this problem, showing birth as something that needs to be managed by a physician, presenting highly dramatized and complicated births, portraying women as out of control, or skewing the birth timeline ("My water broke. I think it's time."). Reality television shows often depict high-drama, medicalized, worst-case scenario scenes that further instill fear.

In the current climate of medicalized and interventive birth, fear, and doubt, it is important to create instead a climate of confidence for women and their families about pregnancy and birth. Encourage women to choose a provider carefully: find a physician or midwife with low rates of intervention. Trustworthy consumer websites such as Lamaze International and Childbirth Connection offer tips on how to choose a provider. Additionally, many clinics offer interview or "meet and greet" appointments where women can meet a provider and inquire about birth outcome statistics and rates of intervention. The location of the birth setting is also important. Women should examine where they want to give birth and choose a setting with low rates of intervention appropriate to their health status and preferences. Active participation and shared responsibility for care is of utmost importance. In so doing, women can participate in childbirth education, evaluate care options, read and ask questions, and co-create their individual birth preferences with their support persons and care provider.

Inclusivity of partners, families, and support persons

Include partners, families, and support persons whenever possible and appropriate. Ask women who their support persons are and encourage their involvement. Use of terms such as "partner" and "support persons" are inclusive of the range of family constellations commonly seen. Specific information related to support of lesbian childbearing couples is available [43]. If women seem to have insufficient social support, recommend doula services including some that may be available at low cost or on a sliding scale, advocate for the provision of doula services in the hospital or birth center setting, and help to foster pregnancy support groups.

A prepared birth partner can offer assistance during labor with physical support and comfort, emotional support, and advocacy. Birth partners can become prepared by attending childbirth education classes along with the mother-to-be, rehearsing techniques such as massage and relaxation, participating in preparing the birth plan, and viewing videos of normal birth. Penny Simkin's book *The Birth Partner: A Complete Guide to Childbirth for Dads, Doulas, and All Other Labor Companions* is an excellent resource for all partners when preparing to support a woman in childbirth [44].

Strategies to help women achieve their preferred birth experience

There are many strategies that health care providers can use to help women achieve their preferred birth experience in a maternity system geared to anticipate and look for problems: shared decision making, evidence-based care, the birth plan, looking critically at the birth setting, and evaluating and influencing nursing support.

Books that focus on the pregnant woman and her desires for her pregnancy and birth can be recommended to women. *Our Bodies Ourselves: Pregnancy and Birth* provides a woman-centered approach to information about pregnancy and birth from selecting a care provider and birth location to care expectations during pregnancy and options for labor and birth [45]. An evidence-based approach with reflections from other women is presented.

Shared decision making

One of the most important methods in helping women to achieve a safe and satisfying birth experience is the shared decision-making model. Often, women and their families are left out of the decision-making process. They may not even know their full array of care options or may not understand the evidence behind the options being offered. Additionally, some providers are not supportive of women's involvement in the decision-making process. Shared decision making involves providing the woman with unbiased and accurate information (evidence-based information, risks and benefits of treatment options), incorporating the woman's individual values and goals, and reaching an agreement together regarding treatment or care. The benefits of shared decision making are increased involvement and greater sense of control, increased satisfaction, and improved outcomes [32]. All women should be encouraged to seek providers that practice evidence-based care and support shared decision making.

Childbirth Connection has engaged in a partnership with the Informed Medical Decisions Foundation for a project called the Maternity Care Shared Decision Making Initiative. The team for this national initiative will develop and test decision aids to help women make decisions about their care that are based on the best available evidence. It is hoped that the project will promote the engagement of providers and women in shared decision making [46,47]. Providers can anticipate and look for these resources in the near future.

Evidence-based care

As defined in the Milbank Report, "Evidence-Based Maternity Care: What It Is and What It Can Achieve" [48], evidence-based maternity care providers use the best available research on the safety and effectiveness of specific practices to help guide maternity care decisions and to facilitate optimal outcomes for mothers and their newborns. Large gaps continue to exist between best evidence and actual maternity care practices in the United States. For example, although continuous electronic fetal monitoring has not been shown to improve outcomes for low-risk women and their newborns, it is used routinely in many U.S. hospitals. The report highlights overused maternity practices that have the potential to increase risk or cause harm as well as underused maternity practices that are beneficial and not known to cause harm.

Overused interventions that should be used judiciously and with careful attention to informed consent include induction of labor, epidural anesthesia for pain relief, delivery by cesarean section, continuous electronic fetal monitoring, artificial rupturing of membranes, and episiotomy.

Underused interventions—practices to use whenever possible and appropriate—include greater use of midwives and family physicians, prenatal multivitamins for prevention of congenital anomalies, smoking cessation interventions, ginger for nausea and vomiting, interventions for preventing preterm birth (smoking cessation, birth-to-conception interval, use of progesterone for those at increased risk for preterm birth, no elective induction of labor before term, Centering Pregnancy group prenatal care, judicious use of cesarean), external version, practices to foster women's satisfaction, continuous labor support, comfort measures in labor, delayed and spontaneous pushing, nonsupine positions for birth, delayed cord clamping, early skin-to-skin contact, breastfeeding, interventions to reduce newborn pain, interventions for postpartum depression, and providing access to vaginal birth after cesarean (VBAC) [48].

The birth plan

The two words "birth plan" can evoke various reactions and feelings among physicians, midwives, and nurses. The use of birth plans began as a list of "I don't want these care measures" or "don't do this to me" items with the potential to be antagonistic to the birth environment. Many clinicians have strong negative feelings toward birth plans and believe that women who write them often end up with complications and ultimately a cesarean delivery. In reality, though, birth plans help women think through their preferences surrounding labor and birth, help women to feel more in control, enhance communication between women and their partners and with care providers, and increase women's satisfaction with the childbirth experience [49].

Instead of using the words "birth plan," encourage the terms "birth wishes" or "birth preferences." Women can be encouraged to thoughtfully create a preference list or wish list, understanding that it is not a rigid, inflexible plan to be followed at all costs but a means of thinking about setting, support persons, and coping measures and communicating with those involved with providing care. This approach helps to create openness to the birth process for women and their families, as well as the midwives, physicians, and nurses providing care. Numerous resources and templates are available for women when creating their birth preferences, and they can be encouraged to bring their preferences in to a prenatal visit(s) to review together with their provider.

Questions for women to consider when creating a birth wish list:

- What will I do to stay confident and feel safe?
- What will I do to find comfort in response to my contractions?
- Who will support me in labor, and what will I need from them? [49]

Two consumer-focused texts that specifically present strategies for developing useful birth plans are *Creating Your Birth Plan: The Definitive Guide to a Safe and Empowering Birth*, by Marsden Wagner with Stephanie Gunning [50], and *Natural Hospital Birth: The Best of Both Worlds*, by Cynthia Gabriel [51]. Both books guide women and their support persons through choosing a care provider and a birth location and considering various care practices and options for labor and birth. Gabriel, a doula herself, recommends a specific process of visualizing or dreaming an ideal labor and birth, planning the most meaningful elements, and finally writing the plan down—a longer version for the woman and her support team and a shorter version for the hospital staff. These books may also be useful for care providers who can then use them in partnership with women as part of the labor planning process during prenatal care.

Birthing environment

The birthing environment has an enormous impact on whether or not a woman experiences a physiologic birth. How a woman feels in the birth environment, how she is able to move about, the support options provided (or not), and method of fetal monitoring for low-risk women all have the potential to disturb the physiologic process. Information about the hospital birth environment is discussed in more detail in chapter 12; out-of-hospital birth is discussed in chapter 13.

Conversations during pregnancy about the philosophy of the selected birth setting and what women can anticipate when they arrive, as well as how women can advocate for themselves in the milieu of the hospital birth setting, are key components of supportive prenatal care. Encourage hospital or birth center tours; explain hospital or birth center options, policies and guidelines (fetal monitoring); and describe available tools and how they can be used for comfort such as tubs, showers, balls, or rocking chairs.

Conclusion

In the current environment of fear and doubt surrounding childbirth, clinicians and women need to work together to regain a culture of confidence. With the media portrayal of birth as highly dramatic and medicalized, along with a birth culture that is highly interventive, it is not surprising that many women fear pregnancy and childbirth. The message that pregnancy and birth are normal life events and that women can achieve a physiologic birth should be everywhere, starting with the preconception period and extending into the next interconception period. The settings where women receive care and give birth should be optimized to support a normal physiologic approach to pregnancy and birth. Group prenatal care may be a beneficial alternative to the traditional model of prenatal care. Providers can use anticipatory guidance and individualized care and can involve women and their families as active partners in care to create a climate of confidence. Finally, promoting evidence-based practices in maternity care and participating in true shared decision-making allows women to feel safe, supported, and confident—knowing that each woman and her health care team are making the best decisions for her and her baby. (See Case Study 3.1.)

Case Study 3.1

Optimal scenario for prenatal care

A woman is seen for a well-woman exam and discusses her reproductive life plan with her health care provider. She had recently stopped using oral contraceptive pills and was hoping to become pregnant. The provider reviewed her current physical activity routine, discussed folic acid supplements, and emphasized the importance of healthy weight and nutrition, as well as discontinuing unhealthy habits such as alcohol consumption. Pregnancy as a normal life event was emphasized.

Months later, the woman has a positive pregnancy test at home and makes an appointment to establish care. It is her first pregnancy, but she had been taking a prenatal vitamin with folic acid since her well-woman exam. She has her first visit with a nurse-midwife at about 8 weeks gestation, where she is able to openly ask questions about her pregnancy and the changes that she is going through. The midwife offers the woman and her partner education regarding nutrition, exercise/activity, the normal physiologic changes of pregnancy, and prenatal testing. As a part of her first visit, she has a gentle, respectful physical exam, lab work performed, and history reviewed. The midwife also discusses how the prenatal visits will be organized throughout her pregnancy, clarifying the woman's preferences.

In the second trimester, the woman has follow-up visits about every 4 weeks with her prenatal care provider. Her visits begin with questions she has about her pregnancy that she has been encouraged to write down since her previous visit. She is provided with resources for childbirth education classes and doula services and encouraged to breastfeed. Normalcy of pregnancy is emphasized. Blood pressure, weight, fundal height, and fetal heart tones are assessed at each visit.

She begins feeling low back pain and hip pain at about 26 weeks. She discusses this with her provider, who takes the time to talk with her about the physiology of low back pain and round ligament pain in pregnancy. The woman and the midwife decide on a plan of care where she will incorporate more stretching and yoga into her exercise routine and use pillows for positioning while sleeping, and she is referred to an acupuncturist who works in the clinic [52].

In her third trimester, she meets with her midwife every 2 weeks. Her hip and back pain have improved and she also discusses with her midwife how she is incorporating more position changes and stretching at work, where she is mostly seated. She brings a notebook with questions and is starting to focus more on labor and the postpartum period. She has signed up for two classes: one about comfort measures in labor and one about breastfeeding. She has also decided on a doula, who will come to the hospital birth center with her and her partner.

During the last month of pregnancy, she comes for visits every week. The midwife encourages her to create a birth preferences list and gives her a template as a reference. She reviews with the midwife the signs and symptoms of early labor and active labor; they plan how she will cope at home during early labor and come to the hospital when she is in active labor. The woman has also expressed the desire to avoid medication in labor and the midwife reviews comfort measures and nonpharmacologic pain relief options such as movement and position changes, massage, and hydrotherapy.

In the last weeks of pregnancy, the midwife also reviews mother and baby-friendly hospital practices such as delayed cord clamping, early bonding and kangaroo care, rooming-in, and support of breastfeeding on-demand. The woman has completed her childbirth education and breastfeeding classes and is feeling confident. She brings her completed birth preferences list and reviews it with the midwife. A copy is made for her medical record and she is encouraged to also bring a copy with her to the hospital. The midwife offers words of support and encouragement: "You *can* do it!"

References

1. Alexander GR & Kotelchuck M. (2001). Assessing the role and effectiveness of prenatal care history, challenges, and directions for future research. *Public Health Reports, 116*(4), 306–316.
2. Novick G. (2004). Centering pregnancy and the current state of prenatal care. *Journal of Midwifery & Women's Health, 49*(5), 405–411.
3. Centers for Disease Control and Prevention. (2010). Births: Final data for 2010. *National Vital Statistics Reports, 61*(1). Retrieved from: http://www.cdc.gov/nchs/data/nvsr/nvsr61/nvsr61_01.pdf. Accessed November 4, 2012.
4. March of Dimes. (2010). Toward improving the outcome of pregnancy III. Retrieved from: http://www.marchofdimes.com/TIOPIII_FinalManuscript.pdf.
5. Centers for Disease Control and Prevention. (2011). Understanding racial and ethnic disparities in U.S. infant mortality rates. *NCHS Data Brief, 74*. Retrieved from: http://www.cdc.gov/nchs/data/databriefs/db74.htm. Accessed April 12, 2012.
6. U.S. Department of Health and Human Services, U.S. Public Health Service. (1989). Caring for our future: The content of prenatal care. Washington, DC: U.S. Public Health Service.
7. Gregory KD, Johnson CT, Johnson TRB, & Entman SS. (2006). The content of prenatal care: Update 2005. *Women's Health Issues, 16*(4), 198–215.
8. Dowswell T, Carroli G, Duley L, Gates S, Gülmezoglu AM, Khan-Neelofur D, & Piaggio GGP. (2010). Alternative versus standard packages of antenatal care for low-risk pregnancy. *Cochrane*

Database of Systematic Reviews, issue 10. Art. No.: CD000934. DOI: 0.1002/14651858. CD000934.pub2.

9. Jordan RG & Murphy PA. (2009). Risk assessment and risk distortion: Finding the balance. *Journal of Midwifery & Women's Health, 53*(3), 191–200.

10. Hatem M, Sandall J, Devane D, Soltani H, & Gates S. (2008). Midwife-led versus other models of care for childbearing women. *Cochrane Database of Systematic Reviews*, issue 4. Art. No.: CD004667. DOI: 10.1002/14651858.CD004667.pub2.

11. American College of Nurse-Midwives, Midwives Alliance of North America, & National Association of Certified Professional Midwives. (2012). Supporting healthy and normal physiologic childbirth: A consensus statement by ACNM, MANA, and NACPM. http://www. midwife.org/ACNM/files/ACNMLibraryData/UPLOADFILENAME/000000000272/ Physiological%20Birth%20Consensus%20Statement-%20FINAL%20May%2018%20 2012%20FINAL.pdf. Accessed November 15, 2012.

12. Lu MC. (2007). Recommendations for preconception care. *American Family Physician, 76*(3), 397–400.

13. Lu MC, Kotelchuck M, Culhane JF, Hobel CJ, Klerman LV, & Thorp JM. (2006). Preconception care between pregnancies: The content of internatal care. *Maternal and Child Health Journal, 10*, 107–122.

14. Preconception and women's healthcare: An interview with Dr. Michael Lu (part one). (2012). Retrieved from: http://www.scienceandsensibility.org/?tag=dr-michael-lu&paged=2. Accessed April 13, 2012.

15. Berghella V, Buchanan E, Pereira L, & Baxter JK. (2010). Preconception care. *Obstetrical and Gynecological Survey, 65*(2), 119–131.

16. Centers for Disease Control and Prevention. (2012). Folic acid recommendations. Retrieved from: http://www.cdc.gov/ncbddd/folicacid/recommendations.html. Accessed November 8, 2012.

17. Baeten JM, Bukusi EA, & Lambe M. (2001). Pregnancy complications and outcomes among overweight and obese nulliparous women. *American Journal of Public Health, 91*(3), 436–440.

18. Zauderer C. (2012). Eating disorders and pregnancy: Supporting the anorexic or bulimic expectant mother. *American Journal of Maternal/Child Nursing, 37*(1), 48–55.

19. Centers for Disease Control and Prevention. (2011). Physical activity: Healthy pregnant or postpartum women. Retrieved from: http://www.cdc.gov/physicalactivity/everyone/guidelines/ pregnancy.html. Accessed November 8, 2012.

20. Floyd RL, Jack BW, Cefalo R, Atrash H, Mahoney J, Herron A, Huston C, & Sokol R. (2008). The clinical content of preconception care: Alcohol, tobacco, and illicit drug exposures. *American Journal of Obstetrics & Gynecology,* supplement to December 2008, 333–339.

21. Vermont Child Health Improvement Program. (2009). Screening for substance use in pregnancy. http://www.med.uvm.edu/vchip/Downloads//ICON%20-%20SCREENING_FOR_ PREGNANCY_SUBABUSE.pdf. Accessed November 10, 2012.

22. Virginia Department of Behavioral Health and Developmental Services. (2012). Screening instruments for pregnant women and women of childbearing age. http://www.dbhds.virginia. gov/documents/scrn-Perinatal-InstrumentsChart.pdf. Accessed November 10, 2012.

23. American College of Obstetricians and Gynecologists. (2012). Opioid abuse, dependence, and addiction in pregnancy. Committee Opinion No. 524. http://www.acog.org/Resources_And_ Publications/Committee_Opinions/Committee_on_Health_Care_for_Underserved_Women/ Opioid_Abuse_Dependence_and_Addiction_in_Pregnancy. Accessed November 10, 2012.

24. Society of Obstetricians and Gynaecologists of Canada. (2011). Substance use in pregnancy. *Journal of Obstetrics and Gynaecology Canada, 33*(4), 367–384. http://www.sogc.org/ guidelines/documents/gui256CPG1104E.pdf. Accessed November 10, 2012.

25. Centers for Disease Control and Prevention. (2004). Surgeon General's report—the health consequences of smoking. Retrieved from: http://www.cdc.gov/tobacco/data_statistics/ sgr/2004/complete_report/index.htm.

26. American Diabetes Association. (2012). Standards of medical care in diabetes—2012. Retrieved from: http://care.diabetesjournals.org/content/35/Supplement_1/S11.full.

27. Barton JR & Sibai BM. (2008). Prediction and prevention of recurrent preeclampsia. *Obstetrics & Gynecology, 112*, 359–372.

28. Bulechek GM, Butcher HK, & Dochterman JC, eds. (2008). *Nursing interventions classification (NIC)*, 5th ed. St. Louis: Mosby Elsevier.

29. Novick G. (2009). Women's experience of prenatal care: An integrative review. *Journal of Midwifery & Women's Health, 54*(3), 226–237.

30. Marvel MK, Epstein RM, Flowers K, & Beckman HB. (1999). Soliciting the patient's agenda: Have we improved? *JAMA, 281*(3), 283–287.

31. American College of Nurse-Midwives. (2012). New survey shows women settling for less. News release. http://www.midwife.org/ACNM-Launches-Our-Moment-of-Truth. Accessed November 4, 2012.

32. Goldberg H. (2009). Informed decision making in maternity care. *Journal of Perinatal Education, 18*(1), 32–40.

33. Childbirth Connection. (2006). The rights of childbearing Women. http://www. childbirthconnection.org/pdfs/rights_childbearing_women.pdf. Accessed November 4, 2012.

34. Massey Z, Schindler Rising S, & Ickovics J. (2006). Centering pregnancy group prenatal care: Promoting relationship-centered care. *JOGNN, 35*, 286–294.

35. Ickovics JR, Kershaw TS, Westdahl C, Magriples U, Massey Z, Reynolds H, & Schindler Rising S. (2007). Group prenatal care and perinatal outcomes: A randomized controlled trial. *Obstetrics & Gynecology, 110*(2), 330–339.

36. Ruiz-Mirazo E, Lopez-Yarto M, & McDonald SD. (2012). Group prenatal care versus individual prenatal care: A systematic review and meta-analyses. *Journal of Obstetrics and Gynaecology Canada, 34*(3), 223–229.

37. Matthews A, Dowswell T, Haas DM, Doyle M, & O'Mathúna DP. (2010). Interventions for nausea and vomiting in early pregnancy. *Cochrane Database of Systematic Reviews*, issue 9. Art. No.: CD007575. DOI: 10.1002/14651858.CD007575.pub2.

38. Vermani E, Mittal R, & Weeks A. (2010). Pelvic girdle pain and low back pain in pregnancy: A review. *Pain Practice, 10*, 60–71. DOI: 10.1111/j.1533-2500.2009.00327.x.

39. Cullen G & O'Donoghue D. (2007). Constipation and pregnancy. *Best Practice & Research Clinical Gastroenterology, 21*(5), 807–818. http://dx.doi.org.ezp1.lib.umn.edu/10.1016/j. bpg.2007.05.005.

40. Hanson L, VandeVusse L, Roberts J, & Forristal A. (2009). A critical appraisal of guidelines for antenatal care: Components of care and priorities in prenatal education. *Journal of Midwifery & Women's Health, 54*(6), 458–468.

41. Lothian JA, Lockwood CJ, & Barss VA. (2012). Preparation for labor and childbirth. In DS Basow, ed., UpToDate. Retrieved from: http://uptodateonline.com. Accessed November 14, 2012.

42. Leap N, Sandall J, Buckland S, & Huber U. (2010). Journey to confidence: Women's experiences of pain in labour and relational continuity of care. *Journal of Midwifery & Women's Health, 55* (3), 234–242. doi: 10.1016/j.jmwh.2010.02.001

43. McManus AJ, Hunter LP, & Renn H. (2006). Lesbian experiences and needs during childbirth: Guidance for healthcare providers. *JOGNN*, 35, 13–23. DOI: 10.1111/J.1552-6909.2006.00008.x.

44. Simkin P. (2008). *The birth partner: A complete guide to childbirth for dads, doulas, and all other labor companions*, 3rd ed. Boston: Harvard Common Press.

45. Boston Women's Health Book Collective. (2008). *Our bodies ourselves: Pregnancy and birth.* New York: Simon & Schuster.
46. Romano A. (2012). The first national maternity care shared decision making initiative. http://informedmedicaldecisions.org/wp-content/uploads/2012/05/First_Natl_Maternity_SDM.pdf. Accessed November 15, 2012.
47. Gee RE & Corry MP. (2012). Patient engagement and shared decision making in maternity care. *Obstetrics & Gynecology, 120,* 995–997.
48. Sakala C & Corry M. (2008). Evidence-based maternity care: What it is and what it can achieve. Co-published by Childbirth Connection, the Reforming States Group, and the Milbank Memorial Fund. Available at: http://www.childbirthconnection.org/pdfs/evidence-based-maternity-care.pdf.
49. Lothian J. (2006). Birth plans: The good, the bad and the future. *JOGNN, 35*(2), 295–303.
50. Wagner M with Gunning S. (2006). *Creating your birth plan: The definitive guide to a safe and empowering birth.* New York: Penguin Group.
51. Gabriel C. (2011). *Natural hospital birth: The best of both worlds.* Boston: Harvard Common Press.
52. Pennick V, & Young G. (2007). Interventions for preventing and treating pelvic and back pain in pregnancy. *Cochrane Database of Systematic Reviews* 2007, issue 2. Art. No.: CD001139. DOI: 10.1002/14651858.CD001139.pub2.

Chapter 4

Supporting a physiologic approach to labor and birth

Lisa Kane Low and Rebeca Barroso

Key points

- Provide individualized instructions to women about when to come in to the birth setting.
- Encourage women to have family present if desired and consider the use of a doula.
- Maintain oral hydration unless the woman is nauseous or vomiting, unable to drink.
- Use intermittent monitoring or auscultation.
- Conduct comprehensive holistic assessments during labor to determine how the woman is coping and her comfort level and for signs of progress in labor.
- Maintain a quiet, supportive physical environment.
- Regularly assess the laboring woman's level of comfort and coping with labor. Consider use of the Utah Coping with Labor Algorithm.
- Encourage freedom of movement in the room and offer options to promote upright positions such as a birth ball, stool, toilet, and/or walking with contractions.
- Allow women to move between a variety of positions to achieve as much comfort as possible and to promote fetal rotation and descent.
- Support women to push spontaneously, only with the contraction, not holding their breath.
- Support women to be in the most comfortable position for them for their birth.
- Provide encouragement or positive statements about women's strength rather than specific direction about how to push or for how long.
- As the baby is born, promote skin-to-skin contact by placing the baby on the maternal abdomen, and delay cord cutting until it has stopped pulsating.

A normal physiologic labor and birth is one that is powered by the innate human capacity of the woman and fetus. This birth is more likely to be safe and healthy because there is no unnecessary intervention that disrupts normal physiologic processes.

Supporting Healthy and Normal Physiologic Childbirth: A Consensus Statement by ACNM, MANA, and NACPM

Supporting a Physiologic Approach to Pregnancy and Birth: A Practical Guide, First Edition.
Edited by Melissa D. Avery.
© 2013 John Wiley & Sons, Inc. Published 2013 by John Wiley & Sons, Inc.

Introduction: What is "normal" childbirth?

The World Health Organization defines normal birth as "spontaneous in onset, low-risk at the start of labor and remaining so throughout labor and delivery. The infant is born spontaneously in the vertex position between 37 and 42 completed weeks of pregnancy. After birth mother and infant are in good condition" [1, p. 4]. In normal birth there should be an evidence-based reason to interfere with the natural process; otherwise the normal physiologic process of labor that results in birth should be left undisturbed or uninterrupted.

This definition of normal birth is the context in which we present a discussion of evidence-based strategies maternity care providers can employ to support women during normal childbirth, avoiding the routine use of non-evidence-based medical interventions. This discussion will be presented from three perspectives. First we describe the supportive roles of maternity care providers, working within the social context of childbirth keeping the woman and her needs central. Second, an overview of techniques maternity care providers can use to promote a physiologic approach to labor and birth is presented, including how to be present, supportive, and responsive to the woman's needs as her labor and birth unfold. Finally, a review of specific routine maternity care practices that can disrupt normal labor and birth are identified, along with alternative approaches to care. Underlying this chapter is the assumption that care providers continuously assess labor progress and when deviations from normal occur, evidence-based care is provided to maintain quality and safety for both the mother and her newborn.

What is a physiologic approach to childbirth?

Natural transitions from pregnancy through the dynamic and powerful process of labor and the act of giving birth are emphasized in a manner that supports a woman's individual labor process, acknowledging the deep psychological and emotional power of transitioning to motherhood. While medical technological advances are often assumed as essential to improved health outcomes, overuse of technology in childbirth has become routine in the United States. Doing less, or only what is needed, should be the focus to support normal, healthy, physiologic childbirth [2]. "What works is not flashy, not expensive, but it's human intensive" [3] and requires health care providers to maintain vigilance in observing and assessing the woman and her fetus during labor and generally "doing 'nothing' well" [4] unless normal becomes abnormal and intervention is then warranted.

Much of the evidence in support of physiologic birth originates in western Europe, where the midwifery model of care is the norm with an ongoing tradition that precedes modern medicine; noninterventive birth remains the norm [5–9]. In a reversal of "pure science" influencing social science, current evidence to promote physiologic labor and birth originates in the psychosocial, anthropological, and childbirth education literature [10–18]. An integration of basic and social sciences is helpful in identifying care practices that can be employed to support a woman during the dynamic process of labor and birth.

The role of health care providers during physiologic labor and birth

The psychosocial and anthropological literature highlights the personal, interpersonal, community, and cultural determinants that interact and reveal a great deal of how an individual woman moves through labor [13,16,19,20]. Within these constructs, members of the maternity care team and family members support the woman in the context of her worldview and social order. A focus on "managing" the labor process is set aside unless obvious deviations from normal occur, requiring some type of action [11,18]. In other words, nurses, midwives, doulas, and physicians are vigilant bystanders with necessary knowledge and expertise to provide evidence-based care and implement interventions should they become medically necessary. A comforting presence that promotes, supports, and sustains physiologic processes is the focus for all members of the maternity care team [21–23].

Members of the maternity care team work together to address the social, emotional, and educational needs of the laboring woman, along with the physiologic needs. They negotiate the complex interplay between providing proactive, anticipatory guidance while also being responsive to the woman's changing needs. Management is reserved for occasions when the maternity care provider identifies the development of a risk condition and must redirect the process because of evidence that something is amiss with the process of labor, the fetus, or the woman [4,14,24,25]. Attention is paid to the environment, creating a space conducive to movement, allowing the woman to be active and assume multiple positions or to rest when desired. Anxieties and fears are addressed, trust and comfort are promoted, and safety is ensured while staying in the background as quietly as possible.

Promoting the natural physiologic rhythm of labor

Labor is a dynamic, complex, and elliptical process, heavily influenced by social and cultural customs and inconsistent with the linear and predictable quantification of labor common in a medical approach to childbirth [26–28]. Many subtle and not-so-subtle physiologic, psychological, and even spiritual changes are perceived by women occurring over a course of weeks, days, and hours to slowly erase the separation from late pregnancy to early labor [29–35]. Despite defining the initiation of labor as dynamic and encompassing physiologic and psychological components, most textbooks turn to quantified definitions using the components of the Bishop score at the onset of labor: presenting part, station, dilatation, effacement, cervical position, and consistency as the key focus [36–38]. Labor onset and progress then become narrowly defined by numerical progression of dilatation, effacement, and fetal descent [39–42]. Although important in evaluating a woman's progress in labor, these measures are not a holistic evaluation of the physiologic, social, and emotional changes that are part of the onset of labor. Labor can instead be likened to a dance; something that begins and progresses individually, rather than the same pattern of progression for all women. The signs of transition from pregnancy to the beginning of labor vary individually from being quite subtle to remarkably sharp as the onset of labor manifests itself as one of the strongest forces of nature [26,27].

Transition to the care environment

The majority of women in the United States move from their home environment to another site for care during the labor and birth process. Transition from home to the birth site is a critical point influencing how a woman and her support persons frame their experience of "normal" labor or not. The shift between the woman's home environment and the "other environment"—more subtle in a birth center and more dramatic in a hospital setting—affects both the rhythm of the labor and her perception of pain [43,44]. The timing of this transition is often described to meet expectations of hospital staff and admission procedures in contrast to focusing on the woman in labor. Instructions about coming to the hospital may be distracting if not consistent with a woman's bodily experience of early labor [45].

Encouraging the woman to trust her sense of when she feels the need to move from her home to a setting where she can be supported by the maternity care team in addition to her family is helpful. Make statements such as "Come into the hospital when you feel like you want to be here instead of at home" or provide general guidelines regarding contraction patterns and associated sensations: "In general, women have contractions that are coming in a pattern and take focus to work through them. It seems like the pattern is not going to stop and it is going to increase." If specific recommendations are provided to women that quantify the timeframe and duration of contractions, a caveat should also be offered, such as "However, every woman's labor is unique, so you may move from home to the hospital (or birth center) when you feel ready, instead of having to meet a set number of contractions in so many minutes."

To realistically prepare a woman, she should understand she may not actually stay in the hospital or birth center setting. Together with her maternity care provider, she may decide that she can return home in early labor and better manage her comfort by not yet being admitted. It can be helpful to normalize that potential to return home as a common check in the labor process, an evidence-based approach to reducing the risk of increased interventions in normal labor [46,47]. Evidence links admission to the hospital during earlier phases of labor with almost twice the risk for increased use of interventions such as augmentation with oxytocin compared to admission during active labor [46,47].

Creating an environment to promote physiological birth

The World Health Organization has identified four evidence-based care practices that promote the process and progression of normal physiologic birth. Lamaze International has identified two additional care practices with similar degrees of scientific evidence supporting their use for normal birth (see Box 4.1) [1].

Physiologic birth is promoted by using less technology, and when necessary, individualizing its use for women with complex health conditions and in circumstances that require added assessment or monitoring. In short, optimal health outcomes during childbirth are accomplished by using evidence-based labor care practices tailored to meeting the unique needs of each woman during childbirth [2,48,49]. Maternity care providers consider the woman's desires and her and her baby's unique health condition in combination with the best available scientific evidence to determine the best

---

Box 4.1   Care practices to support physiologic birth

1. Labor should begin on its own (1, p. 4).
2. Laboring women should have continuous support from others throughout labor (1, p. 12).
3. Women should not give birth on their backs (1, p. 35).
4. Mothers and babies should not be separated after birth and should have unlimited opportunity for breastfeeding (1, p. 35).
5. There should be no routine interventions during labor and birth.
6. Laboring women should be free to move throughout labor.

Lamaze International, 2012

Box 4.2   Enhancing labor admission and ongoing care

- Minimize the number of personnel engaging the laboring woman.
- Provide uninterrupted time to get acquainted with the birth room before others enter that same space.
- Keep environmental stimuli to a minimum.
- Allow the laboring woman to choose the quantity and quality of light and sound in her space.
- Don't turn back the covers on the bed, as if the woman should immediately enter the bed, vs. being admitted to the full room with multiple options.
- Vital signs can be obtained quietly between several contractions, never during a contraction.
- Ask assessment questions between contractions while maintaining eye contact with the woman.
- Avoid overly focusing on the paper or computer health record where information is being recorded.

---

approach to her care during labor and birth. All maternity care providers impact a woman and her family, thus the team must have a common goal to promote care that supports physiologic birth [50].

Labor admission process

Specific strategies to individualize care and promote an atmosphere conducive to the unfolding of physiologic labor can be used. These simple practices alone challenge the usual hospital admission practices by encouraging the woman to be up and around instead of in the bed and sitting or lying down. Routines such as obtaining maternal vital signs and ongoing intermittent assessment of fetal well-being can be redesigned to cause less disruption to the process of labor. (Techniques are listed in Box 4.2.)

These measures convey a message of importance to the woman. Questions are asked but are inserted around the unfolding process of labor, allowing the woman to make labor her primary focus. This approach also establishes a relationship between the maternity care providers and laboring woman, particularly the nurse who will be with her during the labor process.

In settings that require an initial fetal monitor tracing, despite evidence indicating that it can disrupt the labor process and lead to increased rates of interventions [51], a portable and silent telemetry unit can be used. Once fetal well-being is established, continuous monitoring should be stopped and intermittent auscultation used. The initial history and physical, including pelvic exam, can be done at the woman's discretion: either quickly at a moment of her choosing or in parts over a period of time. When a woman is in very active labor, with limited time between contractions, the midwife, physician, or nurse can prioritize those items critical to providing safe, immediate care to the woman and fetus. Establishing the fetal position and presentation, confirming fetal well-being, and obtaining maternal vital signs can take priority while other assessments are completed as time allows.

Clinicians need to balance obtaining information that is medically necessary versus simply completing paperwork tasks; limiting duplicate questioning by multiple providers supports the woman so she can focus on the work of labor. Health care team members work collaboratively to gather important data and information needed by all while minimizing repeated disruptions for the laboring woman. Extraneous conversations, not focused on the woman in labor, should be minimized. Noise from beepers, alarms on equipment, and even the movement of equipment in and out of the birthing room space should be reduced or done quietly.

Progressing in first stage labor

To promote the normal process of more advanced labor, the focus of the maternity care team may become more active in supporting the laboring woman, assuring that she is well hydrated, nourished with high-quality foods that appeal to her [52], and encouraging rest as much and as deeply as possible between contractions. As labor continues, a key role for nurses and other providers is to remind the woman of this balance so that she can retain the necessary energy to work with her progressing labor contractions.

Advancement in labor is often explained to women as contractions that become longer, closer together, and more intense over a period of time [45] and described by care providers in terms of quantifiable changes in dilatation, effacement, and station [37,53–55]. Yet vaginal examination for cervical dilatation, effacement, and descent is only one limited element of assessing a woman's progress in labor. Frequent vaginal exams may disrupt the labor physiology by causing discomfort or anxiety for the woman or requiring her to assume a supine position that can be uncomfortable or result in supine hypotension. A more comprehensive approach to evaluating a woman's progress in labor includes assessment of her overall well-being including emotional, psychological, and physical changes in addition to the more objective elements indicative of progress.

When assessing a woman's progression in labor, maternity care providers first observe the woman in the space where she is laboring. How is she responding to those around her, does she appear relaxed between contractions, is she able to rest? What is her mood? Is she fearful, expressing anxiety, or is she speaking calmly, engaging in discussions beyond a focus on her labor? Progress may be manifested by her gradual or sudden withdrawal into the hard work at hand that consumes more of her energy and attention as she progresses toward birth. Assessing how a woman is responding to labor over time is a key focus instead of just observing the frequency of contractions or assuming a cervical examination is the only tool to assess labor progress.

An additional level of assessment includes palpating the contractions [56]. The nurse, midwife, or physician assesses contraction strength by placing her/his hand, with the woman's permission, on the fundus to feel the intensity of the uterine tightening; is it soft, firm, or very firm during the contraction? Are there changes in intensity over time? As labor progresses, increasing firmness is generally felt when contractions are palpated. Beyond the firmness of the contraction, frequency and duration of the contractions are evaluated over time. The combination of a progressive increase in frequency and duration is considered rather than one over the other. Observing a woman over a period of at least 30 minutes, noting how she responds to her contractions, allows a more holistic assessment of how a woman is experiencing labor.

Additional labor observations include the woman's movement in the room and how she interacts with others. Is she able to move from one position to another or is it a challenge to change or assume new positions because of the intensity of her contractions? Has the woman changed from being more mobile to now being in bed or sitting? In general women become more internally focused, almost withdrawn as they focus on the intensity of labor over time [57]. Contrary to popular media representations of women in active labor, there is typically not an entire personality change for an individual woman, but she may demonstrate a sense of increased intensity, resulting in what might be perceived as shortness with those around her. This should be interpreted as conserving her focus and energy for the labor process, rather than focusing on those around her.

Assessing coping during labor

For many women, as labor intensifies, the perception of discomfort may be more pronounced as maintaining comfort becomes more challenging. Increased tension and discomfort may indicate progress and can also interfere with the labor. Is the woman able to maintain a relaxed appearance during her contractions or is tension increasing? Are her shoulders elevated or is she squeezing other's hands during the contraction? Look for evidence of tension in her face, shoulders, general posture, and even in her voice as she goes through a contraction. A health care provider can offer support by placing a hand on a tense shoulder, encouraging slower breathing, offering suggestions such as dropping her shoulders, opening her mouth, relaxing her forehead. Combining specific suggestions with touch can help promote comfort and allow the clinician to assess how the woman is coping with increased labor intensity.

A common practice in the hospital setting is to assess a woman's level of pain using a scale of 1 to 10. A laboring woman would be asked to rate her pain using the descriptors of zero being no pain to 10 being the worst pain she has ever experienced. The McGill pain scale [58] is intended to be used universally across all settings and conditions of pain. However, in the context of labor, assessing comfort or coping may be a more helpful focus. It is not the actual experience of pain but the manner in which the woman is able to work with the pain that is the key indicator of whether or how the pain needs to be treated in labor [59–61]. A systematic approach to assessing a woman's coping with labor is outlined in Figure 4.1. Using the University of Utah Health System Coping with Labor Algorithm, maternity care providers can assess a woman's ability to cope with labor [62]. A woman is asked, "How are you coping with your labor?" Based on her response, the

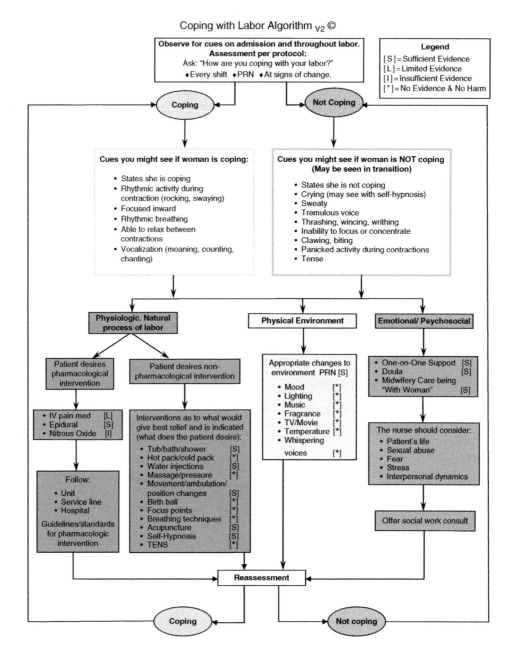

Figure 4.1 Coping with Labor Algorithm.

health care provider offers options to support her physical and emotional coping so that her labor can progress physiologically. In the Coping with Labor Algorithm the steps outlined in response to the woman's sense of coping are divided into the key areas that can influence her overall comfort and well-being; physiologic process of labor, physical environment, and psychosocial/emotional support. Under each of these key areas are suggested options for enhancing the woman's sense of comfort, including the level of evidence that supports that particular intervention. The health care provider can use this guide to offer options and alternative approaches to address an individual woman's desires and needs, while also supporting an evidence-based approach to the type of care being provided. Through this approach the health care provider can aid the woman in achieving a level of comfort that allows her to focus on the work of labor; it is not simply a process of eliminating pain.

Promoting comfort during labor

Throughout labor, health care providers can offer simple options while keeping careful watch of maternal, fetal, and labor well-being. For example, rather than the usual approach of asking someone if she would like to have a sip of water, the health care provider can simply say "Water?" or "Drink?" while holding up the water container. To encourage movement that can promote progress in labor the woman can be encouraged to ambulate by simply saying "Walk?" while pointing to a clear path. In early labor, discussions about possible positions and why a woman might want to select each can be helpful. During active labor a simpler approach helps a woman maintain her focus, remain relaxed as labor progresses, and gives her permission to respond in simple terms like "Yes," "No," or "Later."

To promote labor progress, encourage a woman to be upright, mobile, and freely move from one position to another, facilitating fetal rotation and descent [57]. Upright positions are typically more comfortable than lying down. The ancient traditional motto "Move the baby by moving the mother" can guide position options for the woman. Suggestions include moving from side to side to aid fetal rotation, using the hands and knees position to promote posterior to anterior rotation, and using an exaggerated Sims position to correct malpresentation or to aid in continued rotation. The health care provider can offer supportive suggestions in contrast to authoritative direction, guided by the woman's desires and responses. Providing information about the reasons for trying a certain position based on an assessment of the fetal position may motivate a woman to change her position in a process of shared decision making while promoting comfort.

Women experience pain during childbirth in a variety of ways ranging from very little to extremely distressing. A woman's confidence about her ability to manage labor, her knowledge about options for maintaining comfort, the support she perceives around her, and other life experiences with pain or trauma all influence her pain experience during childbirth. The duration of her labor, her fatigue, and her ability to rest between contractions also impact her experience of pain and discomfort. Maintaining mobility and the continuous presence of a support person are two key evidence-based approaches to maintaining comfort and managing the pain of childbirth [63,64]. Social support provided by a doula or trained support person, in addition to family members, can improve outcomes for the mother and her newborn, including shorter duration of labor, less use of epidural and pharmacologic pain management techniques, less risk for a cesarean birth, greater satisfaction with the birth experience, and increased success with breastfeeding [63]. The Coping with Labor Algorithm is an evidence-based approach to

Table 4.1   Nonpharmacologic comfort measures and techniques.

Options and measures to increase comfort and reduce pain	
Tools to support upright positions	**Tools to promote relaxation**
Birthing ball	Hydrotherapy (shower, tub)
Birthing stool	Massage
Hanging, holding someone's shoulders	Reflexology
Keeping head of bed >45° elevated	Breathing techniques
Sitting on the toilet	Visualization/hypnosis
Techniques to reduce back pain	**Environmental tools**
Acupressure/acupuncture	Maintain low lighting
Sterile water papules	Speak in low tones
Positioning (hands and knees)	Create space for movement
Exaggerated Sims position	Adjust number of people as needed
Counterpressure	Use of aromatherapy as indicated

assess the woman's status and work through multiple care options that promote comfort and reduce pain as necessary [60].

Maternity care providers should be knowledgeable about the full range of pharmacologic and nonpharmacologic support and pain relief options that are safe during childbirth. Nonpharmacologic approaches are less likely to disrupt physiologic labor and more likely to support labor progress [59,65]. Table 4.1 lists options to support women while promoting relaxation and not interfering with the normal progression of labor.

Monitoring maternal and fetal status during labor

By observing the woman in labor, maternity care providers can assess the intensity and frequency of contractions, her response to labor changes over time, and her comfort level as these changes unfold. A woman's energy level, presence of fatigue, and emotional well-being can also be assessed as additional indicators of labor progress. Observations should be made over an extended period of time rather than during a single contraction. Vaginal examinations augment the information obtained through observations versus being the only information used to assess labor progress. A vaginal examination is only performed when the information gained is necessary in making a clinical decision changing the current care being provided to the woman.

Unless signs of maternal and/or fetal compromise are present, maternal vital signs are monitored utilizing the current recommendations outlined by professional maternity care organizations [66,67] and fetal heart rate per intermittent auscultation guidelines outlined by the American College of Nurse-Midwives [68]. Acknowledging the evidence about continuous electronic fetal monitoring (EFM), the three major professional associations of maternity care providers—the American College of Obstetricians and Gynecologists (ACOG), American College of Nurse-Midwives (ACNM), and Association of Women's Health, Obstetric and Neonatal Nurses (AWHONN)—caution

Box 4.3   Technique for performing intermittent auscultation*

1. Perform Leopold's maneuvers to identify the fetal presentation and position.
2. Assist the laboring woman into a position that maximizes the provider's ability hear the heart rate over the fetal thorax or back while also preserving the woman's comfort.
3. Assess uterine contractions by palpation.
4. Determine the maternal pulse rate.
5. Place the fetoscope or Doppler on the woman's abdomen, over the fetal thorax or back.
6. Determine the baseline fetal heart rate by listening between contractions.
7. Verify that the maternal pulse differs from the fetal heart rate if necessary.
8. Count the fetal heart rate after a uterine contraction for 30–60 seconds every 15–30 minutes in active labor and every 5 minutes in second stage of labor.
9. Note increases or accelerations or decreases or decelerations from the baseline rate by counting and recording the fetal heart rate using a multiple-count strategy such as counting for 5–15 seconds three to five times to note increases or decreases in the counts.

*Adapted from [68].

their members about the routine use of EFM. Despite these evidence-based recommendations, over 94% of women reported being monitored continuously when they were in labor [69]. Studies confirm that routine use of EFM, particularly for low-risk women, offers little clinical benefit while increasing the risk of surgical interventions in birth [51,70]. Compared to intermittent auscultation of the fetal heart rate, EFM provides *no* reduction in the overall risk of perinatal death or cerebral palsy [68]. At the same time, overinterpretation of EFM tracings leads to higher rates of cesarean section and assisted vaginal delivery [71,72]. Continuous EFM also limits a woman's ability to remain mobile during labor [73]. Intermittent fetal monitoring can be performed in a nondisruptive manner between contractions, while supporting labor progress by not limiting movement (see Box 4.3) [68].

Assessing progress in labor

As previously described, the frequency of contractions, intensity of discomfort, level of fatigue, and ability to be upright and mobile, as well as how supported a woman feels, all intersect to influence her progress in labor. Traditional models of assessing labor progress have assumed a linear rate of dilation over time once a woman was in active labor. As a result, time and rate of dilation have been linked in essentially a one-to-one relationship. A common expectation for women in active labor (greater than 4 cm dilatation) has been to progress at a rate of 1 cm per hour. When a woman's progress did not match this standard, interventions were frequently initiated to increase the rate of progress. More contemporary research conducted with multiple populations has challenged this prevailing assumption [42,74,75]. Variable change over time has been documented as being normal, particularly in the earlier part of active labor [76]. It is important to maintain the principle that every woman's labor is unique. Allowing for a wider range in the rate of dilation and experience of contractions during normal labor is essential.

A new partograph, or method of documenting labor progress over time, has been developed to assist maternity care providers move away from traditional expectations of

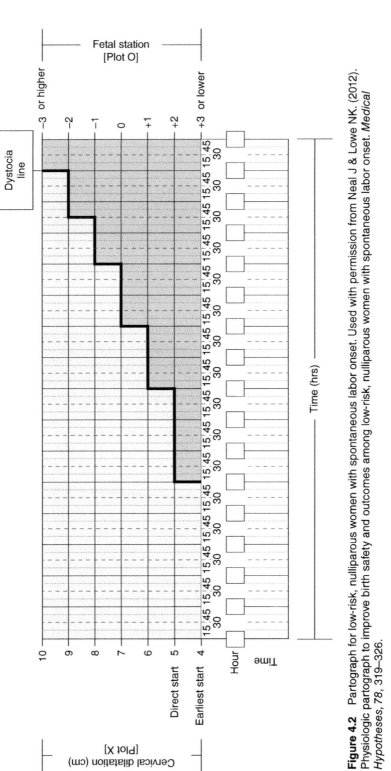

Figure 4.2 Partograph for low-risk, nulliparous women with spontaneous labor onset. Used with permission from Neal J & Lowe NK. (2012). Physiologic partograph to improve birth safety and outcomes among low-risk, nulliparous women with spontaneous labor onset. *Medical Hypotheses, 78*, 319–326.

labor progress [76]. The partograph has long been advocated to maintain appropriate surveillance of labor progress. The new partograph (Figure 4.2) offers an alternative for documenting labor progress in low-risk nulliparous women based on principles that acknowledge the range in cervical change over time.

- Principle 1: Active labor onset must be accurately diagnosed before the rate of cervical dilatation (cm/h) is used to assess labor progression.
- Principle 2: Expectations of cervical dilatation (cm/h) for the population must be appropriately defined.
- Principle 3: Cervical dilatation rates progressively accelerate throughout the majority of active labor.
- Principle 4: The time duration necessary for the cervix to dilate from one centimeter to the next is more variable in earlier active labor than in more advanced active labor [76].

In summary, there is a critical need to reevaluate assumptions about normal progress in labor. Individual variations found in more contemporary models can replace older assumptions about the linear pattern and pace of labor and promote a physiologic approach to labor and birth. All influences on the pace of labor progress are considered, including use of epidurals, continuous versus intermittent monitoring, freedom of movement, comfort level, and presence of support.

Tailoring interventions to promote physiologic birth

In the context of normal physiologic birth, there is a tendency to frame strategies commonly used in labor management such as intravenous fluids, artificial rupture of membranes, or pharmacologic methods of pain relief as inappropriate and disruptive. Evidence-based approaches to supporting physiologic labor are congruent with doing less rather than using fewer specific technological approaches. However, there are circumstances where a woman may require additional resources or therapeutic options during labor to encourage progress and maintain her well-being beyond the approaches already discussed. A key principle in deciding what to do in a particular situation is to move from least invasive to more invasive options over time as indicated by the woman's desires and status in labor. Equally important for the woman who develops complications is to remember to continue to support normal aspects of her labor and birth while managing the complication and carefully continuing to assess maternal and fetal status.

It is important not to identify any one intervention as wrong but to utilize a framework of making decisions with the laboring woman and her support persons in a respectful and collaborative manner that maintains an individualized approach in support of normal physiologic birth. For example, mobility can facilitate progress and promote fetal descent, but a woman may also become fatigued if she is unable to rest at some point. A warm bath can promote relaxation and labor progress but prolonged periods of time (periods extending beyond 2 hours) may reduce the efficiency of contractions and labor progress [59]. Getting in and out of the tub after periods of time or resting after periods of walking are examples of creating a balance of specific practices. The same is true of more advanced interventions. Artificial rupture of membranes can increase the risk of infection over time.

However, if a woman has been in labor for an extended period of time, is fatigued, and is not making progress for several hours, rather than more advanced interventions such as epidural anesthesia or Pitocin augmentation of labor, a woman and her provider may decide that amniotomy is the desired initial intervention.

The use of each care practice or intervention must be considered in the context of the individual woman's labor status and progress, the risks and benefits of the intervention balanced with consideration of whether other more appropriate, evidence-based options may better support labor progress. The maternity care provider always questions how an intervention may augment or disrupt the normal physiologic process of labor. Information regarding the risks, benefits, evidence, available alternatives, and potential effects of each intervention should all be reviewed with the woman to allow her to make an informed choice that will accomplish the desired outcome.

Entering and progressing through second stage labor

Anatomically, second stage labor is defined as complete dilatation of the cervix (10 cm) to complete expulsion of the fetus. While the second stage of labor is specifically defined, the true demarcation between the final dynamics of first stage and the beginning of second stage labor is less distinct. Subtle changes signaling second stage may appear in the final phases of active labor or there may be a lull in the frequency and intensity of contractions at the end of first stage labor. This can be misconstrued as labor slowing down, and in fact can be a common variation in normal labor [57,77].

Physiologically, second stage labor is defined as the onset of the urge to bear down until birth of the baby, with the station of the presenting part predicting the onset of pushing instead of complete dilatation. Ten centimeters of dilatation is commonly used as the marker of second stage labor; many maternity care providers encourage maternal pushing efforts as soon as a woman is complete. In contrast, the physiologic process of second stage labor is initiated when the vertex or presenting part of the fetus has descended to a point where it stimulates an involuntary urge to bear down [56]. The urge to push typically occurs at approximately plus one station, or the when the pressure of the presenting part stimulates pelvic floor nerves [78]. Prior to this pressure sensation, a woman may be completely dilated but not feel an urge to push. Allowing for a period of passive descent of the presenting part and not encouraging maternal pushing efforts prior to the spontaneous urge to push are consistent with the physiologic processes of labor and birth [79]. Passive descent is particularly important during second stage labor in the presence of an epidural, which reduces the sensations to bear down, possibly requiring longer passive descent. Allowing passive descent—in other words, not encouraging active pushing effort until spontaneous urge—can help a woman conserve her energy, reducing the liklihood of maternal fatigue or an instrumental delivery. The value of using passive descent or delaying active pushing effort is unclear [80], yet the process is consistent with physiologic principles and does not increase fetal or maternal negative health outcomes [81,82].

The physiologic process of second stage depends on mechanisms that promote synchrony between descent of the fetal head and stretch of the pelvic floor with maternal

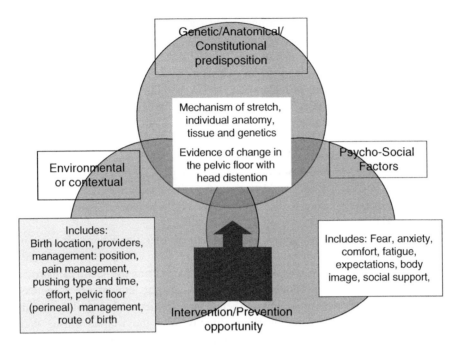

Figure 4.3   Factors that influence second stage labor.

effort. It is a dense process with anatomic and psychological contributors [78]. The dynamic nature of second stage requires changes in process, typically directed by nurses and other maternity care providers supporting the woman when these sensations begin. Multiple processes, including modifiable and nonmodifiable factors (Figure 4.3), combine to affect second stage labor progress for each individual woman. Maternity care providers continue to make assessments and respond to the cues of the woman to determine how active a role is required. When a woman initiates pushing, decisions about the degree of direction offered, the type of pushing effort (Valsalva versus non-Valsalva), and position of the woman [78,79,83] are tailored to the unique circumstances of each woman's labor. Maternal fatigue, the woman's expressed pain or fear, routine practice or experience of the maternity care provider, the woman's use of pain-reduction medication, and fetal status are all considered [79,83–85].

Supporting a woman during pushing

Evidence supports self-directed, spontaneous pushing efforts as optimal to improve pelvic floor outcomes [86,87]. This approach is consistent with the physiologic approach to giving birth [78]. Spontaneous pushing during second stage labor, where the woman begins to bear down instinctively in response to physical cues and sensations, has been shown to improve health outcomes for both the mother and newborn compared to directed or Valsalva pushing [88]. Benefits include fewer perineal lacerations [89] and, in particular, reduced risk of negative urogynecological changes including incontinence [86,87,90]. Yet a national survey confirmed that over 75% of U.S. women experience directed or valsalva pushing encouragement during second stage labor [69]. In addition, when a woman has epidural anesthesia, even providers who generally encourage spontaneous pushing begin to use more directed approaches [91] presumably to counter the reduced sensation from the epidural which can slow progress in second stage labor.

Encouraging maternity care providers to adopt woman directed, spontaneous pushing remains challenging [92]. As early as 2000, AWHONN issued clinical guidelines advocating for spontaneous pushing as the preferred model of care. AWHONN subsequently strengthened the guidelines in 2008, recommending only using spontaneous pushing and denouncing directed pushing. The American College of Nurse-Midwives endorsed spontaneous pushing as a best practice consistent with physiologic birth [93], and a national survey of certified nurse-midwives and certified midwives (CNMs and CMs) indicated spontaneous pushing is the dominant method advocated by midwives during second stage [91].

Assuming fetal descent is progressing and the fetus is tolerating labor well, there is no need for maternity care providers to direct maternal pushing efforts. However, there are some circumstances when a woman may request assistance from the health care provider. Limited progress over time, extreme fear or pain with pushing, or evidence of increasing maternal fatigue or changes in fetal well-being may influence the approach used by the nurse, midwife, or physician working directly with the woman during second stage [83,85]. In these situations, a more directive role for the health care provider may be warranted [91,94,95]. There is no guide for when this change in approach should be implemented. In studies examining how maternity care providers support women in labor, changes in approach during second stage labor were driven by clinical considerations [79,83–85].

In some circumstances, maternity care providers may use an approach described as supportive direction [79,83], a blended approach of supporting maternal efforts plus adding responsive direction when a woman asks for help or information. This strategy has not been examined in clinical trials. It is a practical alternative to using only one or the other approach, offering a middle ground between "directed" and "spontaneous" approaches. The provider maintains a supportive rather than directive role. For example, if the laboring woman says, "Am I doing it right, am I making progress?" the health care provider can ask, "How is it feeling, do you have a sensation of the baby moving?" and may also offer position changes such as "If this position is not feeling comfortable we can try another option" rather than a directive "You need to hold your breath longer."

Positions for birth

Similar to encouraging a woman to be upright and mobile to promote progress in labor, she is also encouraged to use varied positions while pushing to support continued descent of the fetus. In general a woman is encouraged not to be on her back or assume a lithotomy position because those position make pushing effort and descent more challenging compared to upright or side lying positions [57]. A similar approach of encouraging the woman to follow her own bodily cues during first stage of labor continues into second stage. Encourage the woman to assume a position that is both

---

Box 4.4   Principles to encourage second stage progress

- Avoid supine or lithotomy positions.
- No one position is best so adjust according to maternal preference, comfort, and labor progress.
- Maintain an upright vs. a recumbent position.
- Use the curve of the pelvis (curve of Carus) by rounding instead of arching the back when bearing down.
- Work with the peaks of contractions to augment the process of bearing down but not beyond the contraction to promote maternal rest.
- Specific positions may be indicated to promote rotation when the baby is in a unique position.
  - A hands and knees position can support rotation when the fetus is in a posterior position.
  - If the fetus needs to rotate from an occiput transverse position, a side lying position can assist in the rotation process.
  - Side lying position may offer increased control and potentially slow the final process of birth in circumstances where a woman may fear the birth is occurring too fast.
  - Squatting position may be used to encourage both rotation and descent by increasing and altering the shape of the available pelvic space.
- Support the woman to work with the physical sensations of second stage such as rectal pressure and perineal stretching by promoting relaxation and breathing instead of pulling back or tensing muscles.

---

comfortable and allows her to bear down as her body indicates. The following principles can be followed to encourage progress in second stage (see Box 4.4).

Maternity care providers continue to offer constant presence and positive encouragement as the woman works through second stage labor. Positive comments such as "You are so strong" or "You are doing so well" reinforce the work that the woman is doing under her own control, without direction. These comments are preferred over directive comments such as "Push," "Harder," or "Longer" or offering multiple commands quickly when she is trying to push. Similar to the first stage of labor, brief, simple remarks are made to offer suggestions in second stage. When assisting the woman to a new position, help her move in stages to slowly accommodate to the change ("Let's start to turn to the left, then after the next contraction, how about seeing if it is more comfortable to place your leg on this pillow," etc.). Encouraging the woman to push longer than her spontaneous urges or advising her to hold her breath longer may increase maternal fatigue without promoting progress and should be avoided.

The final phase of pushing to accomplish birth

Health care providers make multiple observational assessments regarding a woman's progress as birth is imminent to guide and individualize the unique needs of each laboring woman. Observational assessments include:

- How is the woman breathing, is she holding her breath?
- Is she using open glottis pushing efforts?
- Is she releasing air instead of holding it in?
- Is she tense, using other muscles that could otherwise be relaxed, like her arms?

- Is she pulling away, working against the sensation or pressure?
- If she is pulling away, is someone talking her through the sensation?

The provider also observes for perineal changes indicating progress as a woman bears down, rather than performing multiple vaginal examinations. Perineal changes that can be assessed over time include:

- Increased bloody show or presence of fluid.
- Bulging that continues to increase over time but generally is not sustained between contractions until the final phase of pushing.
- Separation of the labia, which begins gradually with the peak of the contraction and increases over time.
- Crowning of the baby's head that is initially only with the peak of the push or contraction and then becomes sustained between contractions.
- Evidence of perineal blanching, indicating a lack of blood supply to the tissue and a potential for tearing.

All of these observations are made in the context of assessing how the woman is progressing and coping overall. What position is working best for her to promote comfort and progress? How is she responding to the others around her, are all members of the maternity care team working together to maintain an optimal environment for her to reach the final phase of pushing to give birth to her newborn?

Care of the woman giving birth

The woman-centered approach by all health care providers continues as labor culminates in the birth. A nondisruptive environment is maintained, despite the potential addition of more personnel to support both mom and baby. At this very intense time, it is important to maintain focus on the woman and not on added providers or the "procedures" of preparing for birth. New personnel should enter into the birth space quietly, eliminating extraneous conversations; all information shared should be essential and provided efficiently. Accessing information outside of the birth space or in written form is helpful so that focus remains on the woman, creating a space around her to support the intense work of giving birth. New providers entering the room should refrain from providing new direction or coaching without a full understanding of what has been working for this woman and her family throughout the labor process.

As the woman pushes and the fetus becomes more and more visible, excitement tends to fill the birth space in the form of coaching or cheering. Statements like "Baby is here, keep going, keep pushing, don't stop" may seem supportive, but in fact may work against promoting the physiologic processes that lead to the final stretch of the perineum. If the woman seems more anxious or is expressing fear or feeling pain, offer comforting statements and encourage her by commenting on how well she is doing. Let her know that a burning sensation can be normal, the intense pressure is her baby's head and is also normal, and that she can use these cues to breathe so that stretch and accommodation can occur. The suggestion of "pushing past the pain" may sound like simple guidance, a sort of "just do it" approach, but in fact, the sensations that the woman is experiencing are her own best guide on how to balance her pushing and breathing efforts. Another option is to ask the woman if she would like to feel the baby's head as it crowns, allowing her to have a greater sense of what is occurring. Some women may prefer a mirror placed where they can observe the progress directly.

The event of birth

As the fetus descends closer, the woman is supported in the most comfortable position. If she has been squatting on the floor, the midwife or physician attending the birth may also need to squat on the floor. The principle is that the midwife or physician is responsive to the woman's needs. Specific positions that may be useful include:

- Hands and knees to promote rotation and reduce back discomfort.
- Side lying to promote rotation and offer a slower pace and control when rapid progress is occurring.
- Squatting, which provides an upright position and control for the woman while offering added space and potential strength in pushing effort to promote rotation and progress.
- High semi-Fowler's, which also allows for a more upright position, allows the woman to see the care provider directly, and can aid in rotation and pushing effort compared to supine positions [79,96–98].

Except for selected unique circumstances such as concern for shoulder dystocia or fetal well-being, the woman is supported to select the position that works best for her to promote progress while maintaining comfort.

As the moment of birth approaches, the goal is to continue to support the woman to respond to her own cues and push as she feels comfortable. Slow, controlled perineal stretching in the final pushing phase is protective against trauma of the genital tract, allowing the woman to "rock" the baby forward by making small progressive increases in the visible bulging, separation, and finally stretching to slowly birth the baby over the perineum. The necessary muscle changes in the pelvic floor and perineal body can occur with minimal trauma. Principles of muscle stretch physiology suggest that slow stretch over time is optimal to allow the muscles to accommodate or adjust to the extension. Stretching too rapidly and not allowing for muscle accommodation may lead to increased risk of trauma or tearing [99]. During this very final phase of perineal stretching the birth attendant may become more directive to slow the birth of the baby by encouraging breathing instead of continued pushing. The most consistent approach to promoting an intact perineum during birth is to have a slow, controlled birth between contractions [24,89]. The provider encourages the woman to "breathe" her baby out instead of actually pushing forward. The final stretch of the perineum and birth of the baby's head can occur under gentle power of the woman's body without added pushing as extension of the baby's head occurs.

Promoting an intact perineum

Routine use of episiotomy is a non-evidence-based practice that has received a great deal of attention in recent years. With increasing evidence that episiotomy can actually increase the risk of lacerations and anal sphincter tears, most providers have stopped performing routine episiotomy [100]. Despite the desire to reduce the use of this practice, limited specific information is available describing the optimal manner to promote birth over an intact perineum and reduce the risk of genital tract trauma. Ongoing observation of the woman and changes to the perineum are useful in identifying progress and may also indicate when specific care practices should be introduced to promote relaxation and reduce the risk of perineal tearing. Specific care practices may include:

- If a woman is very tense and fearful as she begins to feel the pressure/burn of perineal stretching, explain the normality of the feeling, maintaining eye contact to encourage relaxation and/or assist her to another position to try to reduce the sensations.
- If fear and anxiety are present for the woman, minimize distractions, maintain a quiet, low-light environment.
- If a woman is in a supine or recumbent position, encouraging a more upright position reduces the risk of perineal tearing.
- If blanching of the perineum is observed encourage the woman to breathe instead of pushing, to support slower perineal stretching.
- Watch for potential areas of tearing, particularly at the apex of the vaginal opening at the top of the perineum and again, encourage slow pushing to promote a more controlled, slow stretch process [101].

In general, there is no specific hand placement or maneuver that has been demonstrated to increase the likelihood of an intact perineum other than encouraging a slow process of stretching, encouraging a woman in her spontaneous self-directed capacity. Perineal massage during pushing has been used to reduce the risk of perineal lacerations and may actually increase the risk of edema and tearing [89]. There is evidence that the use of a warm compress, placed against the perineum during end stage pushing, reduces the risk of third- and fourth-degree lacerations [102]. A warm compress using a washcloth, or gauze squares soaked in warmed water, can be placed against the perineum between and during contractions. It is unclear if use of a compress promotes the likelihood of an intact perineum [102]. Other strategies have included helping a woman give birth between contractions when the baby's head appears to be extending. Encouraging her to breathe rather than push when the vertex is highly visible promotes a slow stretch.

  As birth becomes imminent, the nurse, midwife, or physician should be communicating her/his observations to the woman, letting her know what is occurring, how close she is to giving birth to her newborn, offering praise and support, and assisting her to maintain control and focus as the intense physical sensations may increase. Maintaining eye contact, encouraging her to breathe, to open her mouth, to relax as much as possible, allowing her legs to be supported in a comfortable position (not exaggerated) are all strategies to encourage a slow physiologic birth. Finally, the provider's hands can be placed in a poised, supportive fashion to receive the baby. Placing fingers into the vagina, adding additional stretching, can increase the risk of lacerations. The use of a hands-off approach can also reduce the incidence of performing an episiotomy [102].

Promoting a positive transition for the newborn

The process of birth is not rushed; instead of the cheering and coaching portrayed in popular media, a calm, quiet environment ensues with the woman focused on giving birth, making the sounds she desires, and those around her responsive and supportive to her needs. As the baby emerges, consistent with supporting normal physiology, the baby is placed on the mother's abdomen or in her arms, skin to skin, umbilical cord intact. The baby begins the transition to extrauterine life, comforted and welcomed by her/his mother.

The ideal placement for the newborn as it is born is on the mother's abdomen, skin to skin, promoting a positive transition from intrauterine to extrauterine life. Skin-to-skin contact promotes thermoregulation of the newborn, reducing physiologic stress and enhances the initiation of breastfeeding [103]. Evaluation of the infant, the assignment of Apgar scores, and initial vital signs can be completed while the infant remains skin to skin with its mother [104]. The umbilical cord is maintained intact until it stops pulsating. Delaying cord clamping is an evidence-based practice that promotes the transition from intrauterine to extrauterine life and offers other additional health benefits [105]. Once the cord has stopped pulsating, clamping and cutting can be completed. Keeping the mother and newborn skin to skin is beneficial and should be maintained to improve the initiation of breastfeeding.

Specific practices that can disrupt normal physiological labor and birth

Throughout this chapter an integrated approach to promoting and supporting the normal physiologic processes of labor and birth has been presented with a focus on not disrupting or disturbing the labor process. This model of care is woman focused and responsive to her needs, in contrast to a health care provider–directed process. Procedures and care practices have been described that are promotive, not disruptive, of normal spontaneous labor and birth. However, in many institutions traditional approaches and practices that do not encourage normal physiologic birth remain. Continuous fetal monitoring for all women, requiring intravenous fluids and prohibiting oral hydration, or limiting freedom of movement are examples of how physiologic labor and birth are disrupted by technology and not supported by evidence. Boxes 4.5 and 4.6 provide examples of practices that promote or disrupt physiological labor and birth. Specific alternatives to disruptive processes are offered for each phase of the labor process. The normal healthy physiologic birth statement by ACNM, Midwives Alliance of North America (MANA) and the National Association of Certified Professional Midwives (NACPM) identifies factors that can disrupt the physiologic processes of normal labor and birth [93]:

- Induction or augmentation of labor.
- An unsupportive environment, i.e., bright lights, cold room, lack of privacy, multiple providers, lack of supportive companions.
- Time constraints, including those driven by institutional policy and/or staffing.
- Nutritional deprivation of food and drink.

- Opiates, regional analgesia, or general anesthesia.
- Episiotomy.
- Operative vaginal (vacuum, forceps) or abdominal (cesarean) birth.
- Immediate cord clamping.
- Separation of mother and infant.
- Any situation in which the mother feels threatened or unsupported.

Box 4.5   Optimal: Promoting physiologic birth

- With strong contractions the woman comes to the hospital with her partner and doula.
- Upon admission to the single maternity care room the woman is able to freely move about with her partner and doula present.
- She sits on a birth ball, rocks in a chair, and drinks juices she chooses.
- Her baby is assessed by intermittent auscultation.
- She becomes more uncomfortable and decides to use hydrotherapy, laboring in the large tub.
- She notes increased pressure and an urge to bear down and decides to move from the tub to the labor bed.
- She chooses a side-lying position as the pressure increases and she begins to spontaneously bear down.
- With her partner and doula at her side she bears down with increasing strength at the peak of the contractions; her nurse continues to auscultate the fetal heart rate and provide support.
- Side-lying position is no longer comfortable so she is assisted to move to a high Fowler's position.
- The baby begins to crown and her midwife supports her to slowly push and breathe her baby over an intact perineum.
- The baby is born, immediately placed on her mother's abdomen, skin to skin, waiting for the cord to stop pulsating.

Box 4.6   Non-optimal: Disrupts physiologic birth

- When contractions are 5 minutes apart the woman is instructed to come to the hospital.
- She is admitted to the single maternity care room with her partner.
- Upon admission a routine IV is placed.
- Continuous fetal monitoring is maintained, requiring the woman to stay in bed.
- A vaginal examination is performed every 2 hours, and no change in cervical dilatation is noted so the membranes are ruptured artificially.
- Still primarily in bed, the discomfort and back pain increase so she asks for pain relief and an epidural is placed.
- After a few hours, she is found to be completely dilated and is directed to begin pushing.
- She is positioned in a semi-Fowler's position with her legs supported by her partner and the nurse.
- Because she does not have any sensation to push, the maternity care team directs her on when and how to push while holding her breath.
- After becoming more exhausted but with the baby not yet fully crowning, the provider offers her an assisted vacuum delivery and she agrees.
- The baby is born, the cord is clamped and cut, and the baby is taken to the warmer for evaluation.

In short, interference with the normal physiologic progression of labor or competing with a woman's ability to work with the labor should be avoided unless there is a specific rationale for doing so. Routine interventions to increase progress are not indicated unless progress has been significantly delayed and/or maternal or fetal well-being is of concern because of a medical complication. Specific practices at the time of birth such as episiotomy, or any particular hand maneuvers such as exerting constant pressure on the posterior vaginal floor, are not indicated and evidence suggests they may actually cause harm [106,107].

Summary

To promote physiologic labor and birth, maternity care providers focus on providing woman-centered care by creating a circle of support for each woman, while also maintaining vigilance in observing her progress through labor. The health care provider role can best be described as "doing 'nothing' well" [4] to avoid the risk of intervening and disrupting labor. The use of any interventions is evaluated against the available scientific evidence in combination with the laboring woman's desires. Through this process, a woman, under her own power, is able to move through the phases of labor and give birth to her newborn in a manner that will support an optimal transition to motherhood.

References

1. World Health Organization. (1996). Care in normal birth: A practical guide. Safe Motherhood. Retrieved from: http://www.who.int/maternal_child_adolescent/documents/who_frh_msm_9624/en/.
2. Childbirth Connection. (2009). Transforming maternity care: Clinical controversies. Retrieved from: http://transform.childbirthconnection.org/blueprint/clinicalcontroversies/
3. Amnesty International. (2010). Deadly delivery: The maternal health care crisis in the USA. Retrieved from: http://www.amnestyusa.org/sites/default/files/pdfs/deadlydelivery.pdf.
4. Kennedy HP. (2000). A model of exemplary midwifery practice: Results of a Delphi study. *Journal of Midwifery & Women's Health, 45*, 4–19. DOI: 10.1016/S1526-9523(99)00018-5.
5. Elliot M. (2006). Midwifery today: Past challenges and achievements inspire present practice. *RCM Midwives, 9*(7), 270–271.
6. Högberg Y. (2004). The decline in maternal mortality in Sweden: The role of community midwifery. *American Journal of Public Health, 94*(8), 1312–1320.
7. Hunter B & Segrott J. (2010). Using a clinical pathway to support normal birth: Impact on practitioner roles and working practices. *Birth, 37*(3), 227–236.
8. Kemp J & Sandall J. (2010). Normal birth, magical birth: The role of the 36-week birth talk in caseload midwifery practice. *Midwifery, 26*(2), 211–221.
9. Kontoyannis M & Katsetos C. (2011). Midwives in early modern Europe (1400–1800). *Health Science Journal, 5*(1), 31–36.
10. Amis D. (2009). Healthy birth practices from Lamaze International. #1. Let labor begin on its own. Retrieved from: http://www.lamaze.org/Portals/0/carepractices/HBP1-formatted.pdf.
11. Davis-Floyd R, ed. (2009). *Birth models that work.* Berkeley: University of California Press.
12. Green J & Hotelling BA. (2009). Healthy birth practices from Lamaze International. #3. Bring a loved one, friend, or doula for continuous support. Retrieved from: http://www.lamaze.org/Portals/0/carepractices/HBP3-formatted.pdf.

13. Kitzinger S. (2011). *Rediscovering birth*, 2nd ed. London: Pinter & Martin.
14. Lothian JA. (2009). Healthy birth practices from Lamaze International. #4. Avoid interventions that are not medically necessary. Retrieved from: http://www.lamaze.org/Portals/0/careprac-tices/HBP4-formatted.pdf.
15. McCourt C, ed. (2009). *Childbirth, midwifery and concepts of time*. Oxford, UK: Berghahn Books.
16. Schwegel J, ed. (2005). *Adventures in natural childbirth: Tales from women's joys, fears, plea-sures, and pains of giving birth naturally*. Cambridge, MA: De Capo Press.
17. Shilling T. (2009). Healthy birth practices from Lamaze International. #2. Walk, move around, and change positions during labor. Retrieved from: http://www.lamaze.org/Portals/0/careprac-tices/HBP2-formatted.pdf.
18. Van Teijlengen E, Lowis GW, McCaffery P, & Porter E, eds. (2011). *Midwifery and the medicalization of childbirth: Comparative perspectives*. Hauppauge, NY: Nova Science Publishers.
19. Jordan B & Davis-Floyd R. (1993). *Birth in four cultures: A cross-cultural investigation of childbirth in Yucatan, Holland, Sweden, and the United States*. Long Grove, IL: Waveland Press.
20. Kildea S. (2006). Risky business: Contested knowledge over safe birthing services for Aboriginal women. *Health Sociology Review*, *15*(4), 387–396.
21. Lummaa V & Clutton-Brock T. (2002). Early development, survival and reproduction in humans. *Trends in Ecology & Evolution*, *17*(3), 141–147.
22. Odent M. (2008). Dispelling the disempowering birth vocabulary. *Journal of Prenatal and Perinatal Psychology*, *23*(1), 5–11.
23. Trevatham WR. (2011). *Human birth: An evolutionary perspective*. Piscataway, NJ: Aldine Transaction Books.
24. Albers LL. (2007). The evidence for physiologic management of the active phase of labor. *Journal of Midwifery & Women's Health*, *52*(3), 207–215.
25. Cragin L & Kennedy HP. (2006). Linking obstetric and midwifery practice with optimal outcomes. *JOGNN*, *35*(6), 779–785.
26. Akrich M & Pasveer B. (2004). Embodiment and disembodiment in childbirth narratives. *Body & Society*, *10*, 63–84.
27. Dahlke LJ. (2009). Essays on childbirth: The why and the how. *Women's Studies*, *38*, 577–596.
28. Simkin P. (1991). Just another day in a woman's life? Women's long-term perceptions of their first birth experience: Part I. *Birth*, *18*(4), 203–210.
29. Dahlen HG, Barclay LM, & Homer C. (2008). Preparing for the first birth: Mother's experi-ences at home and in hospital in Australia. *Journal of Perinatal Education*, *17*(4), 21–32.
30. Farley C & Widmann S. (2001). The value of birth stories. *International Journal of Childbirth Education*, *16*(3), 22–25.
31. Freeman J. (2005). Birth stories. *Midwifery Matters*, *107*, 9–11.
32. Hayden JM, Singer JA, & Chrisler JC. (2006). The transmission of birth stories from mother to daughter: Self-esteem and mother-daughter attachment. *Sex Roles*, *55*, 373–383.
33. McHugh N. (2001). Storytelling and its influence in passing birth culture through the genera-tions. *Midwifery Matter*, *89*, 15–17.
34. Page RE. (2003). An analysis of APPRAISAL in childbirth narratives with special consideration of gender and storytelling style. *Text*, *23*(2), 211–237.
35. Savage JS. (2001). Birth stories: A way of knowing in childbirth education. *Journal of Perinatal Education*, *10*(2), 3–7.
36. Creasy RK, Resnick R, Iams JD, Lockwood CJ, & Moore TR. (2008). *Creasy & Resnick's maternal-fetal medicine: Principles and practice*, 6th ed. Philadelphia: Saunders-Elsevier.

37. Cunningham C, Leveno K, Hauth J, Rouse D, & Spong C. (2010). *Williams obstetrics*, 23rd ed. New York: McGraw-Hill.
38. Gabbe SG, Niebyl JR, Galam H, Jauniaux ER, Landori M, Simpson JL, & Driscoll D. (2012). *Obstetrics: Normal and problem pregnancies*, 6th ed. Philadelphia: Elsevier-Saunders.
39. Cesario SK. (2004). Reevaluation of Friedman's labor curve: A pilot study. *JOGNN*, *33*(6), 713–722.
40. Gross MM, Drobnic S, & Keirse MJ. (2005). Influence of fixed and independent factors on duration of normal first stage of labor. *Birth*, *32*(1), 26–33.
41. Lavender T, Hart A, Walkingshaw S, Campbell E, & Alfirevic Z. (2005). Progress of first stage of labour for multiparous women: An observational study. *BJOG*, *112*(2), 1663–1665.
42. Neal JL, Lowe NK, Patrick TE, Cabbage LA, & Corwin EJ. (2010). What is the slowest-yet-normal cervical dilation rate among nulliparous women with spontaneous onset of labor? *JOGNN*, *39*(4), 361–369. DOI: 10.1111/j.1552-6909.2010.01154.x.
43. Leap N, Dodwell M, & Newburn M. (2010). Working with pain in labour: An overview of the evidence. *New Digest*, *49*, 22–26.
44. Maher J. (2007). The painful truth about birth?: Contemporary discourses of caesareans, risk and the realities of pain. Presented at the Australian Sociological Association (TASA) 2007 Conference. Retrieved from: http://www.tasa.org.au/conferences/conferencepapers07/papers/19.pdf.
45. Low LK & Moffatt A. (2006). Every labor is unique: But "call when your contractions are 3 minute apart." *MCN*, *31*(5), 307–312.
46. Bailit JL, Dierker L, Blanchard MH, & Mercer BM. (2005). Outcomes of women presenting in active versus latent phase of spontaneous labor. *Obstetrics & Gynecology*, *105*(1), 77–79.
47. Holmes P, Oppenheimer LW, & Wen SW. (2001). The relationship between cervical dilatation at initial presentation in labour and subsequent intervention. *BJOG*, *108*(11):1120–1124.
48. Berghella V, Baxter J, & Chauhan S. (2008). Evidence-based labor and delivery management. *American Journal of Obstetrics and Gynecology*, *199*(5), 445–454.
49. Romano A & Lothian J. (2008). Promoting, protecting, and supporting normal birth: A look at the evidence preserving normal birth. *JOGNN*, *37*, 94–105. DOI: 10.1111/J.1552-6909.2007.00210.
50. Kennedy HP, Grant J, Walton C, Shaw-Battista J, & Sandall J. (2010). Normalizing birth in England: A qualitative study. *Journal of Midwifery & Women's Health*, *55*(3), 262–269.
51. Gourounti K & Sandall J. (2007). Admission cardiotocography versus intermittent auscultation of fetal heart rate: Effects on neonatal Apgar score, on the rate of caesarean sections and on the rate of instrumental delivery—a systematic review. *International Journal of Nursing Studies*, *44*(6), 1029–1035.
52. American College of Nurse-Midwives. (2008). Providing oral nutrition to women in labor. Clinical Bulletin No. 10. *Journal of Midwifery & Women's Health*, *53*, 276–283. DOI: 10.1016/j.jmwh.2008.03.006.
53. Bradley RA. (2008). *Husband-coached childbirth: The Bradley Method of natural childbirth*, 5th ed. New York: Random House.
54. Gaskin IM. (2003). *Ina May's guide to childbirth*. New York: Random House.
55. Markhoff H & Mazel S. (2008). *What to expect when you're expecting*. New York: Workman.
56. Varney H, Kriebs J, & Gegor C. (2004). *Varney's Midwifery*, 4th ed. Sudbury, MA: Jones and Bartlett.
57. Simkin P & Ancheta R. (2011). *The labor progress handbook*, 3rd ed. Malden, MA: Blackwell.
58. Melzack R & Wall PD. (1988). *The challenge of pain*, 2nd ed. New York: Penguin Books.
59. Jones L, Othman M, Dowswell T, Alfirevic Z, Gates S, Newburn M, Jordan S, Lavender T, & Neilson JP. (2012). Pain management for women in labour: An overview of systematic reviews. *Cochrane Database of Systematic Reviews*, issue 3. Art. No.: CD009234. DOI: 10.1002/14651858.CD009234.pub2.

60. Gulliver B, Fisher J, & Roberts L. (2008). A new way to assess pain in laboring women. *AWHONN Nursing for Women's Health, 12*(5) 404–408.
61. Schuilling KD & Sampselle C. (1999). Comfort in labor and midwifery art. *Image: Nursing Scholarship, 31*(1), 77–81.
62. Roberts L, Gulliver B, Fischer J, & Cloyes KG. (2010). The Coping with Labor Algorithm: An alternate pain assessment tool for the laboring woman. *Journal of Midwifery & Women's Health, 55*(2), 107–115.
63. Hodnett ED, Gates S, Hofmeyr GJ, Sakala C, & Weston J. (2011). Continuous support for women during childbirth. *Cochrane Database of Systematic Reviews, 16*(2): CD003766. Review. PMID: 21328263.
64. Lawrence A, Lewis L, Hofmeyr GJ, Dowswell T, & Styles C. (2009). Maternal positions and mobility during first stage labour. *Cochrane Collaboration Review, 2*. DOI: 10.1002/14651858. CD003934.pub2.
65. Lowe N. (2004). Context and process of informed consent for pharmacological strategies in labor pain care. *Journal of Midwifery & Women's Health, 49*(3), 250–259.
66. Agency for Healthcare Research and Quality. (2007). Intrapartum fetal heart rate monitoring: Nomenclature, interpretation, and general management principles. Retrieved from: http://guidelines.gov/content.aspx?id=14885.
67. Association of Women's Health, Obstetric and Neonatal Nurses. (2008). Fetal heart monitoring. Retrieved from: http://www.awhonn.org/awhonn/binary.content.do?name=Resources/Documents/pdf/5_FHM.pdf%20.
68. American College of Nurse-Midwives. (2010). Intermittent auscultation for intrapartum fetal heart rate surveillance. Clinical Bulletin No. 11. *Journal of Midwifery & Women's Health, 55*(4), 397–403.
69. Declercq ER, Sakala C, Corry MP, & Applebaum S. (2006). *Listening to mothers II: Report of the Second National US Survey of Women's Childbearing Experiences.* New York: Childbirth Connection.
70. Grimes DA & Peipert JF. (2010). Electronic fetal monitoring as a public health screening program: The arithmetic of failure. *Obstetrics & Gynecology, 116*(6), 1397–1400.
71. Alfirevic Z, Devane D, & Gyte GM. (2006). Continuous cardiotocography (CTG) as a form of electronic fetal monitoring (EFM) for fetal assessment during labour. *Cochrane Database of Systematic Reviews, 19*(3): CD006066.
72. Barber EL, Lundsberg LS, Belanger K, Pettker CM, Funai EF, & Illuzzi JL. (2011). Indications contributing to the increasing cesarean delivery rate. *Obstetrics & Gynecology, 118*(1), 29–38.
73. Zwelling E. (2010). Overcoming the challenges: Maternal movement and positioning to facilitate labor progress. *MCN: The American Journal of Maternal/Child Nursing, 35*(2), 72–78.
74. Zhang J, Troendle J, Mikolajczyk R, Sundaram R, Beaver J, & Fraser W. (2010). The natural history of the normal first stage of labor. *Obstetrics & Gynecology, 115*(4), 705–710. DOI: 10.1097/AOG.0b013e3181d55925.
75. Zhang J, Landy HJ, Ware Branch D, Burkman R, Haberman S, Gregory KD, & Uma M. (2010). Contemporary patterns of spontaneous labor with normal neonatal outcomes. *Obstetrics & Gynecology, 116*(6), 1281–1287.
76. Neal J & Lowe NK. (2012). Physiologic partograph to improve birth safety and outcomes among low-risk, nulliparous women with spontaneous labor onset. *Medical Hypotheses, 78,* 319–326.
77. Palmer J. (1996). Physiological pushing in the second stage of labour: The future for midwifery care. *Australian College of Midwives Inc. Journal, 9*(3), 15–19.

78. Roberts JE. (2002). The "push" for evidence: Management of the 2nd stage. *Journal of Midwifery & Women's Health, 47*(1), 2–15.

79. Roberts J & Hanson L. (2007). Best practices in second stage labor care: Maternal bearing down and positioning. *Journal of Midwifery & Women's Health, 52*(3), 238–245.

80. Tuulis M, Frey HA, Odibo AO, Macones GA, & Cahill AG. (2012). Immediate compared with delayed pushing in the second stage of labor: A systematic review and meta-analysis. *Obstetrics & Gynecology, 20,* 660–668. DOI: http://10.1097/AOG.0b013e3182639fae.

81. Brancato R, Church S, & Stone P. (2008). A meta-analysis of passive descent versus immediate pushing in nulliparous women with epidural analgesia in the second stage of labor. *JOGNN, 37,* 4–12. DOI: 10.1111/J.1552-6909.2007.00205.

82. Simpson KR & James DC. (2005). Effects of immediate versus delayed pushing during 2nd-stage labor on fetal well-being: A randomized clinical trial. *Nursing Research, 54*(3), 149–157.

83. Roberts JE, Gonzalez C, & Sampselle C. (2007). Why do supportive birth attendants become directive of maternal bearing down efforts in second stage? *Journal of Midwifery & Women's Health, 52,* 134–141.

84. Bergstrom L, Richards L, Morse J, & Roberts J. (2010). How care givers manage distress in second stage labor. *Journal of Midwifery & Women's Health, 55*(1), 38–44.

85. Sampselle CM, Miller J.M., et al. (2005). Provider support of spontaneous pushing during the 2nd stage labor. *JOGNN, 34*(6), 695–702.

86. Bloom SL, Casey BM, Schaffer JI, McIntire DD, & Leveno KJ. (2006). A randomized trial of coached versus uncoached maternal pushing during the second stage of labor. *American Journal of Obstetrics and Gynecology, 194,* 10–13.

87. Schaffer JI, Bloom SL, Casey BM, et al. (2005). A randomized trial of the effects of coached vs. uncoached maternal pushing during the second stage of labor on postpartum pelvic floor structure and function. *American Journal of Obstetrics and Gynecology, 192*(5), 1692–1696.

88. Association of Women's Health, Obstetric and Neonatal Nurses. (2008). *Nursing care and management of the second stage of labor,* 2nd ed. Washington, DC: AWHONN.

89. Albers L, Sedler K, Bedrick EJ, Teal D, & Peralta P. (2005). Midwifery care measures in the second stage of labor and reduction of genital tract trauma: A randomized controlled trial. *Journal of Midwifery & Women's Health, 50*(5), 365–372.

90. Prins M, Boxem J, Lucas C, & Hutton E. (2011). Effect of spontaneous pushing verses Valsalva pushing in the second stage of labour on mother and fetus: A systematic review of randomized trials. *BJOG, 118*(6), 662–670. DOI: 10.1111/j.1471-0528.2011.02910.x.

91. Osborne K & Hanson L. (2012). Directive versus supportive approaches used by midwives when providing care during the second stage of labor. *Journal of Midwifery & Women's Health, 57*(1), 3–11.

92. Simpson KR, Knox GE, Martin M, George C, & Watson SR. (2011). Michigan Health & Hospital Association Keystone Obstetrics: A statewide collaborative for perinatal patient safety in Michigan. *Joint Commission Journal on Quality and Patient Safety, 37*(12), 544–552.

93. American College of Nurse-Midwives, Midwives Association of North America, & National Association of Certified Professional Midwives. (2012). Supporting healthy and normal physiologic childbirth. Retrieved from: http://www.midwife.org/ACNM/files/ACNMLibraryData/UPLOADFILENAME/000000000272/Physiological%20Birth%20Consensus%20Statement-%20FINAL%20May%2018%202012%20FINAL.pdf.

94. Bianchi A & Adams E. (2009). Labor support during second stage labor for women with epidurals. *Nursing for Women's Health, 13*(1), 39–47.

95. Sprague A, Oppenheirmer L, McCabe L, Graham I, & Davies B. (2008). Knowledge to action: Implementing a guideline for second stage labor. *MCN: The American Journal of Maternal/Child Nursing, 33*(3), 179–186.

96. Adachi K, Shimada M, & Usui A. (2003). The relationship between the parturient's positions and perceptions of labor pain intensity. *Nursing Research, 52*(1), 47–51.

97. Hunter S, Hofmeyr GJ, & Kuller R. (2007). Hands and knees posture in late pregnancy or labor for fetal malposition (lateral or posterior). *Cochrane Database of Systematic Reviews*, issue 4, Art. No.: CD001063.

98. Gupta JK, Hofmeyr GJ, & Shenmar M. (2012). Position in the second stage of labour for women without epidural anaesthesia. *Cochrane Database of Systematic Reviews, 19*(5): CD002006. DOI: 10.1002/14651858.CD002006.pub3.

99. Low LK. (2010). The final stretch: Range of normal perineal changes during second stage labor in first vaginal birth. *Journal of Midwifery & Women's Health, 55*(5), 482.

100. Agency for Healthcare Research and Quality. (2005). The use of episiotomy in obstetrical care: A systematic review. Retrieved from: http://archive.ahrq.gov/clinic/tp/epistp.htm.

101. Meyvis I, Rompaey BV, Goormans K, Truijen S, Lambers S, Mestdagh E, & Mistiaen W. (2012). Maternal position and other variables' effects on perineal outcomes in 557 births. *Birth, 39*(2), 115–120.

102. Aasheim V, Nilsen AB, Lukasse M, & Reinar LM. (2011). Perineal techniques during the second stage of labour for reducing perineal trauma. *Cochrane Database of Systematic Reviews, 7*(12): CD006672.

103. Moore ER, Anderson GC, Bergman N, & Dowswell T. (2012). Early skin-to-skin contact for mothers and their healthy newborn infants. *Cochrane Database of Systematic Revirews, 16*(5): CD003519.

104. Haxton D, Doering J, Gingras L, & Kelly L. (2012). Implementing skin-to-skin contact at birth using the Iowa model: Applying evidence to practice. *Nursing for Women's Health, 16*(3), 220–229; quiz 230. DOI: 10.1111/j.1751-486X.2012.01733.x.

105. Mercer J & Erickson-Owens D. (2006). Delayed cord clamping increases infants' iron stores. *Lancet, 367*(9527), 1956–1958.

106. Hastings-Tolsma M, Vincent D, Emeis C, & Francisco T. (2007). Getting through birth in one piece: Protecting the perineum. *MCN: The American Journal of Maternal/Child Nursing, 32*(3), 158–164.

107. Mayerhofer K, Bodner-Adler B, Bodner K, Rabl M, Kaider A, Wagenbichler P, & Hussein P. (2002). Traditional care of the perineum during birth: A prospective, randomized, multicenter study of 1,079 women. *Journal of Reproductive Medicine, 47*(6), 477–482.

Section 2

Interventions and approaches

Chapter 5

Promoting comfort: A conceptual approach

Kerri D. Schuiling

Key points

- Comfort is important to everyone.
- Comfort is a valued holistic outcome.
- Comfort can exist in spite of great pain.
- Comforting can diminish pain.
- Relieving pain does not necessarily increase comfort.
- Enhancing comfort during labor and birth may enable women to find the strength needed to work with their body's physiology during labor and birth.

Tears roll down your face
I see pain within your eyes
My arms comfort you

Dina Montgomery

Introduction

Comfort is a holistic phenomenon and a basic human need that is welcomed by most individuals because of the sense of ease or relief that it brings. In fact, a lack of comfort (discomfort) is one of the primary reasons individuals seek health care [1]. Research suggests that comfort is more than the absence of pain [2,3] and that its presence may prove to be beneficial for individuals seeking care. Theories about comfort suggest that it is strengthening, health producing, and may help to bring about subsequent positive outcomes [3–6].

It is important for clinicians to understand comfort theory and how to operationalize its concepts when providing care to women during pregnancy and childbirth. Comfort interventions are nonpharmacologic and, when used effectively, can enhance a woman's labor physiology and support normal childbirth. Supporting the physiologic processes of

---

Supporting a Physiologic Approach to Pregnancy and Birth: A Practical Guide, First Edition.
Edited by Melissa D. Avery.
© 2013 John Wiley & Sons, Inc. Published 2013 by John Wiley & Sons, Inc.

labor and birth by promoting comfort has the potential to promote normal birth. In the absence of complications, comfort measures are preferred over the routine use of invasive techniques that may be unnecessary and lead to a broader cascade of interventions.

The Philosophy of the American College of Nurse-Midwives promulgates the belief that every person has the right to self-determination and active participation in health care decisions [7,8]. Further, the philosophy statement includes "therapeutic use of human presence and skillful communication" and "watchful waiting and nonintervention in normal processes," concepts consistent with providing comfort. Common components of midwifery care for women in labor include providing comfort and encouraging women to use self-identified comfort measures. Interventions that promote comfort support a birthing woman's ability to be an active participant in her birth, connected to her body, her emotions, and to the experience [3]. These concepts are formally described by midwives related to maternity care and can be applied by all health professionals working with women during pregnancy, labor, and birth. This chapter will provide a theoretical perspective on the idea of providing comfort to support normal pregnancy and birth to help clinicians provide support to women during this important time in their lives.

Historical context of comfort

Comfort is not a new concept in health care and is commonly referred to as a component of the art of nursing. Carper [9] described the art of nursing as a feeling experience visible only through actions taken to comfort and provide care for the patient. It is reasonable to posit that comfort as an *art* is an integral part of the midwifery model of care, an approach that can be used by all clinicians as a mechanism of support for women during childbirth.

Comfort is most visible in the nursing literature where it is documented as an important aspect of nursing care. The nurse provided comfort to patients primarily through physical comforting techniques and modifying the environment. Harmer emphasized that nursing care is concerned with providing a "comfortable environment" and that the personal care of the individual includes making him "feel comfortable" [10, p. 4] and Van Blarcom [11] identified the "giving of comfort" as an important aspect of the nurse's duty.

From 1930 to 1959 comfort became less the focus of patient care and instead was used as a strategy for achieving quality care. During this time providing pain relief became the primary goal of patient care. Interestingly, care recipients, not clinicians, were blamed if they did not experience pain relief because it was believed that they must not have followed the prescribed treatment plan. By the 1960s comfort and pain relief became subsumed under other concepts such as caring, and comfort was addressed primarily in a physical context [12].

From the mid-1980s through the 1990s comfort, as an important aspect of nursing care, once again began to appear more frequently in the nursing literature. Interestingly, however, comfort was often described in relation to factors that deprive one of comfort such as fatigue, nausea, and pain [13]. Furthermore, some authors suggested that comfort could have meaning only when it was contrasted with discomfort because it seemed that comfort was recognizable only when the patient left a state of discomfort and entered a state of comfort [14]. However, other theorists posit that comfort is more than the absence of pain and that by enhancing comfort individuals are better able to successfully use health-seeking behaviors (HSB) [15,16]. Comfort theory has regained an important role in the philosophy of nursing care and is often a phenomenon of interest in studies about the provision of care [16].

Kolcaba's theory of comfort

Katherine Kolcaba developed a holistic definition of comfort [2,5,6,17–19]. A concept analysis of comfort as it is used in ordinary language revealed four meanings: (1) cause of relief, (2) state of ease and peaceful contentment, (3) relief, and (4) whatever makes life pleasurable [5]. The etymologic derivation of comfort, *comfortare*, is Latin and means to strengthen greatly [5,20]. Although the meaning "to strengthen" is not widely used, it seems to have relevance, especially within the context of birthing women. Childbirth research about processes of care that include comfort measures during childbirth suggests that comfort can be strengthening during labor and enable women to use less analgesia [21].

Kolcaba's theory of comfort is bi-dimensional and includes technical senses as one dimension and contexts of experience as the second dimension [17]. The three technical senses of comfort are (1) relief, (2) ease, and (3) transcendence. Relief occurs when a comfort need has been met and the individual returns to normal functioning. The sense of ease represents a state of calmness or contentment and is required for effective performance. Transcendence is a state of feeling self-motivated to overcome problems [15]. These three technical senses were derived from etymological and conceptual analysis and represent the first dimension of comfort.

Clearly each of the technical senses is affected during pregnancy and childbirth; therefore clinicians need to include them in their assessments of pregnant women. Identifying which sense(s) is impacted will help the clinician formulate an intervention that is specific to the particular comfort need of each woman. Simple techniques such as listening to a woman's concerns and providing needed information can be comforting. Reassuring women about the normalcy of their pregnancy can ease concerns that may occur along the way. Woman-centered care and support throughout pregnancy and labor, including specific care techniques to support normal labor progress, can provide the tools women need to feel confident in their ability to progress through pregnancy, labor, and birth.

The second dimension of comfort consists of four contexts of experience that were synthesized from the literature on holism (1) physical, (2) sociocultural, (3) psychospiritual, and (4) environmental. The physical context of experience refers to body sensations; the sociocultural context is about introspection and relationships with self, family, and society; the psychospiritual context relates to one's belief about the meaning of life and awareness of one's self including one's sexuality; the environmental context is about one's surroundings and includes temperature, light, noise, color, and anything else that is in that person's immediate surroundings [15,16].

The second dimension and its contexts of experience enable clinicians who provide care to birthing women to identify during the prenatal period those specific experiences that bring comfort to an individual woman when she is in pain. During prenatal visits, it is important to discuss the woman's relationships with her family members and ask her to identify who may be most supportive to her during labor. Assessing spiritual beliefs and what activities support those beliefs can also be discussed prenatally. For example, some women use prayer as a coping mechanism during childbirth, suggesting it brings them a sense of comfort. It is also useful to have the woman tour the birthing unit prior to giving birth. This will allow for a discussion about the importance of adapting that environment to support her needs during labor. For example, some women may want to use music and imagery during labor, and therefore if a CD player or radio is not part of the birthing room, she could bring her own CD player with music she preselects. Often a few changes can make the labor environment more supportive and individualized, thus increasing a woman's sense of comfort. It is important to appreciate that it is the woman who provides the meaning of labor and it is she who defines for clinicians what measures will bring her comfort. Use of a well-developed birth plan can document the various comfort measures a woman believes will be helpful to her during labor as well as ways her family and support persons can participate in the process.

Kolcaba [22] provides a holistic definition of comfort that encompasses a health and wellness perspective: "comfort is the immediate state of being strengthened by having the needs for relief, ease or transcendence addressed in the four contexts of holistic human experience: physical, psychospiritual, sociocultural, and environmental." Although this definition is complex, thinking carefully through the possibilities for providing or enhancing a woman's comfort in each of the three senses, through each of the four experience contexts, may enhance a clinician's deliberations about how to maximize a woman's comfort during pregnancy as well as during the process of labor and birth.

Integral to Kolcaba's [2] theory of comfort are HSBs as conceptualized by Schlotfeld [23]. Health-seeking behaviors are a wide range of acquired activities that may be voluntary or involuntary, conscious or unconscious, and internal or external [22,24]. In order to use HSBs the individual needs to have some knowledge of them and a desire to pursue the specific activities [22]. Comfort resulting from HSBs is a holistic outcome accounting for whole person responses [6]. Examples of internal HSBs particular to labor would include cortisol levels, healing, and inflammatory responses. Common external HSBs during labor may include ambulation, freedom of movement, use of imagery, and meditation.

Kolcaba's [2,16,22] theory of comfort can easily be used by clinicians caring for women during birth. Childbirth is a naturally occurring and usually desired, whole person event. Clinicians providing comforting interventions during labor may enable transcendence from physical pain and, therefore, empower a woman in finding her agency (capacity to exert her own power) and ability to master the labor process. Transcendence is the ability to rise above one's pain or problems. Patterson and Zderad theorized that comfort occurs when patients control and plan their destiny, which frees them to be all that they can be in a particular time and in a particular situation. Transcendence differs from the other technical senses of comfort because it necessitates the woman's participation and is dependent on performance and potential to overcome pain or disability [17]. During childbirth, a woman may wish to remain upright and ambulatory even though when she is upright her labor pain increases. However, if maintaining locus of control is of primary importance to her and she is supported in her decision to remain ambulatory, having the control to make her own decision may provide her with a greater sense of strength and enable her to rise above (transcend) the pain of contractions.

Kolcaba's theory of comfort consists of three parts. Part 1 entails the process of comforting with enhanced comfort as the outcome, suggesting that the actions of good clinicians are comforting to patients. If comfort measures applied by clinicians are effective the patient will feel more comfortable than prior to the action [16].

Part 2 entails the relationship between comfort and HSBs and the subsequent desirable internal or external outcomes. Part 2 has the potential to provide researchers/scientists with a framework for pursuing the evidence for specific practices that may result in improved outcomes. Childbirth provides a valuable model for conducting research about part 2 of the theory because the experience of giving birth is holistic and comfort measures are commonly used by midwives, doulas, family members, and maternity nurses to support women during labor. Identifying subsequent healthy outcomes that result from comfort measures employed during labor would contribute to the development of evidence-based guidelines for the care of laboring women. Using comfort measures that are nonpharmacologic and yet effective may have the potential to decrease costs related to maternity care.

Part 3 of the theory focuses on institutional integrity, which includes the institution's values, financial stability, and wholeness of health care organizations. If patients experience comfort during their care experience and have positive subsequent outcomes, institutional integrity is positively affected because theoretically variables such as length of stay and patient satisfaction would probably be improved. For example, if a maternity unit is within an institution that subscribes to using comfort theory, the clinicians would use comfort measures with women during labor and birth. If positive outcomes occur during labor and birth as a result of applying comfort theory, then it is highly likely women would be more satisfied with their birthing experience in that institution.

The theory of comfort and how each of the concepts impact the three parts of the theory are depicted on the Comfort Line website (http://www.thecomfortline.com/index.html).

Pain and comfort during childbirth

Few would disagree that for most women pain is a critical concern during childbirth [26] and that clinicians would be remiss (if not negligent) if pain relief were not part of the care provided to women in labor. Labor pain differs from other types of pain in that it is intermittent and is not part of a pathologic process but, rather, is part of a normal physiologic process leading to birth [1]. Pain in the context of helplessness, suffering, and loss is different from pain in the context of coping resources, comfort, and a sense of accomplishment [27].

Women express and manage labor pain and cope with their labor based on a number of individual and other factors. Lowe notes: "The experience of pain during labor is not a simple reflection of the physiologic processes of parturition. Instead, labor pain is the result of a complex and subjective interaction of multiple physiologic and psychosocial factors on a woman's interpretation of labor stimuli" [28, p. 82].

The experience of labor pain is therefore unique [29] and connected to each woman's perception [28]. How she views the pain, whether as a strengthening event, a challenge to be met, or as noxious stimuli, and how she manages the pain, affects her perception of the birth event. Mastery of the process can lead to an increased sense of self-esteem and personal strength [28].

The pain of childbirth generally begins with mild contractions that build in intensity over time. Their gradual increase in strength and intensity allows a woman to adapt and identify coping mechanisms that enable her to work with and be an active participant in the labor and birth process. However, the majority of efforts directed at managing labor pain focus on obliterating the pain versus moderating and keeping the pain within the woman's compass of control. Although epidural analgesia provides effective pain relief for many women, and certainly is an important and necessary form of pain relief for some women, reports link epidurals with a number of adverse effects both during labor and postpartum [30,31]. It is important then for women to be educated about all forms of pain relief and equally as important to educate women about interventions that promote comfort. Relieving pain does not necessarily bring about comfort [1]. Comfort during childbirth is critically important, and therefore it cannot be assumed that pain relief necessarily enhances comfort for all women. Both are important components of care.

Epidurals, however, remain a popular choice of pain relief for women in labor. Childbirth Connection's national survey of women's childbearing experiences (Listening to Mothers II) found that 76% of the mothers surveyed (n = 1,573) used epidural or spinal anesthesia during labor [32]. This statistic has changed little from the first Listening to Mothers study in which almost two-thirds of mothers surveyed used epidural analgesia. In the 2002 study 26–41% of the women were unable to respond about the associated side effects of epidurals [33].

Lundgren and Dahlberg's [34] phenomenological study about women's birth experiences identified four themes from women's narratives: (1) pain is hard to describe and is contradictory, (2) trust in oneself and one's body, (3) trust in the midwife and husband, and (4) transition to motherhood. The women described pain as a natural process of childbirth and that the ability to cope with the pain, to be strong during the process, came from within the woman. The experience of pain and the experience of strength gave meaning to the transition to motherhood; it brought the woman closer to her baby. Many of the women described labor as *listening to and going into their own body*, revealing labor as a holistic experience. They further indicated that they avoided labor pain by *hiding in their own bodies*. This description aligns with comfort's sense of transcendence.

Pain can have a protective function in assisting individuals to recognize themselves as harmed and needing to take refuge. Studies of pregnant women have identified that neuropeptides (beta endorphins and enkephalkins) may modulate pain during labor, thereby enabling the woman to work with the process of labor [35]. More recently it has been suggested that transcutaneous electrical nerve stimulation (TENS) works to reduce labor pain because it stimulates the release of endorphins or other endogenous opiates that have a similar action to medications such as morphine and codeine [36,37]. By blunting, but not obliterating, the perception of pain, a woman is able to continue to react to noxious stimuli, allowing for continued self-assessment of well-being. She is able to use the pain of labor as a guide indicating a need to change positions, to ambulate, to recognize that progress is occurring. Managing labor pain by obliteration removes the woman from control of her labor, of her birth. In a sense, it can decentralize her from the very process in which she is (or should be) the center. A power imbalance may be created that systematically relieves the woman of her agency in the birthing process and gives control over to the attending clinicians.

Contemporary health care seems to project a negative view of all pain that carries over to pain in childbirth, even though it is widely accepted that labor pain is different from other types of pain. In a medical model context, pain is believed to be ominous and a warning sign of illness or injury. Conversely, Yerby [29] provides a poignant explanation for the usefulness for discomfort and pain during labor:

> [I]t warns that birth is imminent and provides the mother time to prepare herself physically and psychologically for it . . . it allows concentration on the task at hand and enables her and her helpers to recognize a deviation from normal. Would any sensation other than pain persuade the vast majority of women to stop what they were doing, however important it felt, and prepare mentally and physically for the imminent birth? [29, p. 45]

It seems that negative cultural views about labor pain have prohibited a shifting of our lens, and considering that pain in labor may have a benefit, interventions need to be identified that enable a woman to work with her body and the nuances of pain so that the information her body is providing can be interpreted. Comfort in labor is a model of health care with the objective of supporting a physiologic process. This is consistent with a midwifery model of care, and differs from the commonly understood medical model with a focus on cure (eliminating the pain of labor). Umansky suggests that childbirth, as currently experienced in the United States, is dehumanizing because it puts the power in the hands of "experts." She further asserts that "modern childbirth defies the quest for self-determination" [38, p. 66]. A focus on removing the woman from controlling her pain essentially fragments her from the birth process. In fact, Martin [39] in her study of how women feel about their bodies in relation to reproductive medicine compellingly argues that women represent themselves as fragmented, lacking a sense of autonomy and feeling carried away by forces beyond their control.

The midwifery care model views childbirth as a natural and normal phenomenon. Within this model pain is recognized as different from pain that arises from pathology. And while pain relief is certainly paramount in providing care to birthing women, midwives recognize that there are many ways to promote pain relief while at the same time promoting comfort that also support a woman's agency in the childbearing process. A midwifery model defines women's bodies giving birth as normal and capable [38]. Common components of midwifery care include encouraging women to self-identify those techniques that bring them comfort and to use self-identified comfort measures as a first approach to pain management.

Nonpharmacologic methods of pain control are often called comfort measures. They assist in blunting, but do not obliterate, the pain of labor. Therefore they enable the woman to be aware of her body's sensations, to interpret the nuances of pain, and to work with the process. Despite reports of the effectiveness of alternative methods of pain control (e.g., freedom of movement, one-to-one support, massage, hydrotherapy); the increase in maternal satisfaction with the birth experience by women who use them; the improved obstetric outcomes; and the reduced cost and risk with these methods, comfort methods receive little attention in the medical literature and are often unavailable to women in North American [32,33,40].

Interventions that are comforting and enhance comfort (a holistic phenomenon and a basic human need) support normal physiologic birth. There is evidence that respect for the innate capability of women to birth without unnecessary intervention is an important predictor of their postpartum health [41,42].

What women bring to birth

Fundamental to holistic healing is the idea that the body, and spirit form an integrated whole and that the individual is deeply connected to herself, her environment and her community [43, p. 102].

Women bring quantitative and qualitative aspects of their lives to birth. A woman's perspective about her body and her pregnancy have as much impact on her childbearing as does her body's physiology. The mind and body are inexplicably linked and in birth their esprit de corps is evident. The variables a woman brings to birth are parts of *her* whole, a gestalt, the whole woman representative of more than the sum of her parts. Each variable interacts with the others, producing a synergistic influence on a woman's health, pregnancy, and birth. The outcome is individual, different, and unique for each woman and for each birth. It is from this woman-centered framework that midwives assist women during birth and are able to provide care that is comforting. The woman provides the midwife with the meaning of labor and defines for the midwife the measures that might bring comfort. Labor is a holistic event. Comfort is a holistic phenomenon.

The midwifery model of care

Comfort and labor may seem to be a paradox. However, when using a midwifery approach to care it becomes evident that comfort can exist during a time known for its great travail. Providing comfort is a common component of midwifery care. Graham included a chapter in his text *Eternal Eve* on the rebirth of midwifery. The chapter focuses on a text written in 1540: *The Byrthe of Mankynde* (T. Raynalde). The text has been translated into German, Latin, and English and has the intention of making clear the role of the midwife in birth.

Also, the midwife must instruct and *comfort* [italics added] the party, not only refreshing her with good meate and drinke, but also with sweet words, giving her hope for a good speedie deliverance [44, p. 144].

Enhancing comfort may provide women with the strength needed to work with the processes of labor. Interventions that increase comfort during labor support the laboring woman's ability to be an active participant in the birth [3]. Promoting and enhancing comfort is integral to the "art" of midwifery care.

Promoting comfort during childbirth does not negate the significance of pain during labor. It does, however, suggest that the scope of comfort is broader than physiologic pain. Comfort theory has greater explanatory power than theories of pain and anxiety [2]. Using comforting interventions does more than bring physical relief of pain. The interventions also strengthen and provide a sense of ease and relief and, in some women, transcendence.

Childbirth is a whole person experience. Women bring myriad variables to their labor and birth. Physical and psycho-social-cultural-spiritual health encompasses many factors that require assessment prior to the onset of labor in order to provide care during birth that is sensitive, effective, and individualized. Caregivers need to ask women to identify those things that comfort them and to identify factors that may make it more difficult for them to achieve comfort during birth. Those factors may include experiences and life situations (culture, violence, abuse) that may impede the ability to achieve a level of comfort. Comforting is incomplete until comfort is brought into being [46]. Utilizing a woman-centered model, caregivers assess the variables that may impact birth from the woman's standpoint. Comfort theory provides a holistic lens for managing pain and enhancing comfort during labor and birth. Comfort theory is health oriented and supports normal birth [1].

Expanding comfort theory and identifying its existence during childbirth has the potential to increase the current knowledge of how to best manage pain in labor and may provide increased options for labor support at less cost and less risk to mothers and babies. A broader appreciation of the use of comforting interventions is needed in order to shift the biomedical paradigm in which epidural anesthetics are provided as a first response to managing pain in labor. More detail on the use of a number of comfort techniques is provided in this book, particularly chapters on continuous labor support, of which comfort is a component, and relaxation. Perhaps by identifying prenatally those measures that can strengthen women during labor and that caregivers can use to enhance comfort during labor and birth, women will recognize childbirth as a challenge to be met with expectations of mastery [3].

Comfort theory has the potential to be helpful in developing evidence-based guidelines for caring for women during childbirth. Understanding the theory encourages clinicians to assess women's individual comfort needs and to use interventions that are specific for each woman. Comfort theory can also support the individual woman as an active participant in her care. Helping her to identify her preferred health-seeking behaviors that she can use during her labor support her role and agency in the process. The institution benefits overall when comfort theory is used because research suggests outcomes are improved with this type of supportive care [45], and care is more cost effective. Thus, the application of comfort theory has a comprehensive benefit for clinicians, the institution, and, most importantly, the women in our care.

References

1. Schuiling KD, Sampselle CM, & Kolcaba K. (2011). Exploring the presence of comfort within the context of childbirth. In R Bryar & M Sinclair, eds., *Theory for midwifery practice*, 2nd ed., pp. 197–214. London: Palgrave McMillan.

2. Kolcaba K. (1994). A theory of holistic comfort. *Journal of Advanced Nursing, 19,* 1178–1184.
3. Schuiling KD & Sampselle CM. (1999). Comfort in labor and midwifery art. *Image: Journal of Nursing Science, 31,* 77–81.
4. Gropper E. (1992). Promoting health by promoting comfort. *Nursing Forum, 27,* 5–8.
5. Kolcaba KY & Kolcaba RJ. (1991). An analysis of the concept of comfort. *Journal of Advanced Nursing, 16,* 1301–1310.
6. Kolcaba K. (1992). Holistic comfort: Operationalizing the construct as a nurse-sensitive outcome. *Advanced Nursing Science, 15,* 1–10.
7. American College Of Nurse-Midwives. (2004). Philosophy of the American College of Nurse-Midwives. Retrieved from: http://www.midwife.org/index.asp?bid=59&cat=2&button=Search&rec=49.
8. American College of Nurse-Midwives. (2012). Our philosophy of care. Retrieved from: http://www.midwife.org/index.asp?bid=18AmA.
9. Carper B. (1978). Fundamental patterns of knowing in nursing. *Advances in Nursing Science, 1,* 13–23.
10. Harmer B. (1924). *Textbook of the principles and practice of nursing.* New York: Macmillan.
11. Van Blarcom C. (1953). *Obstetrical nursing,* 3rd ed., rev. New York: Macmillan.
12. McIlveen K & Morse J. (1995). The role of comforting in nursing care: 1900–1980. *Clinical Nursing Research, 4,* 127–148.
13. Funk S, Tornquist E, Champagne M, Copp L, & Wiese R. (1989). *Key aspects of comfort: Management of pain, fatigue and nausea.* New York, NY: Springer Publishing Co.
14. Morse J, Bottorhoff J, & Hutchinson S. (1995). The paradox of comfort. *Journal of Advanced Nursing Science, 44,* 14–19.
15. Apostolo JL & Kolcaba K. (2009). The effect of guided imagery on comfort, depression, anxiety, and stress of psychiatric inpatients with depressive disorders. *Archives of Psychiatric Nursing, 23,* 403–411.
16. Kolcaba K. (2003). *Comfort theory and practice: A vision for holistic health care and research.* New York: Springer.
17. Kolcaba K. (1991). A taxonomic structure for the concept of comfort. *Image: Journal of Nursing Scholarship, 23,* 237–240.
18. Kolcaba K. (1995). The art of comfort care. *Image: Journal of Nursing Scholarship, 27,* 287–289.
19. Kolcaba K. (1995). Comfort as process and product, merged in holistic nursing art. *Journal of Holistic Nursing, 13,* 117–131.
20. Morse J, Bottorhoff J, & Hutchinson S. (1994). The phenomenology of comfort. *Journal of Advanced Nursing Science, 20,* 189–195.
21. Simkin P. (1995). Reducing pain and enhancing progress during labor: A guide to non-pharmacologic methods for maternity care givers. *Birth, 22,* 161–171.
22. Kolcaba K. (2012). The comfort line. Retrieved from: http://www.thecomfortline.com.
23. Schlotfeld R. (1975). The need for a conceptual framework. In P Verhonic, ed., *Nursing Research,* pp. 3–25. Boston: Little, Brown.
24. Glazer G & Pressler J. (1989). Schlotfeld's health seeking nursing model. In J Fitzpatrick & A Whall, eds., *Conceptual models of nursing practice,* pp. 241–253. Englewood Cliffs, NJ: Prentice-Hall.
25. Patterson J & Zderad L. (1988). *Humanistic nursing.* New York: NLN.
26. King T. (2002). Labor pain in the 21st century. *Journal of Midwifery & Women's Health, 47,* 6.
27. Lowe N. (2002). The nature of labor pain. *American Journal of Obstetrics and Gynecology, 186S,* S16–S24.

28. Lowe N. (1996). The pain and discomfort of labor and birth. *Journal of Obstetric, Gynecologic and Neonatal Nursing, 25*, 82–92.

29. Yerby M. (2000). *Pain in childbearing.* London: Bailliere Tindall.

30. American Congress of Obstetricians and Gynecologists. (2002). Obstetric analgesia and anesthesia. ACOG Practice Bulletin No. 36. (Reaffirmed 2010.)

31. Lieberman E & Donoghue C. (2002). Unintended effects of epidural analgesia during labor: A systematic review. *American Journal of Obstetrics and Gynecology, 186S*, S31–S68.

32. Declercq ER, Sakala C, Corry MP, & Applebaum S. (2006). Listening to mothers II: Report of the Second National U.S. Survey of Women's Childbearing Experiences. Retrieved from: www.childbirthconnections.org/listeningtomothers/.

33. Declercq ER, Sakala C, Corry MP, Applebaum S, & Risher P. (2002). Listening to mothers: Report of the First National US Survey of Women's Childbearing Experiences. Retrieved from: http://childbearingconnection.org/pdf.asp?PDFDownload=LtMreport. Accessed December 7, 2011.

34. Lundgren I & Dahlberg K. (1998). Women's experience of pain during childbirth. *Midwifery, 14*, 105–110.

35. Cahill C. (1993). Beta-endorphin levels during pregnancy and labor: A role in pain modulation? *Journal of Advanced Nursing, 18*, 424–436.

36. Rodriguez MA. (2005). Transcutaneous electrical nerve stimulation during birth. *British Journal of Midwifery, 13*(8), 522–526.

37. Bedwell C. (2011). Why do women use TENS equipment and how effective is it? *British Journal of Midwifery, 19*(6), 348–351.

38. Umansky L. (1996). *Motherhood reconceived: Feminism and the legacy of the sixties.* New York: New York University Press.

39. Martin E. (1992). *The woman in the body: A cultural analysis of reproduction.* Boston: Beacon Press.

40. Marmor T & Krol D. (2002). Labor pain management in the United States: Understanding patterns and the issue of choice. *American Journal of Obstetrics & Gynecology, 186S*, S173–S180.

41. Roberts J & Woolley D. (1996). A second look at the second stage of labor. *Journal of Nurse-Midwifery and Women's Health, 25*, 415–423.

42. Sampselle C & Hines S. (1999). Spontaneous pushing during birth: Relationship to perineal outcomes. *Journal of Nurse-Midwifery and Women's Health, 44*, 36–39.

43. Boston Women's Health Collective (1998). *Our bodies, ourselves for the new century.* New York: Touchstone.

44. Graham H. (1950). Rebirth of midwifery. In H. Graham, ed., *Eternal Eve*, pp. 138–144. New York: Heinemann.

45. Hodnett ED, Gates S, Hofmeyr GJ, Sakala C, & Weston J. (2011). Continuous support for women during childbirth [PDF]. *Cochrane Database of Systematic Reviews*, issue 2. Art. No.: CD003766. DOI: 10.1002/14651858.CD003766.pub3.

46. Kolcaba K. Personal communication, July 12, 2000.

Chapter 6

Continuous labor support

Carrie E. Neerland

Key points

- Be sure that *all* laboring women have continuous support during labor.
- Adopt AWHONN guidelines for nurse staffing for care of women in labor.
- Protect the physical and emotional space of labor to support women during labor.
- Offer a variety of comfort measures to women in labor.
- Be fully present when providing labor support.

> *A woman giving birth to a baby thrives when she's at the center of a circle of love.*
> **Marsden Wagner (with Stephanie Gunning)**

Introduction

Labor support spans centuries and cultures and it is well understood that women benefit from and desire such care during childbirth. In the United States prior to the 1900s, most women gave birth in their homes, where they had the support of knowledgeable women such as mothers, grandmothers, neighbors, friends, and midwives. As childbirth moved to the hospital setting, women became more isolated during the process of birth and it was not until the 1960s and 1970s that fathers were allowed in the delivery room. In our current health care system, women receive varying degrees of labor support depending on the birth setting, the kind of support available, and the support women seek on their own. In this chapter we discuss the concepts of continuous labor support and presence, the benefits of this approach, and how it can be used to provide optimal care to women in labor.

Continuous labor support and presence are both valuable components of supporting physiologic labor and birth. Continuous labor support is the continuous presence of an individual offering support to the woman in labor. The literature on continuous labor support has identified the following components: physical comfort measures, emotional

Supporting a Physiologic Approach to Pregnancy and Birth: A Practical Guide, First Edition.
Edited by Melissa D. Avery.
© 2013 John Wiley & Sons, Inc. Published 2013 by John Wiley & Sons, Inc.

support and continuous presence, facilitation of communication and advocacy, information and advice, and guidance and support for the woman's partner [1,2]. Continuous labor support may be provided by a health care provider, registered nurse, doula, family member or friend, or a combination.

Presence is an element of continuous labor support, and as presented later in this chapter, is more of a practice style or an art form. While continuous labor support is the *what* of the labor support equation, presence is the *how*.

Continuous labor support: An evidence-based practice that supports normal physiologic birth

Importance and evidence

As the cesarean section rate has climbed to one-third of all births in the United States, it is paramount that women's health care providers, health care organizations, and hospitals reexamine the care that is provided during labor and birth. Continuous labor support is an intervention that supports normal physiologic birth and has numerous benefits while having no adverse affects.

According to the recent Cochrane review "Continuous Support for Women during Childbirth," women who had continuous labor support were more likely to have a spontaneous vaginal birth and their labors were shorter. They were also less likely to have a cesarean section, instrumental vaginal birth (vacuum or forceps), intrapartum analgesia, or regional analgesia (epidural); to report dissatisfaction with their childbirth experience; or to have a baby with a low 5-minute Apgar score. No adverse or harmful affects with continuous labor support have been reported in any study [3]. The Milbank Report titled "Evidence Based Maternity Care: What It Is and What It Can Achieve" also highlighted continuous labor support as an underutilized intervention or practice to use whenever possible and appropriate, as the practice has been shown to improve outcomes with no adverse or harmful effects [4].

The World Health Organization has identified four care practices that promote, support, and protect normal birth [5]. Lamaze International has recommended two additional practices including continuous labor support. Lamaze asserts that women with continuous labor support have greater confidence, are more able to work with their labor, and are less likely to use medication in labor or have interventions [6]. Childbirth Connection (previously Maternity Center Association), Doulas of North America, the American College of Nurse-Midwives, and the Association of Women's Health, Obstetric and Neonatal Nurses all endorse continuous support for women in labor.

Who should provide labor support?

The Listening to Mothers II survey in 2006 [7] revealed that 96% of women surveyed reported having received some type of supportive care during labor and birth. The definition of supportive care is similar to continuous labor support in that it includes physical comfort, emotional support, and providing information. Labor support persons reported by the women surveyed varied: 82% were supported by a husband or partner, 56% by nursing staff, 38% by a family member or friend, 34% by a physician, 8% by a midwife, and 3% received support from a doula (3% other). Of women who received doula care, 100% felt supported in labor by their doula, while 89% felt supported by their husband or partner, 66% felt supported by their midwife, 44% felt supported by their family practice physician, and 37% by their obstetrician [7].

The Cochrane review found that effects of continuous support were strongest when the support person was neither a hospital employee nor a person in the woman's social network. Compared to women with no continuous support, women with continuous support provided by someone not employed by the hospital or in their social network were 28% less likely to have a cesarean birth, 31% less likely to receive Pitocin, 9% less likely to use any type of pain medication, and 34% less likely to express dissatisfaction with the childbirth experience. However, continuous support from a husband or partner, family member, or friend was more effective than not having continuous support [3]. The bottom line is this: continuous labor support in any form is more beneficial than not providing continuous labor support.

The specific birth setting has a major impact on the type and quality of labor support available for women. Multiple barriers can impact the ability of nurses, physicians, and midwives to provide continuous labor support. Midwives and physicians may have other time demands and responsibilities or may not be interested in providing labor support. Nurses might also have competing responsibilities such as caring for multiple women at one time or additional duties that do not allow them to provide continuous support. The attitude and culture of the birth environment can also influence labor support. Nurses who intend to provide continuous support may not be supported by their nursing colleagues or managers and are sometimes even chided for providing that level of care [8].

Nursing

Nurses have many demands on their time, particularly if nurse-patient ratios are high. Patient acuity also impacts how nurses are able to care for women during labor. In recent years, there has been in increase in the rates of induction, cesarean sections, and medical and obstetric complications. Patient care scenarios with increased acuity and intervention place additional demands on nurses' time due to the use of technology, increased need for documentation, and frequent assessments.

Nurse staffing has a significant impact on the availability of continuous labor support. Nurses are sometimes asked to care for two or even three women in labor at the same time, making continuous labor support nearly impossible as they move from room to room, unable to give their undivided attention to one woman. Many nurses, along with the Association of Women's Health, Obstetric and Neonatal Nurses (AWHONN), assert that continuous labor support provided by a registered nurse (RN) is an important part of labor care. AWHONN's position statement on nursing support of laboring women states: "that continuously available labor support from a registered nurse is a critical component to achieve improved birth outcomes. The RN assesses, develops, implements, and evaluates an individualized plan of care based on each woman's physical, psychological and socio-cultural needs, including the woman's desires for and expectations of the laboring

---

Box 6.1   Role of nurse in labor and birth

- Assessment and management of the physiologic and psychological processes of labor.
- Facilitation of normal physiologic processes, such as the women's desire for movement in labor.
- Provision of physical comfort measures, emotional and informational support, and advocacy.
- Evaluation of fetal well-being during labor.
- Instruction regarding the labor process.
- Role modeling to facilitate family participation during labor and birth.
- Direct collaboration with other members of the health care team to coordinate patient care.

---

process. Labor care and labor support are powerful nursing functions, and it is incumbent on health care facilities to provide an environment that encourages the unique patient-RN relationship during childbirth" [9]. Components of the role of the nurse in labor and birth [9] are highlighted in Box 6.1.

In 2011, AWHONN published new perinatal nurse staffing guidelines. "Guidelines for Professional Registered Nurse Staffing for Perinatal Units" reflects the changes that have occurred in perinatal nursing in the past several decades, such as increased rates of induction, cesareans, and other interventions. The guidelines recommend one-to-one RN-to-woman ratio for women in labor who have medical or obstetric complications, are receiving oxytocin, or choose minimal intervention in labor (e.g., decline analgesia or anesthesia) [10].

Modification of environment and culture

There are multiple ways in which health care providers can advocate for continuous support for women in labor. Because continuous labor support is an evidence-based practice, health care providers can offer education for managers and staff through in-services, grand rounds presentations, or poster presentations. Health care facilities, executives, and other health care providers with decision-making authority should be offered the information about the evidence and ways staff can provide continuous labor support in order to help create an organizational environment supportive of such practices. Health care providers involved in direct patient care can provide modeling for other staff and student learners and reinforce the importance of continuous labor support. Many nurses may not have received education about how to provide labor support; therefore, formal education programs about providing continuous labor support including specific techniques should become part of required ongoing training. Additionally, health care providers can provide information to interested women about how to find and choose a doula.

Challenges for women in finding support

Women may experience barriers and challenges in finding a labor support person. They may lack adequate social support, such as a teen or a woman who is not partnered, or they may lack the financial resources to hire a doula. All women should be asked prenatally whom they are planning on for labor support and should be educated about the benefits of continuous labor support. If a woman desires a doula, local resources can be presented. Some hospitals and birth centers offer doula services to women. It is important that clinicians are aware of available local resources. Some insurance plans do cover doula services, and women can be encouraged to contact their insurance company. Finally, some doulas will work with women on a sliding scale fee arrangement or at no charge if the doula is relatively new and gaining experience. The woman should be encouraged to meet with the doula prior to labor and birth so that they can get to know one another and discuss the woman's expectations as well as clarify the services the doula offers.

Review: The labor process and the fear-tension-pain cycle

The initiation of the complex process of human labor is still not completely understood. Labor initiation is thought to be an intricate interaction of fetal, maternal, and placental mechanisms. The chief physiologic force during labor is that of uterine contractions, but many physical changes and discomforts occur throughout the various phases and stages of labor such as low back pain, pressure and stretching of the pelvic ligaments, cervical stretching pain, pressure on the muscles of the pelvic floor, and stretching of the vaginal canal and tissues. Many psychological or emotional changes can occur during labor such as excitement, fear, anxiety, helplessness, exhaustion, discouragement, or empowerment.

The interplay between the physical and emotional factors may affect the birth process [11]. Dr. Grantly Dick-Read, a British obstetrician who is often considered the father of the "natural childbirth" movement, hypothesized that with increased fear, a woman's body becomes more tense, and with more muscle tension, pain increases [12]. His hypothesis is supported by what we know today about cathecholamines and the fight-or-flight response. Catecholamines, or the hormones dopamine, epinephrine, and norepinephrine, are produced by the adrenal gland. These hormones are released in response to stress and cause physiologic changes that prepare the body for intense physical activity (fight-or-flight response). This reaction of the sympathetic nervous system causes increased heart rate and blood pressure, decreased gastrointestinal motility, and constriction of blood vessels. During labor, norepinephrine and epinephrine increase, which can influence uterine vasoconstriction, with individual variation among women [13]. Thus, increased fear and tension may lead to decreased uterine blood flow and potentially impede labor progress and further contribute to difficulty in coping with labor.

How well is she coping? Pain versus suffering

Penny Simkin, physical therapist and childbirth educator, makes the distinction between pain and suffering. Although the words "pain" and "suffering" are often used interchangeably, Simkin notes that pain is an unpleasant physical sensation, while suffering is an emotional state of distress; may include feelings of fear, helplessness, loneliness, or anguish; and may or may not be related to physical pain [14]. Although some women may choose epidural anesthesia in labor to relieve their pain, they may still suffer in an emotional or psychosocial way. Fear of what is next, history of abuse, current family or relationship stress, or feelings of loneliness may surface during the labor process. Clinicians can be sure to remember that there are variations in individual pain thresholds during labor, coping methods, and emotive behaviors.

When women are able to draw upon tools or comfort measures within themselves and their support persons to cope with the pain and discomforts in labor, they often feel more in control and have greater satisfaction with the birth experience [15]. Signs that a woman is coping with labor include explicitly stating she is coping, rhythmically moving with contractions, focusing inward, using breathing/rhythmic breathing, ability to relax in between contractions, or using vocalization (moaning, counting, chanting).

Signs that a woman is not coping with labor may include crying, panicked reactions during contractions, thrashing, writhing, inability to relax between contractions, tense muscles, clawing, biting, and inability to focus or concentrate. Continuous labor support, comforting presence, and specific comfort measures can be utilized to assist a woman who is having a difficult time coping. Gulliver et al. created the Coping with Labor Algorithm, which allows the care provider to assess the woman in a way that incorporates culture and beliefs about labor and labor pain and then provides suggestions to enhance coping based on the woman's response. This algorithm is presented in more detail in the chapter on labor and birth [16].

Elements of labor support

Components of continuous labor support have been identified as physical comfort measures, emotional support and continuous presence, facilitation of communication and advocacy, information and advice, and guidance and support for the woman's partner. Here, we discuss the following elements of labor support: comfort measures and physical support, the environment and "holding the space," emotional support, reassurance, and information and advice. A discussion of "holding the space" is included, as it addresses comfort within the physical environment of the hospital and how the environment can have an impact both physically and emotionally. Additionally, the topic of reassurance on its own is relevant, as the current culture surrounding birth in the United States has become focused on the use of technological interventions with much less emphasis on simple support measures.

Comfort measures and physical support

Women in labor are experiencing an intensely physical event. There are many ways to offer comfort and provide physical support during labor. Please refer to related chapters for complete descriptions of some of these comfort measures during labor. A list of possible comfort measures for labor is provided in Box 6.2.

Box 6.2   Comfort measures for labor

- Encouraging movement and positioning.
- Touch/massage.
- Hydrotherapy.
- Intradermal water blocks.
- Acupuncture and acupressure.
- Hypnosis.
- TENS unit.
- Aromatherapy.
- Heat/cold.
- Relaxation and breathing.
- Music and audioanalgesia.
- Environment: lighting, music, temperature, aromatherapy, whispering, minimizing noise.

The environment: Holding the space

The hospital is a busy and foreign place to most people, full of strange sights and sounds. A laboring woman may come in contact with many staff throughout the process of labor, childbirth, and postpartum including nurses, nursing assistants, registrars, medical students, phlebotomists, nursing students, residents, physicians, and midwives. Frequent intrusions, vaginal examinations, common procedures, electronic fetal monitoring (EFM), and confinement to the bed can all cause stress for the woman in labor. These disturbances can potentially have adverse effects on the woman's ability to cope with labor as well as the progress of labor.

"Holding the space" is a concept that means protecting the physical and emotional space of the woman in labor [17]. The care provider is a guardian or protector of the space, working to minimize unnecessary interruptions and noise, keeping the environment comfortable for the woman, and advocating for the woman as needed. Ultimately, the goal is to keep distractions to a minimum so that the woman's focus is not interrupted time and again, thus she is allowed to keep her focus, rhythm, and coping intact.

Holding and protecting the space can be achieved in a number of ways. First, space can be protected by managing the number of people in the room and how they interact and communicate. Only those that are directly involved with providing care or who have permission should be in the room. If a student is to be involved directly or wishes to observe, it is paramount that permission is obtained from the laboring woman. Special attention should be focused on how those in the presence of a laboring woman are communicating and what they are communicating. At times, hospital staff or support persons might engage in discussion about topics unrelated to what is happening in the room and may even talk over the patient. This is disrespectful to the woman and may interrupt her focus and efforts to cope with her labor. The care provider can model supportive behavior by refocusing the attention back to the woman in labor and by not engaging in discussions that are not about the care of the laboring woman. A student may be assigned specific activities to support the woman, with permission, thus extending the care of the regular staff and providers and increasing the experience of the students/learners. In addition, it is appropriate for the care provider to ask the woman who she prefers to have in the room with her and ask people to leave if the woman desires.

Second, protecting the space can be aided by organizing necessary procedures and care tasks to minimize interruption. Attempt to group care tasks together, such as taking vital signs, to reduce disruption. If there are required care measures or procedures, perform them between contractions, if possible, so that the woman is not distracted by the extra touch, sounds, or discomfort. Consideration is also given to the use of time between contractions, which is crucial resting time and can become difficult for the woman if there is always something that needs to be done.

Third, controlling the physical environment is also part of holding the space. Keep lights low and avoid harsh lighting directly on the woman, keep external and hospital noises to a minimum, and use soft voices. Music, aromatherapy, and adjusting the temperature in the room can be utilized and adapted according to the woman's preference. If there is adequate space, consider moving the bed to the side of the room so that it is not the main focus within the labor room.

Emotional support

The environment and physical surroundings are not the only parameters that need to be addressed to support a woman in labor. Her inner emotional and psychological needs also need to be met so she feels safe, confident, respected, and ultimately well cared for. A woman's emotional state in labor can be assessed by observation or by asking. By observation, one can evaluate how well a woman is coping by watching how she is breathing with contractions, how she is moving with contractions, how she may be vocalizing with labor, and what she is doing during the rest periods in between contractions. Many women will readily offer up how they are feeling, especially in the earlier phases of labor. Other women, however, may remain stoic or turn inward, even though they might be feeling extremely uncomfortable. In this way, it is not always possible to understand how a woman is feeling merely by observing. It *is* appropriate to ask a woman how she is feeling and coping with labor but it should be done in a respectful and sensitive manner. Many women reach an inward almost trance-like state, an instinctive state that Simkin refers to as reverie, where the neocortex, or thinking part of the brain, shuts off and the more primitive parts of the brain (the midbrain and brainstem) take over [18]. Interruptions such as questions, unexpected touch, lights, or people coming and going can activate the neocortex and inhibit the primitive parts of the brain, making it more difficult for the woman to find or return to her reverie. Do not ask questions during contractions and interfere with the woman's concentration and coping efforts. Instead, ask between contractions. "What were your thoughts during that contraction?"

Reassurance

Reassurance and praise play a large part in supporting a woman during labor and in maintaining the normalcy of birth. Offer calm, sensitive words of reassurance when appropriate, reminding the woman that she is doing a great job and that her body is doing what it is supposed to do. Suggestions include: "You are doing a great job of working through those contractions"; "You are doing a great job of relaxing in between contractions"; "Your body really knows what to do"; "Your body is working in just the right way and you are working with it"; "You are really listening to your body." Reassurance can also be offered in physical ways as well: by touch, holding hands, offering a smile or a hand to hold [19]. When offering reassuring words during a contraction, use a calm, firm voice so that the woman is able to hear you and does not have to avert her focus to ask what was said.

Additionally, when listening to the fetal heart tones intermittently by Doppler or with continuous EFM (if required), offer information to the woman and her support person(s) about the heart beat in an objective way. "The baby's heart beat is normal. We will listen again in about 15 minutes." "The monitor shows us the baby's heart rate is normal and reactive, which means that the baby is doing well." If continuous EFM is needed, some women are reassured by hearing the heartbeat from the monitor. Be respectful of her comfort and ask for permission before turning the volume down or off.

Information and guidance

The importance of reassurance and praise for a woman in labor has been presented. Equally important is offering women information and advice during the labor process. As the laboring woman is working with her contractions, she may become tired, may feel she is less able to cope with the contractions, or might wonder how she is progressing. The care provider should offer appropriate guidance regarding what the woman and her support person(s) can do to help with coping and aid comfort. This includes specific coping tools or methods that the woman can employ for pain relief such as heat, massage, or hydrotherapy. Advice or suggestions on coping methods such as position changes, breathing methods, and relaxation can be provided by staff and family members.

Information should be offered to the woman and her support person(s) about how she is progressing in labor including any procedures that are being performed. Minimize vaginal and other exams if possible and let the woman know the findings of the vaginal exam as soon as it is performed and she is able to listen. In early labor, be sure to describe effacement as well as dilatation and what that means. In active labor, effacement becomes less important and information should be offered as to the process of dilatation and descent.

If any procedures or tests need to be performed, explain the reason for the procedure or test, any choices about the procedure or test, how it is to be performed, and obtain consent prior to the test or procedure. Not only is it the woman's right to be informed, but if she understands and can anticipate a procedure, it will help to decrease her fear and anxiety.

What is presence?

Presence is defined by Merriam-Webster as "the fact, condition, or quality of being present." It can also be defined as "a person's bearing, personality, or appearance." The origin of the word "presence" is from the Latin word for presence, *praesen*, and is derived from *prae* meaning "in front" and *sens* meaning "being" [20]. Presence is central to the practice of midwifery and supporting women during childbirth. Midwife scholars refer to presence as being "with woman," which is the literal translation of the word midwife. Further, the concept of being "with woman" is defined as "the provision of emotional, physical, spiritual and psychologic presence/support by a midwife as desired by the laboring woman" [21]. Of course nurses, physicians, and other support persons also have the skills to be "with woman." The essential elements of presence have been identified by Hunter as (a) knowledge and professional expertise, (b) sensitivity, (c) personal attention, (d) nurturance, (e) support and guidance, (f) advice and information, and (g) a trusting, flexible, reciprocal, and caring relationship.

In supporting normal birth, the act of being "with woman" or presence is vital. Presence is not only about the physical space or environment but about creating a caring, respectful setting where the woman always comes first. Presence is a process that begins when the clinician first steps into the birthing environment. Learning as much about the woman before entering her space is valuable so as not to bombard the laboring woman with questions about her history and her labor, as this can be disruptive to her coping processes. Obtaining information in advance can also help to prevent repeated questions that were already asked by nursing staff. In addition, reviewing the birth plan (if one was prepared) prior to entering the room can help the caregiver to understand the woman's wishes for her labor and birth and enable further conversation as her labor progresses. Attention to the birth plan demonstrates respect for the woman's work and thoughtfulness when approaching her birth.

Presence does not mean that the clinician must leave his or her personality at the door when entering a birthing room but rather adapting in a calm, respectful, and sensitive manner (the woman is already adapting to the hospital or birth center space). Being present in labor includes courtesy and respect. Many women in labor feel vulnerable and exposed—they are in a foreign place, often wearing only a hospital gown or t-shirt, and are coping with the discomforts of labor. Respect the woman's privacy and space by knocking lightly on the door and asking permission to enter. Introduce yourself to the woman and her support person, and do so between contractions if possible. When assisting the woman during position changes or performing a physical exam, respect her privacy and keep her as covered as she wishes. Finally, ask the proper pronunciation of the woman's name and use language interpreters if needed, speaking directly to the woman when working with an interpreter. These suggestions, while simple, can be forgotten when staff are busy and are important to creating a woman-centered environment.

Hands-on, physical assessment is obviously essential in labor. Approaching the assessment in a non-hurried, gentle manner, and with permission, shows the woman respect and caring and nurtures the mutually trusting relationship. Ask permission to palpate contractions and perform as much of the physical exam and pelvic exam as possible in between contractions.

The clinician uses presence as a tool to assess and to simultaneously provide a sense of normalcy and calm [22]. If the woman is lying down or sitting, it is appropriate for the provider to ask permission to sit with the woman. This shows personal attention and respect for the woman by being on the same level or "with" the woman versus standing over or above her. A provider will use presence to quietly and calmly observe what is happening in the room and assess how the woman is coping and how her support persons are working with her.

With electronic documentation available in most hospitals today, vital signs and fetal monitoring strips can be reviewed prior to entering the room. If this option is not available, the fetal monitor tracing or computer console should *not* be the first thing that a provider examines upon entering the room (unless an urgent or emergent situation). Doing so places the woman's work and expertise behind that of the technology. An unnecessary focus on the fetal monitor can also shift the support person's attention to the technology and away from the woman. Gently refocus the support person's attention to the woman. This refocus can be done by saying something such as, "The monitor gives us an idea about how often the contractions are happening and how long they last, but it cannot tell us how strong they are. Only the woman can tell us how strong they are." Again, continuous fetal monitoring should be reserved for situations where it is deemed necessary, as it has not been shown to be beneficial in low-risk labor and birth [23–25].

The art of doing "nothing" well

Presence continues throughout the labor process with quiet yet vigilant observation and assessment. If the woman is progressing normally and coping well, then praise and reassurance are offered. If the woman or her support person is in need of advice or guidance, it is given in a positive, reassuring way. Kennedy described midwifery as "the art of doing 'nothing' well" and, at times, presence means doing "nothing" [19]. It is an approach to care that supports the normalcy of birth and involves watchful waiting and intervening only when necessary.

Using a positive presence or being "with woman" during labor has many benefits. First, women feel well supported. Second, women have enhanced self-esteem and increased feelings of control and confidence in labor. This leads to an improved ability to "handle" childbirth. Third, using presence provides positive modeling to other staff and support persons. Finally, using presence as a tool for vigilant assessment conveys a sense of calm and normalcy. This helps to create an environment of trust in a woman's body and her ability to give birth, a tuned in-ness and positivity about the labor process.

Summary

From the evidence, it is clear that women benefit from continuous labor support with decreased rates of intervention and cesarean section; however, many of those involved in the care of laboring women are often burdened with competing interests such as caring for multiple women and other demands of the clinical environment. Increased education efforts, culture change, and lobbying for continuous labor support can help to make continuous labor support a part of the labor support equation for *all* women.

The hospital can be a busy and intimidating environment for women and their families, and any health care provider can use several simple measures to provide a calm, supportive presence (the *how* of the labor support equation). At times, that means simply "doing nothing" but being present in the room and letting the process unfold. Watchful waiting is a significant paradigm shift for many in the current fear-based culture in maternity care. Providing a supportive environment, however, can be modeled and taught in nursing schools, medical schools, and midwifery programs in order to move from a culture of fear to a culture that is confident and supportive of women, trusting in women's bodies.

References

1. Hodnett E. (1996). Nursing support of the laboring woman. *JOGNN*, *25*(3), 257–264.
2. Simkin PP & O'Hara MA. (2002). Nonpharmacologic relief of pain during labor: Systematic reviews of five methods. *American Journal of Obstetrics and Gynecology*, *186*(5), 131–159.
3. Hodnett ED, Gates S, Hofmeyr GJ, Sakala C, & Weston J. (2011). Continuous support for women during childbirth [PDF]. *Cochrane Database of Systematic Reviews*, issue 2. Art. No.: CD003766. DOI: 10.1002/14651858.CD003766.pub3.
4. Sakala C & Corry M. (2008). Evidence-based maternity care: What it is and what it can achieve. Co-published by Childbirth Connection, the Reforming States Group, and the Milbank Memorial Fund. Available at: http://www.childbirthconnection.org/pdfs/evidence-based-maternity-care.pdf.
5. Chalmers B & Porter R. (2001). Assessing effective care in normal birth: The Bologna Score. *Birth*, *28*(2), 79–83.
6. Hotelling B, Amis D, Green J, & Sakala C. (2004). Care practices that promote normal birth #3: Continuous labor support. Lamaze International Education Council. *Journal of Perinatal Education*, *13*(2), 16–22.
7. Declercq ER, Sakala C, Corry MP, & Applebaum S. (2006). Listening to mothers II: Report of the Second National U.S. Survey of Women's Childbearing Experiences. Retrieved from: www.childbirthconnection.org/listeningtomothers/.
8. Payant L, Davies B, Graham I, Peterson W, & Clinch J. (2008). Nurses' intentions to provide labor support to women. *JOGNN*, *37*(4), 405–414.
9. Association of Women's Health, Obstetric and Neonatal Nurses. (2011). AWHONN position statement: Nursing support of laboring women. *JOGNN*, *40*, 665–666. Available at: http://www.awhonn.org/awhonn/content.do?name=05_HealthPolicyLegislation/5H_PositionStatements.htm.
10. Guidelines for Professional Registered Nurse Staffing for Perinatal Units Executive Summary. (2011). *Nursing for Women's Health*, *15*, 81–84. DOI: 10.1111/j.1751-486X.2011.01603.x.
11. Simkin P & Ancheta R. (2011). *The labor progress handbook: Early interventions to prevent and treat dystocia*, 3rd ed. Oxford: Wiley-Blackwell.
12. Dick-Read G. (2013). *Childbirth without fear: The principles and practice of natural childbirth.* London: Pinter & Martin.
13. Lederman RP, Lederman E, Work BA Jr, & McCann DS. (1978). The relationship of maternal anxiety, plasma catecholamines, and plasma cortisol to progress in labor. *American Journal of Obstetrics and Gynecology*, *132*(5), 495–500.
14. Simkin P. (2011). Pain, suffering, and trauma in labor and subsequent post-traumatic stress disorder: First of two posts by Penny Simkin, PT, CCE, CD (DONA). Available at: http://www.scienceandsensibility.org/?p=2145.
15. Hodnett ED. (2002). Pain and women's satisfaction with the experience of childbirth: A systematic review. *American Journal of Obstetrics and Gynecology*, *186*(5), 160–172.
16. Gulliver B, Fisher J, & Roberts L. (2008). A new way to assess pain in laboring women: Replacing the rating scale with a "coping" algorithm. *Nursing for Women's Health*, *12*(5), 404–408.

17. Seibold C, Licqurish S, Rolls C, & Hopkins F. (2010). "Lending the space": Midwives perceptions of birth space and clinical risk management. *Midwifery*, *26*(5), 526–531.
18. Simkin P. (2008). *The birth partner: A complete guide to childbirth for the dads, doulas, and all other labor companions*, 3rd ed. Boston: Harvard Common Press.
19. Kennedy HP. (2000). A model of exemplary midwifery practice: Results of a delphi study. *Journal of Midwifery & Women's Health*, *45*(1), 4–19.
20. Merriam-Webster.com. (2012). S.v. "presence." Retrieved from: http://www.merriam-webster.com/dictionary/presence. Accessed August 2, 2012.
21. Hunter LP. (2009). A descriptive study of "being with woman" during labor and birth. *Journal of Midwifery & Women's Health*, *54*(2), 111–118.
22. Kennedy HP & Shannon MT. (2003). Keeping birth normal: Research findings on midwifery care during childbirth. *JOGNN*, *33*(5), 554–560.
23. Wood SH. (2003). Should women be given a choice about fetal assessment in labor? *American Journal of Maternal/Child Nursing*, *28*(5), 292–298.
24. American College of Nurse-Midwives. (2010). ACNM Clinical Bulletin Number 11. Intermittent auscultation for intrapartum fetal heart rate surveillance. *Journal of Midwifery & Women's Health*, *55*(4), 397–403.
25. American College of Obstetricians and Gynecologists. (2009). ACOG Practice Bulletin: Clinical Management Guidelines for Obstetrician-Gynecologists Number 106. Intrapartum fetal heart rate monitoring: Nomenclature, interpretation, and general management principles. *Obstetrics & Gynecology*, *114*(1), 192–202.

Chapter 7

Techniques to promote relaxation in labor

Kathryn Leggitt

Key points

- Relaxation techniques can be a safe and effective means of coping with labor pain, decreasing the use of medication and epidural.
- Women often learn relaxation techniques in childbirth education classes but may have difficulty putting what they have learned into action or may have not attended class.
- Simple guided imagery scripts, personal music selections, and position changes can be helpful in labor to promote relaxation.
- Remember the labor room environment and adjust the setting to promote relaxation by reducing bright light, noise, and incorporating support persons into the labor support process.
- Relaxation techniques described here remain valuable even if a woman is restricted to bed due to a complication or if she has used an epidural, but may need to be modified.
- A variety of relaxation techniques may be considered, as each woman is unique in her application of these techniques.

Relaxation means releasing all concern and tension and letting the natural order of life flow through one's being.

Donald Curtis

Introduction

Assisting women to relax and release tension during labor is a key part of providing labor support. Family members and other support persons also appreciate guidance so they can be an active part of assisting their loved one progress in labor. In this chapter specific techniques to promote relaxation in labor such as language use, music, imagery, positioning, and use of heat and cold are reviewed. Examples of simple phrases, guided imagery, and physical support that all providers may use in supporting women during labor and birth are provided.

Supporting a Physiologic Approach to Pregnancy and Birth: A Practical Guide, First Edition.
Edited by Melissa D. Avery.
© 2013 John Wiley & Sons, Inc. Published 2013 by John Wiley & Sons, Inc.

Why relaxation?

Isn't it our very first line of action, when interacting with a woman who first presents in labor struggling to cope? "Relax," we tell her. "Let your shoulders go, try to breathe." But why do we do so?

All pain serves a purpose; as a signal from an injured area to the brain it is generally a warning that something is amiss. During times of pain or stress, the body's "fight-or-flight" response is activated. Heart and respiratory rates increase, and blood flow increases to organs that may need to take action: the heart and muscles. The pain is a warning to try to fix things: run away, eat, rest, remove your hand from the flame, or ice your inflamed ankle. Relaxation achieves the opposite physiologic actions from pain: heart and respiratory rates decrease, catecholamine levels decrease, and blood pressure decreases. The exciting thing about relaxation is that it is a learned behavior that can be achieved by an individual, and once achieved, even if only partially achieved, it produces the above physical effects. Researchers of pain and pain management have long noted that the actions of physical and mental relaxation, both alone and when combined with pharmacologic interventions, reduce pain and perception of pain [1–4].

The pain of labor serves a slightly different purpose. Unlike most other pain, normal labor pain is not a signal that something is wrong. Rather, it is a signal that something is about to happen, giving the laboring woman an opportunity to arrange herself, her surroundings, and her support person(s) to promote the safe birth of her infant. Additionally, labor pain is not continuous, as is the pain of injury, but comes and goes, often with pain-free intervals between contractions. Nevertheless, labor is perceived by most women as extremely painful, and often emotionally stressful as well, as a woman realizes that motherhood is no longer an aspect of her future but will be happening in a few hours. Can techniques that promote relaxation be expected to make a difference in the face of this acutely painful experience? Thankfully, the answer most researchers find is "Yes" [5,6]. On a practical note, women who use relaxation techniques to cope with labor will have varying degrees of success, as unique as the laboring woman herself.

Not only does relaxation help reduce a mother's experience of pain in labor; conversely, increased pain and tension might impede the progression of normal labor. Recall Dick-Read's "fear-tension-pain" cycle, a graphic but simple description used to promote his method of natural childbirth and that describes the physiologic effects of pain [7]. In his model, women without knowledge of the process of childbirth experienced fear when labor began, their fear manifested as increased tension, which in turn led to increased pain, in an ongoing cycle leading to more fear and ultimately more pain. Consider the corollary to the body's response to pain, with increased heart rate and respiratory rate, increased blood flow to the heart and muscles of action, and decreased blood flow to "nonessential" organs such as the uterus. Like any muscle, the uterus works best when well oxygenated! Normal labor progress can be thus be impeded by tension and pain [8].

But, one might ask, why bother with relaxation? Effective means of pharmacologic pain relief are at the ready for laboring women, including the use of the epidural, which often makes labor an almost pain-free experience. Interventions for relief of labor pain must be considered from the perspective of safety for both the mother and her fetus.

While intravenous medication and spinal or epidural anesthesia are used daily without complication, as health professionals we must remember that they are not risk free. We counsel women before administering medication or an epidural about the potential side effects and risks: respiratory depression in the newborn, dysfunctional labor pattern, urinary retention, infection [9–11]. By using relaxation techniques, many women are able to use safe, effective means of coping with labor pain without exposing themselves or their fetus to the potential risks and side effects of the use of pharmacologic interventions. If pharmacologic interventions are ultimately used, the dosage and time of exposure may be reduced.

Childbirth education

The application of relaxation techniques within the context of pregnancy and childbirth was first introduced in formal childbirth education classes in the 1960s. Women and their partners received instruction about birth, relaxation and breathing techniques, and labor support (coaching) in group classes outside of the hospital [12]. The significance of childbirth preparation extended further than the content of the classes: unmedicated childbirth gained more acceptance, the doors of the labor room were literally "opened" to those providing labor support, and relaxation techniques were introduced as a legitimate coping strategy for pain management. The breathing techniques used to support relaxation in labor represent one of the first mind-body therapies used within a health care setting. The partnership between the laboring woman and her "labor coach" also legitimized the labor support role, demonstrating that one-on-one support also promoted relaxation.

Promoting relaxation

Childbirth classes are an ideal venue for teaching pregnant women and their support person(s) many of the relaxation techniques that will be reviewed below. When women have attended classes, they often arrive in labor already using the techniques they have learned. However, many women do not attend childbirth classes, and furthermore, most care providers can recall examples of women who have gone to class but nevertheless present in labor despairing, "I forgot everything" or "That breathing stuff doesn't work!" Thus it is up to the innovative labor nurse, midwife, or physician to adapt these methods "on the fly" when a woman is in labor. Unfortunately, promoting relaxation cannot be done while completing an admission database or performing a history and physical and entering admission orders. It requires focused attention on the part of the provider and being with the laboring woman. The provider can assure the woman that she/he wants to help her and will do so as quickly as possible. A basic assessment of the current well-being of the mother and her fetus should be performed, and then, if all is well, the "paperwork" of her admission may be set aside to spend focused time with the mother and her partner. Try a relaxation technique for a contraction or two, perhaps beginning with progressive relaxation between contractions and continuing it through the contraction, moving on to other techniques as needed. When the woman responds to a relaxation practice, encourage her partner to continue where you left off, and then resume the paperwork between her contractions.

The use of language is so important in promoting relaxation, reducing fear, and promoting a feeling of safety in labor. Obstetrician and hypnotherapist Jacki Irland notes that all laboring women are in an altered state of consciousness similar to a hypnotic trace, and as such, their subconscious and conscious minds are hyperacute to the things providers say. By remaining calm, using supportive words, and assuring the woman that all is well, we can go a long way to promoting relaxation [13]. Consider these examples:

> Allyson arrives in labor, this is her first baby, and her cervix is 6cm dilated on admission. Her membranes are ruptured and she is having variable decelerations of varying depths with each contraction. Her provider might say, "You have to stay on the monitor, because the heart rate keeps dropping." On the other hand, the provider could tell her "Overall, your baby looks well on the monitor. Often, after the water breaks, we can see the heart rate go down during a contraction. Your baby's getting a really strong hug! This is common, but I will watch closely. I'm not worried now; I will tell you if I am."

> Latoya has been laboring normally with her third baby, and as she approaches full dilatation, her membranes rupture spontaneously with meconium-stained fluid. Her provider could tell her, "There's meconium in the fluid, the baby could breathe in that meconium and have complications." Alternatively, the provider could say, "The baby's had a bowel movement before birth. Did you know that's pretty common? Usually it doesn't mean anything, but we get to have another nurse at your birth because every once in awhile a baby can try to make a little mess with that poop!"

In each of the above examples, one can easily see that one approach can promote fear and anxiety for the laboring woman, while the other can promote a feeling of safety, even in the face of a complication. Even common expressions can inadvertently promote anxiety in laboring women. This author has been humbled by this realization more than once. Imagine my surprise at frightening a woman who had reached complete dilatation when I told her "Your cervix is all gone."

Women often labor with supportive (or sometimes not so supportive) family or friends present. Take a few moments, when introducing a relaxation technique, to show a woman's support people how they can help her to use a specific practice. While labor nurses, midwives, and physicians can provide the support, and often will if a woman's family does not seem able to help, getting her family involved helps to promote their relationship and bonds.

Music

Music researchers have measured the effects of music on the brain, the central nervous system, and vital signs and noted its powerful effect on emotions. This emotional effect is used by advertisers, film directors, and mothers of cranky children worldwide [14,15].

It should be noted, however, that while the childbirth literature has not consistently found music to be effective in specifically relieving labor pain, it has been found to promote relaxation [16–18]. Levitin devotes a chapter of his book to the processing of music by the brain, noting that music affects all areas of the brain, including the language centers in the frontal and temporal lobes, the cerebellum's "timing circuits," and the portions of the "reptilian brain" in the cerebellum and amygdala where we experience our emotional response to music. Music, and memories of music, and indeed of certain sounds, can produce a multitude of emotions [14,15].

However, using music to promote relaxation can be tricky, as musical tastes are unique and varied and not always what one might stereotypically expect from a given individual. The familiar music associated with a massage or a pedicure in a spa, while soft and soothing, is typically Euro-centric and might not be as appealing to women from other cultural backgrounds. One might even run the risk, if the wrong music is chosen, of promoting irritation instead of relaxation!

Short of loading an MP3 player with countless playlists of songs that might appeal to a woman, how can a busy labor nurse or care provider begin to incorporate the use of music? A small investment on the part of the provider or workplace in simple equipment, such as small speakers that could universally be connected to an iPod, other MP3 player, cell phone, tablet, or laptop, will provide the flexibility to use a music source provided by the birthing unit or a music source that the woman brings from home.

Start by purchasing recordings of relaxation music, loading them onto an iPod or other MP3 player, and then playing them on the speakers in the labor room. If you are feeling more creative, make your own playlist by thinking of music that makes you feel relaxed while listening. What qualities do you find in this music? Generally, this music will have a slower beat, perhaps being enjoyed "in the background" without paying particular attention to it. The selections might include rhythmic, percussive drumming. Try one of the free smart music streaming services, such as Pandora or Spotify, and choose an example song you find relaxing to seed a "channel." Take note of the songs and artists that the music streaming service plays for you. Particular selections you've discovered can be added to your "relaxation playlist" and shared with laboring women.

Another option would be to have your workplace invest in a few "tablet" computers. Again using a streaming service like Pandora or Spotify, personalize the music for each woman using a tablet; simply ask her what she would like to listen to and then seed a new personal "channel" for her based on her own tastes. If no other source of music is available, most hospitals do have a "relaxation channel" on their television service, with preprogrammed music and relaxing images.

Progressive relaxation

Progressive relaxation is a primary technique for relaxation, presented in numerous formats in childbirth class, in yoga classes, and taught by therapists. By focusing from head to toe on specifically relaxing each part of the body individually, using calm and even breathing throughout, a deep sense of relaxation can be achieved, with the associated physiologic benefits already described [8]. When the abdominal muscles, specifically, are relaxed, the sensation of pain from contractions can be reduced because the uterus is not contracting against already contracted abdominal muscles.

Women can use progressive relaxation techniques on their own by using self-talk. They could record a preprinted relaxation script and play the recording during pregnancy and labor. Purchasing numerous prerecorded scripts and listening to them in labor is another option. However, many women will present in labor without having prepared specific relaxation recordings. Fortunately, guiding someone through progressive relaxation is simple and can easily be done by any care provider.

Start by encouraging the woman to sit or lie in as comfortable a position as possible, with every part of her body supported by the surface on which she is sitting or lying. She should not have to support her own arms, legs, or head. No body part should rest on another, so if she is sitting, let her rest her arms on the arms of the chair and uncross her legs. If she is lying on her side, her top leg should not be resting on her bottom leg but rather flexed to the front and supported by pillows. Remind her that she may have a contraction during the relaxation technique, and that she should continue to try to maintain her slow steady breathing through the contraction. Try to gauge the frequency of her contractions, and plan a little relaxation exercise that can ideally be completed between contractions. Here is a sample that should fit in between even frequent contractions:

> "Breathe in slowly, breathe out slowly. Begin at the top of your head, and bring warmth and relaxation to those muscles. Soften the muscles of your forehead and face, let your jaw be loose. Let your shoulders slump and soften, let your arms soften; let even your fingers be loose and soft. Breathe deeply and let the muscles of your chest relax, breathe out slowly. Let your belly be loose. Picture your baby, warm and comfortable within. Breathe in, breathing warmth and relaxation to your hips, your thighs, and your legs. Breathe out, let even your feet and toes be soft and relaxed. Gently inhale and exhale, sweeping your body with your breath. Each time you exhale, sink further into this relaxed feeling."

When you have finished slowly completing the script, sit in silence with her. Soon, a contraction will start. Recognize this, and softly continue the relaxation exercise:

> "Your contraction is beginning. Let your uterus do its work. Continue to inhale, and exhale. Your hands stay loose and soft, your face stays loose and soft, your belly muscles above the uterus stay loose and soft. Inhale and exhale. Your hands stay soft, your shoulders stay soft. Inhale and exhale. Soft hands, soft shoulders, soft belly. Your contraction is halfway over; you're on the down side now. Soft hands, soft belly. Inhale and exhale. Almost done. Soft face, soft shoulders, everything loose. You are doing fine."

Take special note when the contraction is over. Many women will increase their breathing rate during a contraction and unintentionally continue to breathe more forcefully after the contraction stops. If this happens, cue the woman to take a breath and hold it for a moment. Then cue her to exhale fully and completely relax when she does so. The exact wording in progressive relaxation is not important. Just start somewhere, use a soft and soothing tone, and watch for signs of tension that may creep back in, and with your voice, encourage relaxation of those muscles.

Breathing techniques

The use of breathing techniques in labor was formerly a hallmark of the Lamaze method [19]. Using patterned breathing can directly promote a semi-hypnotic state, improve relaxation, and may additionally serve as a means of distraction from the sensation of pain during contractions. By practicing breathing techniques ahead of labor, breathing can become an automatic response to pain, and relaxation can be triggered as a conditioned response to breathing. However, patterned breathing, like progressive relaxation, can also be taught during labor [20–22]. One disadvantage of patterned breathing is that, if applied with enthusiasm or not modified between contractions, hyperventilation with associated symptoms of tingling fingers or lips can occur.

The original implementation of patterned breathing advocated different types of breathing for the various stages of labor; however, any breathing pattern that is helping a woman gain relaxation and cope with contractions may be used.

Slow deep breathing is just as implied and was traditionally recommended for the beginning stages of labor. Using this breathing pattern, a woman inhales slowly at the start of a contraction and relaxes completely as she lets that breath go. She repeats slowly inhaling and exhaling for the length of the contraction, focusing on relaxation with each exhalation. She may vocalize with the exhalation, focusing on low deep sounds such as "ohhh" or "haahhh."

Light accelerated breathing was traditionally recommended as labor progressed. Using this breathing pattern, each contraction begins with a slow deep breath and a slow exhalation focusing on relaxation. Through the contraction, however, the breath is light and shallow, becoming faster as the contraction intensifies, peaking at a rate of perhaps one breath per second, and then becoming slower again as the contraction subsides, and ending with a slow deep breath and slow exhalation.

Transition breathing is a form of light accelerated breathing, but periodically the light breaths are interspersed with a breath with more forceful exhalation. Several light breaths are taken in a row, with the mother making a sound such as "hee" with each exhalation. After three or four light breaths, she takes a fuller breath with a slower exhalation, making a different and more forceful sound, such as "hoo." This pattern of breathing may be used when more distraction from the pain of labor might be useful, and it can be used to avoid breath holding and spontaneous pushing prior to complete dilation. Like the preceding breath patterns, this pattern begins and ends with a slow deep inhalation and exhalation.

Imagery

Imagery uses the ability of the mind to pretend and remember and promotes relaxation by creating a specific scene with a positive relaxing association in one's mind. It is almost always used in conjunction with progressive relaxation [23]. Like progressive relaxation, sample guided imagery exercises are numerous in childbirth preparation materials. A few to consider investigating are *The Childbirth Kit*, which comes complete with preprinted glossy photos of relaxing images with scripts for each one [24], or *Easing Labor Pain* [25]: Alternatively, a personal imagery can be created as follows.

> After using a progressive relaxation exercise with a woman, as she has entered a relaxed state, ask her to imagine herself in a special place, either a place she has been before or a place that she images, where she feels relaxed and safe. Ask her to tell you about the place that she has imagined. Help her to take the image further, by fleshing out the details in her image. Try to involve each of her senses: sight, touch, sound, and smell. If she has described, for example, her cozy bed at home, ask her to feel the softness of her pillow supporting her head, to take in the color of her comforter, and to feel how warm it makes her muscles. Have her picture the cherished items on her nightstand or dresser that she has kept as a memento of a loved one or a special event. Ask her to imagine the sounds she might hear in her room: the hum of the furnace fan in the background, the sound of a squirrel running along the roof, her family's voices in the next room. Ask her to bring to mind soothing odors that she might notice in her room, a cup of tea on the nightstand, breakfast being prepared in the kitchen, the clean smell of her freshly shampooed hair, or her partner's aftershave on his pillow. Have her imagine the room in daylight, and then talk her through a transition to a gentle, cleansing rain that she can watch through her window while staying warm and cozy inside.

Other more specific shorter imageries could also be used during the course of a contraction. A woman could be asked to imagine the colors of a rainbow, one by one, filling her mind, each for a few seconds. She could be asked to imagine herself floating securely in warm water and to imagine that she is riding up a gentle wave as a contraction builds, then riding down safely to float again as the contraction subsides. She could imagine being outdoors on a hot day and feeling a refreshing cool breeze as each contraction begins, buffeting her gently during the contraction and subsiding as the contraction is over. There is, literally, no end to the imagination.

Heat and cold

The use of heat or cold therapy has not been studied as a method of promoting relaxation but instead has been examined as a means of pain relief [26]. The use of heat increases blood flow to muscles, can relieve muscle spasms, and can promote relaxation [27]. Heat and cold applications also provide an alternative sensory experience that competes with the experience of pain [28]. Heat can be provided by warmed blankets, rice packs, or specifically designed electric or quick-heating chemical packs. Institutions generally have specific approved heat therapy guidelines, which may or may not include the warming of rice packs in a microwave. Cold can be provided by washcloths dipped into a basin of ice water, quick-cool chemical packs, or fans. The long-time practice of using a hot wet towel wrapped in a chux and heated in a microwave has contributed to patient burns and should not be used. Additionally, hot or cold applications should be avoided on body parts that may have decreased sensation after an epidural, to avoid inadvertent burning or freezing injuries.

The area of heat or cold application could include the whole body, by use of warm blankets or a fan, or involve a specific body area or areas, such as warm packs on the low abdomen, back, or perineum or cold applications to the face or neck during second stage labor [27].

Physical positioning

Imagine trying to become relaxed or maintain a relaxed state while in an uncomfortable physical position. When choosing positions to promote relaxation in labor, particular emphasis should be placed on encouraging positions that promote the progress of normal labor and avoiding positions that can deter normal labor. Specific positions that have been studied include the use of the Sims position, sitting, and squatting [16,29,30], and most nurses, midwives, and physicians use a variety of positions to promote relaxation and help women cope with pain in labor. When laboring women are encouraged to find their own position of comfort, most choose upright positions in early labor and lie down as labor progresses. These positions change the relationship between a woman's pelvis, her fetus, and gravity [28]. Other positions that may be encouraged include a hands and knees position, lunging, forward leaning on a bed or ball, dangling with support of another person, or squatting [29]. Conversely, the supine and low Fowler's position often adopted by laboring women because they find movement challenging, and by medical personnel because of ease in fetal monitoring, can increase sensations of pain, decrease relaxation, and slow the progress of labor, because compression of the vena cava decreases oxygenation of the uterine muscle and can lead to fetal compromise. These positions should be avoided [8]. Even when fetal monitoring is necessary, or a woman is confined to bed because of pregnancy complications or anesthesia use, side lying or Sims positions are preferred [27,30].

Fetuses in the posterior position or a malpositioned fetal head can cause increased back pain during labor. A forward-leaning position is a time-honored choice to promote comfort and relaxation, relieve pain, and encourage repositioning of the fetus. A woman can be supported in a forward-leaning position by sitting on a physical therapy ball and leaning forward onto a bed, by kneeling on the bed facing and leaning forward onto the raised head of the bed, by resting on her knees and elbows, or, if standing, by leaning forward on a countertop, a wall, or her partner. Although not particularly relaxing, lunging can also be tried, either during or between contractions. If a woman has difficulty lunging on a flat surface, go with her to the stairwell and try going up stairs, two at a time [27]. Combining positioning with heat or cold can provide additional pain relief.

After a period of activity or frequent position changes in labor, women sometimes need to be reminded to take a break for restoration of their energy. Promoting labor progress means that activity should be balanced with rest; and positions that encourage relaxation are those that simply require the woman to do nothing, such as lying down or resting in a rocker.

Hydrotherapy

The use of water and water immersion to promote relaxation has been increasingly reported [31–33] in the literature (refer to chapter 9). However, full immersion in water may not be possible in many labor units. Simple hydrotherapy options can be adopted for use when a tub is not available at the facility or not available to the woman because of labor complications. A woman can find relaxation in the shower, even if telemetry monitoring is being used, particularly if she is provided with a stool or physical therapy ball to sit on while in the shower. Water can be directed onto her back or her abdomen, whichever she finds more soothing. If a woman is confined to bed, a footbath could be prepared, including the use of essential oils noted for relaxation (refer to chapter 10). During second stage labor and as the baby is crowning, many women find the application of warm wet compresses soothing and to promote relaxation of the perineum.

Miscellaneous relaxation aides

Consider the environment in the labor room. While most facilities don't have the financial resources to Feng Shui their patient rooms, relaxation can be promoted by dimming the lighting, maintaining a comfortable temperature, and decreasing noise and distractions [27]. Try to keep the room uncluttered, removing unnecessary equipment, closing cabinet doors. Remove malodorous items from the room promptly [34]. Remind or assist women in maintaining physical hygiene; remove drying mucous or blood from her skin, bring her a toothbrush, help her wash her face if she has been perspiring, or tie back her hair if she is warm.

Pay attention to the effect that the woman's support person(s) can have on her ability to relax. If several visitors are talking animatedly amongst themselves or watching television loudly but not helping the laboring woman, talk to them and engage them in activities that support rather than detract from relaxation. Suggest they try a back or foot massage or teach them to talk their laboring woman through a mental imagery.

When women are facing complications that might require frequent blood pressure monitoring, continuous fetal monitoring, intravenous lines and pumps, or epidural lines and pumps, consider the effects of these activity-restricting interventions on a woman's ability to relax. Ask her if she would find it more relaxing to leave the blood pressure cuff in place so that you don't have to disturb her, or to have you place it each time the blood pressure needs to be taken. Demonstrate to her how to move and find comfortable positions despite IV lines and pumps and reinforce the importance of doing so. Use pillows liberally if she is confined to bed to fully support her abdomen, back, and extremities [30].

Emotional relaxation

While the primary focus in this chapter has been on physical relaxation for a laboring woman, the provider should never lose sight of the importance of a woman's emotions on the progress of her labor [35]. Sometimes a woman is able to voice negative emotions such as fear, distrust, or memories of previous painful events during her labor, but often she is unable to find words to express these feelings. Use your judgment. It may be helpful for her to express negative emotions if she is able, and if you can just listen without judgment or a need to "fix" the problem she describes. However, labor is generally not a time to uncover long buried fears and emotions, so don't push if she cannot readily identify why she feels distress. Instead, the relaxation techniques presented above can also be used to facilitate emotional relaxation and a sense of calm. This may be particularly true with the use of imagery. When using hypnosis, for example, hypnotherapists rely on the use of words to create imagery and the subconscious mind's inability to separate imagery from reality, and take advantage of the calm, relaxing, safe feelings evoked in imagery to promote relaxation [36].

Mindfulness in relaxation

Mindfulness has been described as "remember[ing] to pay attention to what is occurring in one's immediate experience with care and discernment" [37]. To provide a simple example, consider the difference one might experience in eating slowly, carefully considering the taste, texture, and quality of each mouthful of food in a meal, as opposed to eating quickly on the way out the door. This same attention may be paid to the practice of relaxation. Mindfulness-based yoga and other relaxation practices have been associated with improved psychological and physical well-being among pregnant women [38]. Yet proficiency with mindfulness can take time to acquire, and might not be achievable for the first time during labor. Care providers who see women prenatally may lay the groundwork for a woman's practice of relaxation by suggesting mindfulness-based workshops, reading materials, or yoga classes.

Additionally, labor nurses, midwives, and physicians can also recognize that many aspects of our work with pregnant and birthing women are stressful. As we tell our postpartum mothers, to be able to care for their children they must first care for themselves. Developing a personal practice of stress reduction and relaxation is a benefit both for the care provider and ultimately to those for whom we provide care.

Summary

Relaxation can be key in promoting the normal progression of labor by enhancing a woman's ability to cope with pain, maintaining her mobility, and can assist in decreasing the use or length of use of interventions that can impede labor progress. A variety of relaxation techniques and practical suggestions for implementation have been presented here, and the reader is also referred to chapters 8 through 11 for additional techniques to promote relaxation and coping in labor.

References

1. Carroll D, Seers K. (1998). Relaxation for the relief of chronic pain: A systematic review. *Journal of Advanced Nursing, 27*(3), 476–487.
2. Good M. (1996). Effects of relaxation and music on postoperative pain: A review. *Journal of Advanced Nursing, 24*(5), 905–914.
3. Good M, Anderson GC, et al. (2002). Relaxation and music reduce pain after gynecologic surgery. *Pain Management Nursing, 3*(2): 61–70.
4. Mandle CL, Jacobs SC, et al. (1996). The efficacy of relaxation response interventions with adult patients: A review of the literature. *Journal of Cardiovascular Nursing, 10*(3): 4–26.
5. Brown ST, Douglas C, et al. (2001). Women's evaluation of intrapartum nonpharmacological pain relief methods used during labor. *Journal of Perinatal Education, 10*(3), 1–8.
6. Smith CA, Levett KM, et al. (2011). Relaxation techniques for pain management in labour. *Cochrane Database of Systematic Reviews, 7*(12): CD009514.
7. Dick-Read G. (1942). *Childbirth without fear.* London: Heinemann Medical Books.
8. Simkin P & Ancheta R. (2011). *The labor progress handbook*, 3rd ed. Oxford: Wiley-Blackwell.

9. Salim R, Nachum, Z, et al. (2005). Continuous compared with intermittent epidural infusion on progress of labor and patient satisfaction. *Obstetrics & Gynecology, 106*, 301–306.
10. Thorp JA, Hu DH, et al. (1993). The effect of intrapartum epidural analgesia on nulliparous labor: A randomized, controlled, prospective trial. *American Journal of Obstetrics & Gynecology, 169*(4), 851–858.
11. Wong CA, Scavone BM, et al. (2005). The risk of cesarean delivery with neuraxial analgesia given early versus late in labor. *New England Journal of Medicine, 352*, 655–665.
12. Romano A & Lothian J. (2008). Promoting, protecting, and supporting normal birth: A look at the evidence. *JOGNN, 37*, 94–105.
13. Irland J. Personal communication, April 2011.
14. Levitin DJ. (2006). *This is your brain on music.* New York: Plume.
15. Sacks O. (2007). *Musicophilia: Tales of music and the brain.* New York: Random House.
16. Simkin P & Bolding A. (2004). Update on nonpharmacologic approaches to relieve labor pain and prevent suffering. *Journal of Midwifery & Womens Health, 49*(6), 489–504.
17. Phumdoung S & Good M. (2003). Music reduces sensation and distress of labor pain. *Pain Management Nursing, 4*, 54–61.
18. Durham L & Collins M. (1986). The effect of music as a conditioning aid in prepared childbirth education. *JOGNN, 15*, 268–270.
19. Savage B. (1987). *Preparation for birth: The complete guide to the Lamaze method.* New York: Ballantine Books.
20. Simkin P. (2008). *The birth partner*, 3rd ed. Boston: Harvard Common Press.
21. Simkin P, et al. (2010). *Pregnancy, childbirth and the newborn: The Complete Guide.* New York: Simon & Schuster.
22. England P & Horowitz R. (1998). *Birthing from within.* Albuquerque: Partera Press.
23. Eller LS. (1999). Guided imagery interventions for symptom management. *Annual Review of Nursing Research, 17*, 57–84.
24. Hale MF & Chalmers L. (1994). *The childbirth kit: Ideas and images to help you through labor.* Redmond, WA: Swanstone Press.
25. Lieberman AB. (1992). *Easing labor pain.* Boston: Harvard Common Press.
26. Fahima F, Behmanesh F, et al. (2011). Effect of heat therapy on pain severity in primigravida women. *Iranian Journal of Nursing and Midwifery Research, 16*(1), 113–116.
27. Adams ED & Bianchi AL. (2008). A practical approach to labor support. *JOGNN, 37*(1), 106–115.
28. Enkin M, Keirse MJNC, et al. (2000). A guide to effective care in pregnancy and childbirth, 3rd ed. New York: Oxford University Press.
29. Mayberry LJ, Wood SH, et al. (2002). Managing second-stage labor: Exploring the variables during the second stage. *Lifelines, 3*, 28–34.
30. Gilder K, Mayberry LJ, et al. (2002). Maternal positioning in labor with epidural analgesia: Results from a multi-site survey. *Lifelines, 6*, 41–45.
31. Cluett ER & Burns E. (2009). Immersion in water in labour and birth. *Cochrane Database of Systematic Reviews, 15*(2): CD000111.
32. Geissbuhler V & Eberhard J. (2000). Waterbirths: A comparative study. A prospective study on more than 2,000 waterbirths. *Fetal Diagnosis & Therapy, 15*(5), 291–300.
33. Geissbuehler V, Stein S, et al. (2004). Waterbirths compared with landbirths: An observational study of nine years. *Journal of Perinatal Medicine, 32*(4), 308–314.
34. University of Minnesota and the Life Science Foundation. (2011). Healing environment. http://www.takingcharge.csh.umn.edu/explore-healing-practices/healing-environment. Accessed December 1, 2011.

35. Sauls D. (2006). Dimensions of professional labor support for intrapartum practice. *Journal of Nursing Scholarship, 38*(1), 36–41.
36. James U. (2009). Practical uses of clinical hypnosis in enhancing fertility, healthy pregnancy and childbirth. *Complementary Therapies in Clinical Practice, 15*(4), 239–241.
37. Black D. (2011). A brief definition of mindfulness. Mindfulness Research Guide, www.mindfulnessexperience.org.
38. Beddoe A, Yang C, et al. (2009). The effects of mindfulness-based yoga during pregnancy on maternal psychological and physical distress. *JOGNN, 38*, 310–319.

Chapter 8

Touch therapies in pregnancy and childbirth

Deborah Ringdahl

Key points

- Simple touch therapy techniques should be taught to those providing pregnancy and labor support, including partners, friends, and family members, in conjunction with prenatal care, childbirth classes, and labor and birth. A group model of prenatal care would be a good learning environment for teaching these skills.
- Educational programs on Therapeutic Touch, Healing Touch, Reiki, and simple massage and touch techniques should be provided for staff and providers working in maternity care in a variety of settings.
- Nursing, midwifery, and physician educational programs should include a theoretical and clinical component that integrates intentional touch in to clinical practice.
- Intentional touch should be considered as the first response to pain and anxiety during childbirth, and specific touch therapies should be incorporated into labor management by nurses and birth attendants.
- Continous labor support should be offered through nursing care, doulas, birth attendants, and other members of the labor support team, incorporating a variety of hands-on techniques and touch therapies with the intention of reducing pain and anxiety and providing comfort and mind-body-spirit support during childbirth.
- The principles of energetic exchange should be considered when providing clinical care. This includes the role of self-care in managing chronic stress and fatigue.
- New models of tertiary and ambulatory health care delivery should be developed that provide access to services that support stress reduction and relaxation techniques, including massage therapy and energy touch therapies.

Touch has memory.

John Keats

Introduction

Long before Ashley Montagu's [1] groundbreaking work on the value of touch, physical touch was used to convey caring, provide comfort, relieve pain, and show support. From birth through death, suffering and pain have been relieved by reaching out with touch to

---

Supporting a Physiologic Approach to Pregnancy and Birth: A Practical Guide, First Edition.
Edited by Melissa D. Avery.
© 2013 John Wiley & Sons, Inc. Published 2013 by John Wiley & Sons, Inc.

connect to the heart and spirit of those in need. The caring and comfort delivered through physical touch is closely tied to the role of healer: throughout history and within many cultures, the laying on of hands has represented the work of both spiritual and professional healers [2]. In the home and in the hospital, hands-on care remains the vehicle for care-giving. Many "old" nursing skills such as giving bed baths and back rubs have provided avenues for human connection, comfort, and support [3]. Within the context of childbirth, the hands of those attending birth represent both skill and compassion, assessing labor progress while supporting the needs of the laboring woman. This chapter will focus on the role that intentional touch therapies play in supporting women through pregnancy, childbirth, and postpartum, including learned labor support techniques, massage therapy, and the energy therapies of Therapeutic Touch, Healing Touch, and Reiki. With the advent of increased awareness of integrative modalities and research to support integrative therapy use, all touch therapies can be reexamined within the context of clinical practice.

The role of touch in contemporary health care

Leder and Krucoff explored the role of touch in contemporary medical practice, noting that allopathic medicine has focused primarily on disease treatment through scientific theories and knowledge, contributing to the prevalence of "objective touch" and "absent touch" [2, p. 322]. Objective data collected through the physical exam and techno-logically mediated diagnostic and treatment modalities reduces the likelihood of experiencing the care, comfort, and compassion that accompanies Healing Touch. The healing properties of touch are described in the context of both complementary and alternative modalities and conventional medical practices, with strong support for using the clinical encounter as an avenue for reaffirming the connection between self and other, body, and world. "Even taking a pulse with care and sensitivity becomes part of an ongoing dialogue between healer and patient, capable of altering the bodily states being examined" [2, p. 325]. Nursing scholarship suggests that the role of healer exists in the creation of a healing environment, which occurs through the intention of the health care provider: "We can become midwives to this process of healing, creating and being safe, sacred space into which the healing might emerge. We can, literally, become the healing environment" [4, p. 28]. The use of intentional touch becomes a part of the energetic exchange of those engaged in healing work.

An ongoing challenge in health care today is to retain a "high touch" practice model in a "high tech" practice environment. A 1978 publication on the doctor-patient relationship discussed the importance of touching in "the context of changing medical technology" [5, p. 1469]. Thirty-five years later, clinical encounters are increasingly impacted by reduced time with health care providers, greater use of nontouch diagnostic testing, and fragmentation in the delivery of care. Prenatal visits are shorter, screening and diagnostic testing has increased, and fewer consumers are attending childbirth education classes. Technology continues to play a prominent role in childbirth, with labor sitting and hands-on labor support replaced by epidural use and centralized monitors. Increasingly, doulas are used to provide labor support while nurses manage medication, vital signs, and technology.

A 2009 Institute of Medicine (IOM) Summit on Integrative Medicine and the Health of the Public identified several aspects of clinical care that have been found to enhance the quality of care and favorably impact outcomes. Of great significance was the finding that one aspect of clinical practice enhanced care and improved outcomes with grade A evidence: empathy and compassion [6]. These findings provide strong support for the value of relationship development, therapeutic presence, and a humanistic approach to health care delivery. Although this evidence is not specific to physical touch, touch serves as an avenue for connection that often transcends traditional barriers and promotes positive relationships. In a study undertaken to measure the psychophysiologic effects of the nonverbal communication of compassion, loving kindness meditation and touch were associated with decreased stress and increased relaxation and peacefulness [7]. The authors concluded, "Extending compassion is not only good care; it also may be good medicine" [7, p. 1].

A variety of touch therapies have been introduced into clinical care over the past several decades, representing a renewed interest in the therapeutic use of intentional touch in clinical practice. Massage therapy, Therapeutic Touch (TT), Healing Touch (HT), and Reiki are all touch therapies that are used to support the healing process. The common thread that exists among these modalities lies in their capacity to reduce stress, promote relaxation, and mitigate pain. In addition to traditional hands-on labor support techniques, these touch therapies provide another vehicle for supporting women through childbirth, enhancing the subjective experience of support, comfort, and caring that represents a humanistic approach to health care delivery.

The role of touch in midwifery, nursing, and medicine

The profession of midwifery has evolved into a clinical specialty that supports scholarship and evidence-based practice but remains grounded in the belief that high-quality care requires human presence, understanding the mind, body, spirit connection, and attention to individual needs. *Varney's Midwifery*, the primary textbook used in midwifery education, contains sections on supportive care during labor, including comfort measures such as positioning changes, relaxation exercises, breathing exercises, and hands-on care such as back rub, abdominal rub, efflueruage, and use of physical touch "to convey caring, comfort, and understanding" [8, p. 789]. Further discussion addresses the importance of individualizing care and considering both midwife and client comfort with touch. Varney also describes the presence of significant others in providing support and comfort, drawing attention to the midwife's role in guiding activities that promote comfort and support.

The Philosophy of the American College of Nurse-Midwives identifies core values of practice, including "therapeutic use of presence" and "watchful waiting and nonintervention in normal processes" [9]. These values also represent competencies that exist as hallmarks of Midwifery, and their practice co-exists as a professional responsibility of midwifery [10]. The ACNM position statement on Appropriate Use of Technology in Childbirth [11] identifies "supportive interventions" as enhancing the normal processes of pregnancy and childbirth. The Cochrane review identifies that therapeutic use of presence and touch during childbirth is associated with reduced interventions and greater satisfaction with the birth experience [12].

Therapies involving touch are particularly congruent with nursing practice: the hands-on work of nursing care provides a natural avenue for touch therapies. Nurses are in a unique position to implement touch therapies in health care settings, as they represent the greatest number of health care professionals, have knowledge of both health and illness, serve as client advocates, and are trusted by consumers [13]. Touch is recognized in the Nursing Interventions Classification Code as a nursing function [14]. The nursing profession has also developed expertise in complementary therapies that promote comfort and reduce pain; Therapeutic Touch and Healing Touch were developed and researched by nurses, and much of the early research on complementary therapies was conducted by nurses [15]. Relief of symptoms such as pain, sleep disturbances, nausea, and anxiety is provided by nurses using a variety of nursing interventions, including music, relaxation techniques, acupressure, massage, and energy touch therapies [16].

During the 1990s, the term "integrative medicine" was coined to better represent the integration of complementary and alternative medicine practices with conventional therapies. Instead of separating out complementary and alternative medicine (CAM) therapies as exclusive avenues to nutritional health, well-being, mind-body connection, and spirituality, it was recognized that supporting optimal health at all levels should be the primary goal for all health providers [17]. Rather than a new specialty area, integrative medicine is an approach to health care delivery that can be incorporated into all areas of medicine: "It provides care that is patient centered, healing oriented, emphasizes therapeutic relationship, and uses therapeutic approaches originating from conventional and alternative medicine" [18]. The principles of integrative medicine provide the foundation for future models of care that incorporate all health-driven modalities, including touch therapies, into primary care, women's health care, and childbirth.

Touch as metaphor for caring: Jean Watson's science of caring

The metaphor of touch easily translates into a care paradigm that illustrates the role of caregiver as an instrument of healing. The hands of the nurse-midwife-physician carry the intention of healing and a caring presence. Jean Watson's theory of caring provides a sound theoretical framework for understanding the caring dimension of hands-on care and the use of touch therapies in providing direct care to women. Watson's ten carative factors represent the framework used by nurses in the delivery of health care that promote integration of mind, body, and spirit [19]. Research suggests that recipients of touch therapies frequently experience an integration of mind, body, and spirit that promotes feelings of well-being [20].

Watson's conceptualization of the reciprocal nature of caring describes a dynamic process that affects both the giver and receiver (patient and clinician). The caring occasion represents a concrete interaction that has a qualitative caring component that results in the experience of mutuality, or transpersonal caring: "The moment has a field of its own that is greater than the occasion itself" [19, p. 5]. Studies on TT, HT, and Reiki suggest that the experience of receiving touch may be similar to the experience of a caring moment and transpersonal caring. For example, researchers exploring the subjective experience of a Reiki session found that recipients of Reiki felt protected, safe, and perceived a positive relationship with the Reiki practitioner [20]. According to Brathovde, "The intentional, compassionate, and restorative touch provided by the Reiki experience affects both practitioner and recipient, and exemplifies what Watson describes as transpersonal caring" [21, p. 97]. Transpersonal caring has the potential for positively impacting both the giver and the receiver.

Use of touch therapies in promoting relaxation and reducing stress and pain

Stress response and relaxation response

When the mind and body experience stress, activation of the hypothalamus results in stimulation of the involuntary (sympathetic) nervous system, increasing the release of adrenaline and noradrenaline, causing an increase in blood pressure, heart rate, respiration, blood flow to the muscles, and metabolism, preparing the body for "flight or fight" [22,23]. This stress, triggered by physical danger, fear, anxiety, has the potential for slowing down labor progress [24]. The relaxation response [22] is the physiologic counterpart to the stress response, resulting in lowered blood pressure, heart rate, respiration, and muscle tension. In many ways, activities that invoke this response serve as an antidote to stress. According to Benson [22], the relaxation response existed in the context of Eastern religious teachings but has more recently been appreciated within meditation, biofeedback, hypnosis, progressive relaxation, and yoga breathing practices. In addition to physiologic changes associated with the relaxation response, an altered state of consciousness emerges, accompanied by feelings of well-being and calm, which can also influence the experience of pain. These subjective feelings have been associated with many practices that elicit the relaxation response, including touch therapies.

Prolonged activation of the stress response has been implicated in the development of many chronic health problems. In the past several decades, a multitude of mind-body therapies have been studied within the context of stress reduction and relaxation for purposes of managing and/or preventing chronic health problems, such as hypertension [25], depression [26], dysmenorrhea [27], anxiety disorders [28], menopausal symptoms [29], epilepsy [30], schizophrenia [31], asthma [32], atopic eczema [33], irritable bowel syndrome [34], and chronic low back pain [35]. These Cochrane reviews provide some evidence that relaxation techniques (primarily progressive relaxation, relaxation tapes, and meditation) impact the ability to cope with chronic low back, menstrual, and gastrointestinal pain, manage anxiety and other mood difficulties related to schizophrenia and epilepsy, and reduce hot flashes and eczema. Additionally, relaxation techniques have been found to reduce the pain of labor [36] and the number of unnecessary cesarean sections [37] and to increase milk volume for lactating women [38].

The role of touch therapies in relaxation

An enlarging body of literature supports the use of touch therapies as stress reduction and relaxation techniques. The majority of studies focus on specific touch modalities, but there is also evidence that intentional tactile touch intervention reduces stress indicators [39]. In a recent review on the effects of back and hand massage on relaxation in older people, statistically significant improvements on physiologic or psychologic indicators of relaxation were found in all studies using slow-stroke back massage and hand massage [40]. An examination of physiologic responses to touch therapy in healthy volunteers showed that 5 minutes of touch massage resulted in decreased sympathetic nervous activity [41]. Researchers investigating the effect of gentle touch on people with mental health disorders or psychological stress found reduction in stress, anxiety, and depression and increases in relaxation and ability to cope [42]. Research studies on Reiki [20,43–59], Healing Touch [43,47,60–74], and Therapeutic Touch [43,47,52,75–87] demonstrate physiologic and psychologic evidence of stress reduction following use of these therapies. To date, the strongest support for the measurable physiologic effect of Reiki was demonstrated in an animal model [88,89].

Pregnancy and stress

Pregnancy represents a period of tremendous physiologic and psychologic adaptation, including hormonal changes, increased nutritional demands, and fears and anxiety related to pregnancy and the uncertainties of childbirth. In fact, an increase in adrenalin and cortisol may serve a protective function by enabling the mother to better cope with the stress and physical changes that accompany pregnancy [23]. Conversely, common discomforts of pregnancy such as first trimester nausea, heartburn, back pain, and fatigue can interfere with daily functioning and contribute to increased stress levels. Many adverse pregnancy outcomes are associated with maladaptive coping mechanisms, such as smoking and alcohol and drug use. Little real attention has been directed toward researching the "normal" stresses associated with pregnancy, although there is considerable research addressing the role of stress in health and illness [90]. The psychological and physical stresses of pregnancy associated with low socioeconomic status, low weight gain, pre-existing health problems, and depression have been correlated with adverse perinatal outcomes such as preterm birth and low birth weight infants [91].

The use of CAM therapies during pregnancy to relieve stress and/or manage the common discomforts of pregnancy is increasing in popularity, in part due to the noninvasive nature of many of these modalities and awareness of the body-mind-spirit connection in health. Therapies that contribute to a relaxation response have the potential for enhancing overall well-being as well as reducing the physiologic effects of chronic stress [23]. Field [92] cited three studies that demonstrated positive outcomes when massage therapy was used during pregnancy: a reduction in pain, anxiety, depression, and leg and back pain and a lower rate of prematurity [93–95].

The causal mechanism for touch therapies in reducing stress, inducing a state of relaxation, and reducing pain has not been established. Little research has been conducted on determining the potential underlying mechanisms for those modalities that elicit a relaxation response [92]. Some authors believe that the reduction in pain associated with massage can be explained through the gate control theory [96–98]. Tactile stimulation may also increase vagal activity, which lowers physiologic arousal and cortisol levels [49,92,96]. There is insufficient evidence to support cortisol reduction as the causal mechanism in the beneficial effects of massage, including a reduction in anxiety, depression, and pain [99]. Kerr, Wasserman, and Moore theorize that sensory reorganization is the mechanism for pain and stress reduction that occurs with touch healing therapies [100].

Labor support techniques

Many hands-on strategies and techniques for labor support have been introduced by authors and practitioners committed to providing low interventive approaches to pregnancy and childbirth. Penny Simkin, a physical therapist specializing in childbirth education and labor support since 1968, is well known for her expertise on comfort measures for childbirth and strategies to support labor progress and the prevention of dystocia. She co-authored *The Labor Progress Handbook* [24], which has been used as a comprehensive educational guide for supporting normal labor progress through nonpharmocological interventions. Included in this handbook is a description of physical comfort measures that are intended to reduce stress and the likelihood of a "labor-slowing fight-or-flight response" [24, p. 33], as well as position changes that promote pelvic mobility. Simkin also describes a variety of hands-on techniques for reducing back pain, including counterpressure, pelvic press, and double hip squeeze. A section on touch and massage also describes and illustrates several techniques useful for enhancing relaxation and relieving pain during labor by focusing on the shoulders, back, hands, or feet [24]. Simkin's "Comfort in Labor" handout describes and illustrates many of these basic techniques [98].

Overview of touch therapies

The National Center for Complementary and Alternative Medicine (NCCAM) defines complementary and alternative medicine as "a group of diverse medical and health care systems, practices, and products that are not presently considered to be part of conventional medicine" [101]. Some of these practices are used in conjunction with conventional medicine and some as an alternative. CAM taxonomy has been used as a way of unifying many unconventional approaches to health care, but there are many differences among CAM practitioners, including educational preparation, state licensure, and national practice standards. Most CAM providers that receive third-party reimbursement have achieved state licensure in their area of specialty, such as chiropractors, naturopathic physicians, acupuncturists, and massage therapists [102]. Some CAM therapies, such as energy touch therapies and aromatherapy, are considered to be within the scope of nursing practice and can be used in conjunction with routine nursing cares [103].

According to the 2010 Complementary and Alternative Medicine Survey of Hospitals [104], 42% of hospitals reported offering one or more CAM therapies, with "patient demand" given as the primary rationale (85%), followed by "clinically effective" (70%). Massage therapy is the top CAM therapy offered in outpatient settings (64%), and second most commonly offered CAM therapy in inpatient settings (44%) (pet therapy ranks first at 51%). Reiki and Therapeutic Touch were offered in 21% of inpatient settings surveyed [104].

Massage therapy

Massage therapy falls within the NCCAM's manipulative and body-based category. It is defined as "the application of manual techniques and adjunctive therapies with the intention of positively affecting the health and well-being of the client" (see Table 8.1) [105]. A variety of styles and techniques accompany massage practice, some that are used primarily for relaxation and others with a clinical focus [106]. Specific massage

Table 8.1 Touch therapies.

Modality	Definition	Origins and training	Professional organization
Therapeutic Touch	A contemporary healing modality drawn from ancient healing practices used to balance and promote the flow of human energy (therapeutictouch.org)	Dora Kunz (intuitive healer) and Dr. Dolores Krieger (RN), 1970 Standardized techniques 3 levels*	Nurse Healers— Professional Associates International Certification
Healing Touch	Use of gentle touch and energy-based techniques to influence and support the human energy system within the body (energy centers) and surrounding the body (energy fields) (Healing Touch International)	Janet Mentgen (RN), 1980 6 levels International certification*	Healing Touch International and Healing Touch Program Certification
Reiki	A Japanese word that means "universal life force energy," Reiki is a hands-on spiritual, vibrational healing practice used to promote balance throughout the human system [182]	Japanese, 1830s, introduced in United States early 1970s 3 levels No uniform teaching standards*	International Center for Reiki Training and other Reiki organizations offer classes No standard certification
Massage Therapy	The application of manual techniques and adjunctive therapies with the intention of positively affecting the health and well-being of the client (American Massage Therapy Association)	Professional schools with licensure Variety of styles and techniques Relaxation and clinical	American Massage Therapy Association State licensing, certification through National Certification Board of Therapeutic Massage and Bodywork (NCBTMB)

*Learning skills for practicing Therapeutic Touch, Healing Touch, and Reiki for use in clinical practice can be achieved by taking classes through the professional organization, usually taught in 1- to 3-day formats.

For patients interested in accessing touch therapy providers for individual sessions, several resources are available through professional organizations that provide information on touch therapy availability within health care institutions and individual providers: The Center for Reiki Research provides a state-by-state listing of hospitals that offer Reiki and the International Center for Reiki Training offers a state-by-state listing of practitioners; Healing Touch International has an online directory that lists Certified Healing Touch Practitioners from around the world, as well as clinics and facilities that use Healing Touch; Nurse Healers—Professional Associates International (TT) provides a listing of qualified teachers and practitioners; the American Massage Therapy Association website provides listings on qualified massage therapists by location, technique, and school (see websites).

strokes relevant to all styles include effleurage, friction movements, pressure stroke, petrissage (kneading), vibration strokes, and percussion strokes [107]. Shoulder massage, hand, and foot massage are techniques that are easy to learn and have been offered in some clinical settings by nurses, massage therapists, and volunteers [107]. According to the Natural Standard professional monograph on massage therapy [108], "the aims of massage therapy are to induce relaxation, relieve stress, improve circulation of blood and lymph, reduce pain, and increase flexibility and general well-being." The trend toward greater use of massage therapy for medical or health reasons is reflected in increases in referrals from physicians, chiropractors, physical therapists, and nurses [109].

Considerable research has been conducted on the outcomes of massage therapy in the past 30 years, primarily examining its effect on chronic health conditions and pain. According to the Touch Research Institute, "Research efforts that began in 1982 and continue today have shown that touch therapy has numerous beneficial effects on health and well-being" [110]. This research institution has conducted more than a hundred studies that have demonstrated positive effects of massage therapy including pain reduction, decreased autoimmune problems, enhanced immune function, enhanced alertness and performance, and enhanced growth in preterm infants. A meta-analysis of massage therapy research showed significant reductions in trait anxiety and depression with multiple applications [111]. Several systematic reviews have examined the use of massage therapy for specific health problems, including low back pain [112,113], chronic constipation [112], diabetes [114], cancer [115–118], depression [91,119], and migraine headaches [120]. A systematic review on insomnia identified the dearth of studies that support several mainstream CAM therapies, including massage use in the treatment of sleeping disturbances [121].

The Cochrane database includes reviews on massage therapy for low back pain [122], neck disorders [123], labor pain [36,124–126], antenatal depression [127], HIV/AIDS [128], and dementia [129]. Although these reviews provide evidence that massage therapy impacts the experience of pain, mood, and other quality of life measures, inadequate number of studies and poor study design prevent the development of strong clinical recommendations. Methodological issues in massage research have been identified, such as inclusion criteria; potential confounders; design rigor; practitioner qualifications effect on efficacy; massage protocol including frequency, duration, total number of treatments, and type of massage; control group issues; and measurement errors [117,130]. Touch therapy research in particular is plagued with the confounding variable of touch and relationship development that may have therapeutic value beyond the particular modality. Goldstone [131] suggests that development of a massage template that provides consistent parameters for practice offers research opportunities for midwives and nurses.

Energy touch therapies

The energy touch therapies of Therapeutic Touch, Healing Touch, and Reiki are catego-rized as biofield therapies, which are "intended to affect energy fields that purportedly surround and penetrate the human body" [132, p. 62]. The subtle and putative nature of biofields limits scientific understanding, but its language resonates with several healing traditions. The concept of subtle energy as a vehicle for stimulating the healing process has been described across cultures as chi, qi, ki, and prana [133]. Although Therapeutic Touch, Healing Touch, and Reiki each have their own history, techniques, and practice standards, they share many similarities. In all three traditions there exists the fundamental assumptions that a universal life force sustains all living organisms [134–136] and that "humans have an energetic, spiritual dimension necessary for sustaining life" that is a part of the healing process [43, p. 221]. "All three of these approaches use a variety of hands-on techniques that are purported to facilitate balance within the body as well as in the biofield that surrounds the body" [137]. The focus is on balancing the energies of the total person and stimulating the body's own natural healing ability rather than on the treatment of specific physical diseases [135,136,138].

The goal of these energy therapies is to assist the recipient in accessing her/his own healing process and to restore wholeness and well-being at the physical, emotional, mental, and spiritual levels [136,139], using centeredness and presence, and for the recipient's "highest good" [132,139,140]. Access to this energy and level of effectiveness is not dependent on the recipient's belief system [134–136]. The major effects of all three energy touch therapies are the initiation of the relaxation response, a reduction in pain and anxiety, and activation of the healing process [132,141,142]. From a physiologic perspective, the biofield therapies of TT, HT, and Reiki appear to affect the autonomic nervous system, "altering the high frequency ratio of heart rate variability, reflecting a greater parasympathetic tone and decreased sympathetic activation" [62, p. 90; 70]. Recipients remain clothed during a treatment session, which may occur while seated or lying down. Lastly, no adverse effects have been noted with any of these modalities.

The touch therapies of TT, HT, and Reiki are described using the language of energy. It is important to note that energy is a concept that is difficult to define and has many meanings that have changed over time [143]. The notion that touch is an energetic exchange between the giver and receiver represents a paradigm shift in our view of health and healing, moving from a causation and mechanistic model of energy to a more relational model that acknowledges that energy has multiple manifestations: "The phenomenon of energy has a qualitative nature and can never be completely knowable, measurable, or ultimately predictable" [143, p. 135]. This particular view of energy may well have its origins in the Aristotelian concept of "energeia," which was used to describe the actualizing of potentials, or "kinesis," the process of change that exists with purposiveness [143, p. 135]. Rogers' [144] science of unitary human beings has been used as a theoretical framework for understanding the experience of Reiki and Therapeutic Touch [139,145–150]. This theory connects scientific principles of energy as matter to the human energy field and energetic interconnections that occur in the environment [151].

Therapeutic touch

Therapeutic Touch is a contemporary interpretation of several ancient hands-on traditions that was developed and standardized in 1972 by Dora Kunz, a gifted healer, and

Dolores Krieger, a PhD prepared nurse. It is defined as "an intentionally directed process of energy exchange during which the practitioner uses the hands as a focus to facilitate the re-balancing of another's energy field in support of healing" [152]. Performing Therapeutic Touch includes a five-step process of centering, assessment, unruffling, rebalancing, and reassessment by placing hands on or near the body with the intention to help or heal, using light touch and/or sweeping hand motions above the skin surface to assess and balance the energy in and around the body (see Table 8.1) [153]. Therapeutic Touch paved the way for practice, research, and scholarship in all energy touch therapies by demonstrating legitimacy within health care, specifically within nursing practice.

Research in the early 1970s showed that patients receiving TT had higher hemoglobin levels than those in a control group without TT [154]. TT received scrutiny in both the practice and research arena, identifying the need for objective evidence to gain professional credibility [142]. Additional research papers focused on the effects of TT on anxiety [77,79,155,156], pain [86,155,157–160], and stress reduction [80,81,83,161]. By 1999, a meta-analysis of thirty-eight research papers [162,163] concluded that TT has a positive and moderate effect [164]. Use of TT for pre-/postoperative patients and oncology patients has also been investigated [75,165–171]. The Cochrane database contains four reviews on TT, suggesting no effect on wound healing [172], inadequate RCTs for evaluating anxiety disorders [173], modest effect on pain relief [174], and some effect on chronic tension headache [175]. Therapeutic Touch, like massage therapy research, is fraught with methodological and study design challenges.

Healing touch

Healing Touch is a combination of hand patterns and sequences developed and compiled in the early 1980s by Janet Mentgen, a nurse. It incorporates many principles of Therapeutic Touch but includes other full body techniques, localized and specific techniques, and specific interventions for identified problems [134]. For example, the "chakra spread" is recommended for use in hospice care or for persons in severe pain, and "magnetic unruffling" was developed to clear the body of congested energy [134]. Similar to Therapeutic Touch, the practitioner directs energy using her or his hands above the individual's body [66]. These techniques are taught through the Healing Touch program in six levels of study (see Table 8.1).

Healing Touch research followed a similar trajectory as Therapeutic Touch, focusing on the clinical benefits of relaxation, pain and anxiety reduction, and a sense of connection and support [70,73,176–179]. Clinical application of Healing Touch research also focuses on chronic health problems and pain management, with research studies demonstrating effectiveness in reducing some of the more stressful aspects of cancer-related problems [42,61,67,180]. Jain and Mills [133] synthesized sixty-six clinical studies that examined biofield therapies in diverse clinical populations and found moderate evidence for biofield's effect on reducing acute pain intensity in cancer. An integrative review of the effects of Healing Touch in clinical practice yielded a critical review of five RCTs [61,65,67,69,181], all supporting the potential clinical effectiveness of Healing Touch improving quality of life in chronic disease management [140]. Similar research concerns about methodology and study design are reviewed, including whether energy research lends itself to conventional scientific methods [65,140].

Reiki

Reiki is a Japanese word that means "universal life force energy"; it is used as a hands-on spiritual, vibrational healing practice to promote balance throughout the human system [182]. Unlike Therapeutic Touch and Healing Touch, which originated within the context of nursing practice, Reiki emerged as a Japanese healing tradition in the mid 1800s and was introduced in the United States in the mid 1970s. Although very similar to TT and HT in application and outcomes, Reiki practice is hands-on and nondirective in nature, with practitioners serving as energy conduits that require an initiation into Reiki energy with less reliance on techniques and hand positions. Unlike TT and HT, Reiki practice does not have a standardized educational or certification program (see Table 8.1).

The trajectory of Reiki practice and research has enjoyed a significant acceleration within the past decade. Increasingly, health care providers are learning how to incorporate Reiki into clinical practice and researchers are developing improved methodology and research designs. The Center for Reiki Research website and the Touchstone Process provide a clearinghouse for disseminating current Reiki research information for practitioners and researchers. The Touchstone Process systematically analyzes published, peer-reviewed studies of Reiki, with results accessible online.

Reiki research outcomes are also focused primarily on reducing stress and pain, increasing relaxation and an overall sense of well-being, particularly in the area of chronic disease and pain management [44,53,55,183–195]. Five systematic reviews on Reiki research representing twenty-four studies and nine RCTs resulted in the following: four studies demonstrated pain reduction, two studies showed decreased depression and anxiety, and one study showed decreased fatigue and quality of life among cancer patients [133,151,196–198]. Vitale concluded, "The field of energy research does not readily lend itself to traditional scientific analysis or strictly linear research methods because paradoxical findings are common" [151, p. 168]. Efforts to strengthen research design and mitigate the confounding effects of human touch have led to the development of "sham" or "placebo" Reiki [199].

Qualitative studies on the experience of receiving TT, HT, and Reiki have demonstrated increased self-awareness [200] and paradoxical findings [20]. Several research studies have also shown beneficial effects of touch therapies for nurses in positively influencing well-being, quality of care, and stress reduction [21,71,85,201–205]. One study suggests that nurses utilizing mind-body techniques for stress reduction are seeking greater spiritual well-being, serenity, calm or inner peace, better mood, more compassion, or better sleep [206]. Application of touch therapies for self-care has considerable value in stress reduction among health providers. Unlike other interventions, those using energy touch therapies receive the benefits of the therapies while performing them on patients. (See Figures 8.1–8.7.)

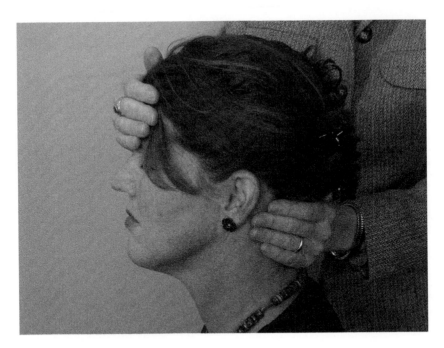

Figure 8.1   Hands on forehead/neck.

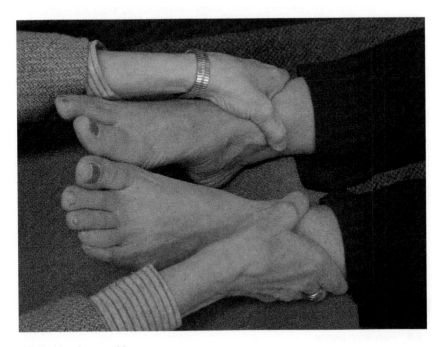

Figure 8.2   Hands on ankles.

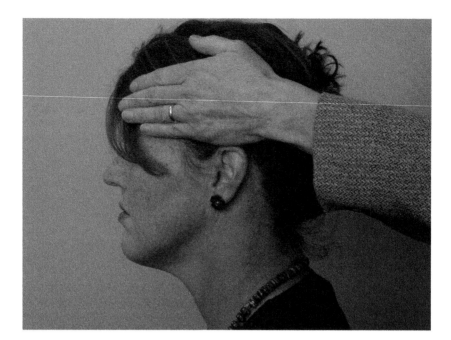

Figure 8.3   Hands on temples.

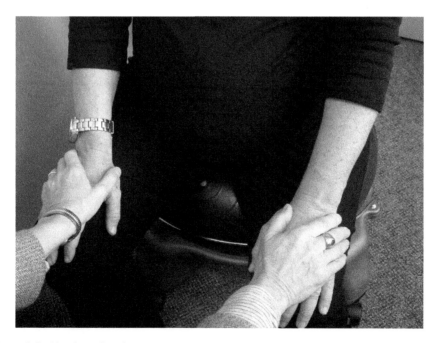

Figure 8.4   Hands on hands.

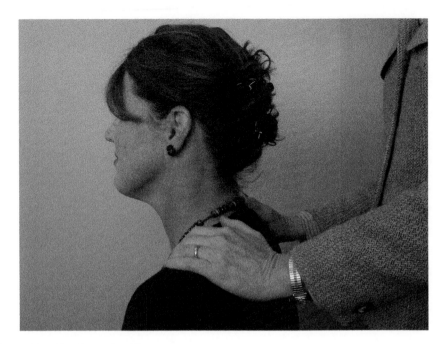

Figure 8.5   Hands on shoulders.

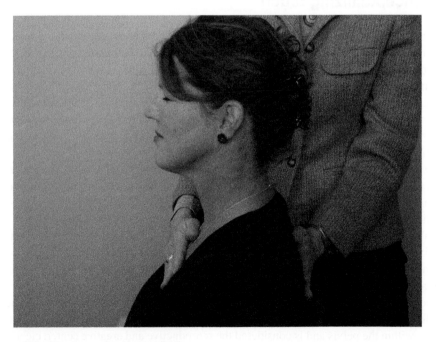

Figure 8.6   Hands on chest/upper back.

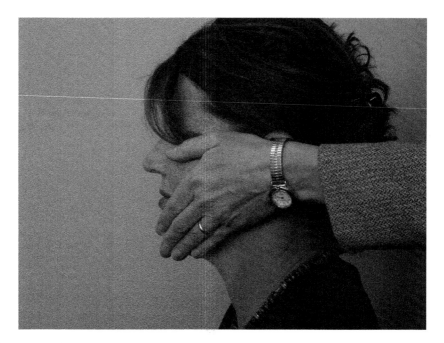

Figure 8.7 Hands on cheeks.

Reconceptualizing touch

The introduction of touch therapies into clinical practice not only adds another dimension to hands-on care but also invites a reconceptualization of intentional touch. All touch therapies provide opportunities to interface energetically with each client, intentionally offering hands-on support. Touch therapy outcomes extend beyond physical healing into the realm of well-being and spiritual connection. The specific properties of each touch therapy may not be well understood from a scientific perspective, but there is considerable resonance with the metaphysical properties accompanying many ancient healing traditions. An example of this can be found in the description of the chakra system as pathways of energy, which developed from the Yoga tradition [207]. The chakra system of Yoga recognizes seven major energetic centers (chakras) that are associated with specific organs and parts of the body. The seven chakras are also identified with nonphysical functions: the first chakra is associated with survival, the second with creativity and sexuality, the third with personal power, the fourth with love, the fifth with communication, the sixth with intuition, and the seventh with knowledge and wisdom [208]. There is a resemblance between the chakra system and Maslow's [209] hierarchy of needs, starting with a foundation of physical survival and ending with self-actualization [210].

The chakra system supports an alternative view to the human body that extends understanding beyond the physical arena. For example, the second chakra, or sacral chakra, resides within the pelvis and is considered the reproductive and creative center, clearly an area of the female anatomy that plays a significant role in reproduction. The fourth chakra, or heart chakra, resides in the chest and represents the energetic center for heartfelt

---

Box 8.1   Light touch sequence for laboring woman

(Approx. 2–3 minutes using each hand position.)

1. General approach: Use touch therapy competencies; apply hands for approximately 2–3 minutes of light touch in each hand position, vary positions and duration based on individual needs.
2. Hands on shoulders (introduction to light touch) (Figure 8.5).
3. One hand on forehead, one hand on upper nape of neck (second chakra, connection to intuition and wisdom) (Figure 8.1).
4. One hand on chest, other hand on upper back (fourth chakra, connection to heart and courage) (Figure 8.6).
5. One hand each on ankle (grounding position, connection to the earth and physical stamina) (Figure 8.2).
6. Hands on shoulders (conclusion to light touch) (Figure 8.5).

---

emotions. Placing hands on the heart can powerfully influence a woman who is moving through a difficult labor (see Box 8.1). Understanding the energetic work of each chakra supports the use of hand positions that balance these energetic centers. The chakra system is incorporated into techniques used in Healing Touch and Therapeutic Touch, but a general knowledge of chakras is useful in all aspects of intentional touch. (See Box 8.1.)

Ethical considerations

In clinical practice, four basic principles of physical touch should be considered: (1) ask permission to touch, (2) provide basic information about what you will be doing, (3) describe anticipated benefits and range of outcomes, and (4) assure the right to decline or discontinue receiving physical touch (see Box 8.2). Nurses, midwives, doulas, and physicians work within their professional roles utilizing an ethical framework provided by their professional organization that identifies general principles of ethical conduct and specialty-specific considerations [10, 211–215]. Adherence to professional boundaries is discussed in the code of ethics for nurses [212], but none of these documents address specific ethical parameters for touch. The Hippocratic Oath, "Do no harm," clearly applies to using touch in ways that could result in harm.

A professional code of ethics also guides practice for massage therapy, Therapeutic Touch, Healing Touch, and Reiki practitioners. In general, these represent statements for standards of conduct that define ethical behavior for each touch therapy including scope of practice, nondiscrimination, sexual impropriety, confidentiality, privacy, informed consent, and high-quality care [105]. The energy touch therapies also include ethics related to intention, healing environment, healing principles, and the nondiagnostic nature of the work [216–219]. In the book *Creating Healing Relationships: Professional Standards for Energy Therapy Practitioners*, Dorothea Hover-Kramer [220] describes parameters for level of competence, record keeping, professional responsibility, boundaries, confidentiality, marketing, and informed consent. General competencies for touch therapies are provided in Box 8.2.

Health care institutions can also develop their own policies, guidelines, and/or competencies for touch therapy use. For example, Reiki practice at a Magnet-designated facility

---

Box 8.2   Touch therapy principles

1. Ask permission to touch before any encounter that involves physical touch, including performing a physical exam or procedure, providing comfort measures, and/or using a specific touch therapy.
2. Describe the areas of the body you will be touching and what sensations the client may experience. If related to a physical exam or procedure, share your findings in simple language.
3. Ask if there is cultural or personal information about touch that should be shared before engaging in physical touch.
4. When using TT, HT, Reiki, or massage or other hands-on comfort measures, (1) provide basic information about what you will be doing; (2) describe anticipated benefits and range of outcomes; (3) ask if there are areas they would prefer not to be touched; (4) let them know you will stop at any time; (5) ask if they prefer to be wakened if they fall asleep; (6) create an environment that promotes feelings of safety. If possible, assure privacy. In a hospital setting, consider putting a sign on the door asking to not be disturbed.

---

in Pennsylvania requires evidence of competency in Reiki practice and adherence to written hospital policy when administering Reiki [146], and a protocol for Reiki use in the operating room was developed at a hospital in New Hampshire following a request to have a Reiki practitioner present during surgery [221].

In an effort to provide guidelines to assure safety and protection of the public using CAM therapies, a diverse group of CAM providers, health care providers, ethicists, legal consultants, health policy specialists, and consumers recently developed ethical guidelines for boundaries of touch in CAM [222]. They provided guiding principles and ethical rules addressing behavior and language regarding inappropriate touch and exposure, as well as the right of the client to discontinue treatment.

Use of touch to provide support during labor/birth

The majority of the literature on touch during childbearing focuses on the use of touch during labor, frequently placed within the context of "labor support." In order to more fully understand this aspect of labor, researchers have examined what constitutes supportive care, the outcomes associated with supportive care, and the role of those providing supportive care during labor, with a recent focus on the role of doula.

In a systematic review of five nonpharmacologic methods for pain relief in labor, Simkin and O'Hara [223] found that continuous nonmedical support by an experienced nurse, midwife, or doula reduced labor pain. They describe labor support as including the following components: (1) physical comforting: touch and massage, assistance with positioning, self-help comfort measures, bathing, grooming, applying warmth or cold; (2) emotional support: continuous presence, reassurance, and encouragement; (3) guidance and emotional support for the woman's partner; (4) information: nonmedical advice, anticipatory guidance, explanations of procedures; and (5) facilitation of communication between the woman and staff, to assist her in making informed decisions [223]. In a survey of postpartum women and their experience of touch during labor, Birch [224] found that 97% found touch during labor to be positive, with preferences for location: 28% found touch to the back to be most therapeutic and 24% found touch to the hands to be most therapeutic. The type of touch perceived as therapeutic varied: 55% chose rubbing and massaging, 28% chose holding, 10% chose pressure, and 7% chose patting.

Laboring women perceive touch as conveying caring and concern, but perception of touch is also influenced by who is providing the touch [97]. Penny [225] found that 94% of laboring women perceived touch as positive when given by a relative or friend, 86% when touched by their husband, 73% when touched by a nurse, and 21% when touched by a physician.

The Coalition for Improving Maternity Services identified education of staff in nondrug methods of pain relief as step seven in the ten steps of mother-friendly care. This step is intended to increase knowledge of nondrug methods of pain relief and reduce unnecessary analgesic and anesthetic drug use [226]. Massage and touch are identified as having no risk of adverse effects and having the following benefits: a reduction in maternal pain, stress, and anxiety and an enhanced ability to cope with labor [223,227]. The use of touch therapies in supporting relaxation and pain reduction can be used in managing the stress and pain that accompanies labor. Lothian, a Therapeutic Touch practitioner and childbirth educator, incorporated TT into her childbirth classes as an alternative method of achieving relaxation [82].

Massage therapy has been the most extensively studied touch therapy for use during childbirth. Two recent Cochrane reviews concluded that massage may be a helpful modality for pain management in labor, but there is insufficient evidence to make clinical recommendations [36,126]. A 1997 study [228] showed a decrease in depressed mood, anxiety, pain, less agitation, shorter labors, shorter hospital stay, and less postpartum depression when massage therapy was performed on the back, head, hips, and feet of laboring women at hourly intervals by their partners. Chang et al. [96] performed the first randomized controlled trial of massage during labor, and showed a reduction in pain during all phases of labor and a reduction in anxiety during the latent phase of labor, as well as an observed reduction in agitation. Women received directional, moderately firm, and rhythmic massage lasting 30 minutes and including abdominal effleurage, sacral pressure, and shoulder and back kneading, first from the primary researcher, who then taught partners to perform the massage [96]. Using a similar study design along with the McGill Pain Questionaire, Chang, Chen, and Huang [229] demonstrated that although massage didn't change the characteristics of pain during labor, it can effectively decrease labor pain during labor.

A systematic review examining continuous labor support, baths, touch and massage, maternal movement and positioning, and intradermal water blocks for back pain relief suggested that all of these methods may be effective in reducing labor pain and improving other outcomes, but additional studies are needed to clarify their effects [223]. Another systematic review on CAM use during labor concluded there was evidence of efficacy with water injections and some evidence that massage was beneficial during labor [227].

A study undertaken to distinguish the effects of massage from the effects of continuous physical presence showed the highest level of satisfaction and greatest reduction in pain among the massage therapy group and the greatest reduction in anxiety among the continous physical presence group [230]. Another study compared the effects of an antenatal massage and relaxation program on reported pain during labor to those receiving relaxation techniques combined with music and found a nonsignificant trend toward lower pain in the massage group [231].

There are many anecodotal stories that support energy touch therapies as useful tools for pain management in labor [232–234], but little research has been conducted in this area. Studies investigating the effect of TT, HT, and Reiki on pain reduction and elicitation of the relaxation response during labor are relevant to this discussion but remain largely hypothetical. For example, the Cochrane review on touch therapies for pain relief in adults (including TT, HT, and Reiki) shows promise for application for labor pain [174], but this research has not yet been conducted.

Application of touch therapies to pregnancy and postpartum

CAM therapies were initially introduced into health care for chronic health problems and managing symptoms related to pain, anxiety, and nausea, often related to cancer and surgical procedures. An additional benefit of CAM therapy use is reducing reliance on pharmaceuticals and their side effects [235], particularly significant when treating conditions during pregnancy, since many medications have an unknown safety profile for their use at that time. Other suggested motivations for selecting CAM therapies during pregnancy are their holistic approach and enhancement of a sense of control and satisfaction with childbearing [236,237]. Research examining the use of CAM therapies for childbearing has significantly increased in the past decade. In a 2010 review of CAM therapy use in maternity care, thirteen of the nineteen studies were published between 2005 and 2010 [238].

A 2011 review on the use of complementary and alternative medicine by pregnant women [239] revealed wide usage of CAM therapies during pregnancy, consistent with demographic data showing that women utilize these therapies more than men [240]. The prevalence of CAM use in pregnancy ranged from 13% to 78%; many women used more than one type of therapy; and the most common modalities used were massage, vitamin and mineral supplement, herbal medicine, relaxation therapies, and aromatherapy [239]. Three studies included touch therapies [237,241,242], demonstrating massage usage during pregnancy ranged from 21% to 50% and Reiki usage was 2%. Another study on CAM use during pregnancy found the most commonly used modalities were herbal therapy, chiropractic, acupuncture/acupressure, massage, homeopathy, and aromatherapy, used for relief of pregnancy-related conditions, including nausea and vomiting, low-back pain, discomfort, or depression [238].

Massage therapy during pregnancy has been studied more than energy touch therapies. Three studies demonstrated effectiveness in the use of massage therapy during pregnancy in reducing depression, anxiety, leg and back pain, and cortisol levels; excessive fetal activity decreased; and the rate of prematurity was lower [93–95]. Massage therapists provided massage therapy for 20 minutes per week for 5 weeks in the study conducted by Field et al. [93], pregnant women with depression were massaged by their significant others over a 16-week period using the same protocol in the study by Field et al. [94], and in the Field et al. [95] study pregnant women diagnosed with major depression were given 12 weeks of twice-weekly massage therapy by their significant other. This last study also resulted in reduced depression and cortisol levels postpartum [95]. Teaching others to touch was relatively easy to achieve; each significant other received one 30-minute session with instructions on how to perform a massage [93–95]. A study conducted on the use of massage and touch therapy for partners of cancer patients concluded that brief instruction is a feasible intervention to increase caregiver efficacy, patient satisfaction, quality of life, and quality of the relationship [243, p. 147], illustrating the importance of teaching touch as another aspect of the professional health provider role.

The benefits of stress reduction and relaxation are not limited to a particular health problem or condition. For this reason, it is useful to consider energy touch therapy application for pregnant and postpartum women, extrapolating from other areas of touch therapy research: reduction of pain and anxiety, particularly in conjunction with the common discomforts of pregnancy that frequently result in fatigue, musculoskeletal pain, anxiety, and/or sleep disturbances. Tiran and Chummun [23] identified numerous antepartal conditions that may be positively impacted by CAM therapies that reduce stress: fatigue, heartburn, nausea, headache, backache, insomnia, mood swings, depression, carpal tunnel syndrome, and elevated blood pressure. Fischer and Johnson [142] identified Therapeutic Touch as an adjunct to midwifery management for a variety of conditions, including morning sickness, anemia, colds and flu, constipation, preterm labor, and pregnancy-induced hypertension. They suggested that couples could learn Therapeutic Touch in childbirth classes, using these techniques to better tolerate common physical complaints of pregnancy, such as ankle edema and low back pain. A clinical practice exchange in the *Journal of Nurse-Midwifery* featured the use of several CAM therapies by certified nurse-midwives (CNMs), including a CNM who practiced Healing Touch for prenatal patients with hyperemesis and back pain, to connect with their unborn baby, to enhance well-being, and to reduce fear of labor [244]. Touch therapies can be used to promote relaxation and reduce the stress of high-risk pregnancies; massage therapy for pregnancy conditions requiring bedrest, energy touch therapies for pain management during procedures such as amniocentesis, and/or any touch therapy that supports rest and sleep when managing pregnancy-related problems. The use of Therapeutic Touch in treating pregnant women with a chemical dependency was found to significantly reduce anxiety [245].

Peck [235] identified several potential benefits of relaxation/guided imagery, massage, and Healing Touch, including feelings of relaxation, feeling "better" in general, enhancement of traditional pain medications' efficacy, elimination of pain, better sleep, facilitation of decision making, ability to think more clearly, reduction in number and intensity of "bad" days, and facilitation of ability to perform certain physical activities and tasks. All of these potential benefits could significantly improve the fatigue and numerous stressors that women experience during the postpartum period. Therapeutic Touch used in conjunction with postpartum home visits yielded several positive results, including feelings of relaxation, connection, and being cared for [246].

Several studies of TT, HT, and Reiki focus on application of these therapies within a perioperative context, noting reduction in pain and anxiety when used pre- and postoperatively [75,147,168,247–254]. Pre-and postoperative use of touch therapies to reduce anxiety and pain also have application within the context of pregnancy, labor, and postpartum, for use before, during, and after invasive procedures such as amniocentesis, epidurals, or cesarean sections.

Models of care

The need for an integrated approach to health care, one that combines the best practices of CAM with the best practices of conventional health care practices, represents a new model of health care delivery [18,255–258]. Increasingly, consumers are seeking alternative pathways to health and embracing a more holistic model of care. The addition of CAM therapies within health care settings represents a response to consumer demand as well as a shifting paradigm within health care. New integrative models of health care are rapidly evolving in tertiary and ambulatory settings, and both allopathic and alternative health care providers are challenged to define their scope of practice in a constantly shifting landscape.

Within hospitals, the introduction of touch therapies into patient care has primarily been initiated through volunteers, but increasingly there is support for embedding these modalities into direct care through educational programs for nurses, midwives, and physicians [146,259,260]. Increased evidence of efficacy and support for integrative nursing practice supports a shift to greater nursing engagement in touch therapies, including informal application in all clinical encounters. (See Case Study 8.1.) Access to integrative services within a hospital setting may also exist through an integrative health team that provides a variety of services through a nurse and physician referral system, such as massage therapy, acupuncture, Healing Touch, Reiki, music therapy, art therapy,

---

Case Study 8.1

The use of touch therapies in labor and birth: Integrating touch into midwifery care
Carissa Scanlan, DNP, CNM

Sue was admitted to the hospital following spontaneous rupture of membranes earlier in the day. She had some mild, irregular contractions but wasn't yet in active labor. She was due in 2 days and this was her first baby. Since she recently broke up with her boyfriend, she was alone today. Sue was excited to meet her new baby but nervous and anxious about when and how labor and birth would proceed. She hoped for an unmedicated water birth. I was the midwife on the labor unit and knew Sue from the clinic. After we talked for a while and discussed options for labor and birth, I told her that I did Reiki and Healing Touch and asked her if she wanted to try it. She agreed. I usually use gentle touch with the intention to support the person's energy so that the person feels centered, grounded, and overall calm and at peace with whatever is happening. I used light touch on each of Sue's chakras (energy centers of the body) to promote balance and openness. Sue visibly relaxed and fell asleep.

Within some hours her contractions became stronger and more frequent. I sat with her and walked with her, supporting her choices for movement and comfort. She was in and out of the birth tub as she preferred. I found myself reaching out to put pressure on her back. We call this "counterpressure," but I know that I was also supporting the second chakra and the uterus, muscles, and bones in this area. My hands would also sometimes go to her hips. I was careful to watch her for cues that my touch was acceptable and helpful and not too much. I also often find it useful to put my hands on a laboring woman's heart (heart chakra). I believe this supports a woman's courage and strength. Sue appeared to react positively to the energy work. She continued with a long, hard, but healthy labor. She pushed well for over 2 hours, as the baby slowly descended. I supported and encouraged her by using different positions and breathing with her, conscious of her need for physical, emotional, and spiritual energy. She was now out of the tub, lying on the bed. As the baby was crowning through several contractions, I helped him make his way out, dried him off, and as he let out a strong cry, I handed baby Joe into his mother's waiting arms.

When women are in active labor, I feel like they have so much going on in their bodies. I want to assist them in coping and experiencing labor and birth and not distract them or make them feel more overwhelmed. I believe that my background and experience with energy work supports moms and babies to have unmedicated and calmer births, especially when labors are long.

and/or reflexology [261]. (See Case Study 8.2.) Ambulatory care models for CAM therapies exist primarily through contracting with CAM practitioners to provide specific services. These services may exist within an integrative care clinic that has a specialty focus, such as oncology or women's health. (See Case Study 8.3.) All of these models represent an integration of allopathic care with complementary therapies that promote a patient-centered holistic approach to health care.

Case Study 8.2

The use of touch therapies on an antepartal unit: An integrative hospital service
Kathryn Kerber RN, MSN, MA, HN-BC. CHTP; Integrative Health Nurse Clinician

In working with pregnant women, antepartally or in labor, I have discovered that women hold the essence of who they are in their chest and heart chakra. The hospitalized pregnant woman struggles with being in the horizontal position. I refer to them as "vertical girls" who have the rug pulled out from under them! Pregnant women often feel out of balance when they are in labor. The symptoms they display are anxiety, fear, restlessness, agitation, and hopelessness, just to name a few. I am immediately drawn to their feet and frequently place my hands around each ankle to provide grounding.

In my practice I use a combination of modalities, and Healing Touch is a part of every modality I provide. I often use foot massage or reflexology with aromatherapy and Healing Touch combined with relaxation breathing. The outcomes have been less anxiety, less fear, decreased restlessness, and overall happier pregnant women who are staying pregnant longer or progressing forward to give birth. They feel empowered to use their breath, which moves the energy from their heart down to their feet. My delight is that "aha" moment when they experience the movement of energy and realize they can use this to feel grounded and centered.

Case Study 8.3

The use of touch therapies in a women's clinic: An interdisciplinary approach
Diana Drake, DNP, RN, WHNP

In the integrative women's clinic, it is not uncommon for a woman to complete her midwife visit and step into the next room for an hour Reiki session to help with insomnia and stress or schedule herself with the acupuncturist for back pain. Among the integrative therapies, Reiki, Healing Touch, and acupuncture are utilized to prevent or manage common pregnancy-related issues that may include fatigue, nausea and vomiting, headaches, pain syndromes, stress, anxiety, depression, sleep issues, and edema. These therapies support the body's natural healing ability and the rebalancing, unblocking, and promoting of healing energy. The woman can self-select or her prenatal provider can recommend a specific therapy. The nurse-midwife, physician, or nurse practitioner collaborates directly with the integrative therapists sharing the same clinic space and at bi-monthly integrative care conferences where all providers share client cases.

Women are also encouraged to attend a preconception or early pregnancy class that focuses on creating a healthy pregnancy experience through a whole-systems approach. In these classes, functional nutrition concepts and energy balancing are introduced as a means of maintaining optimal health and providing individual strategies for prevention. A Reiki therapist and an acupuncturist offer women a hands-on experience, and as the pregnancy progresses, the small group class provides continuing support and tools throughout prenatal care, postpartum, and lactation. Some of the therapies are also offered in the adjacent hospital and birthing unit.

Table 8.2   Application of MT, TT, HT, Reiki during pregnancy, childbirth, postpartum.

Pregnancy	Childbirth	Postpartum
Nausea	Labor support	Anxiety/depression
Constipation	Labor pain	Fatigue
Low back pain	Anxiety	Relaxation/stress reduction
Relaxation/stress reduction	Pre- and post-procedures	Improved sleep
Anxiety/depression		Breastfeeding
Childbirth preparation:		Headache/migraine
relaxation techniques		
Improved sleep		Surgical recovery
Headache/migraine		
Fatigue		
Pre- and post-procedures		

Summary and recommendations

One of the characteristics of patient-centered care is that it "provides physical comfort and emotional support" [18, p. 280], which is particularly congruent with the outcomes associated with touch therapies. Each case study illustrates the role that touch therapies play in providing comfort and support, reducing the normal stressors that accompany pregnancy and childbirth. Touch as a noninvasive strategy for reducing pain, stress, and anxiety has numerous applications within the context of childbearing and great potential for supporting these normal processes. (See Table 8.2 for a summary of applications of touch therapies during pregnancy, childbirth, and postpartum.) Introducing a wider range of touch therapies into practice may be the next step in redefining supportive interventions in pregnancy, labor/birth, and postpartum care.

Expanding the practice of intentional touch is an integration of "old" hands-on caregiving skills with "new" integrative touch therapies. Reexamining the value of human touch can serve to reconnect us to our healing roots; the hands as a metaphor for caring remind us that we are instruments of healing [262]. Reconceptualizing touch as a vehicle for energetic exchange, facilitation of energetic balance, and support for the healing process adds yet another dimension to the hands-on work of providing care. Specific touch therapies may invite a more conscious engagement in using hands with intention and healing purpose while generating energetic self-awareness and providing guidance in self-care practices.

References

1. Montagu A. (1971). *Touching: The human significance of the skin*. New York: Harper and Row.
2. Leder D & Krucoff MW. (2008). The touch that heals: The uses and meanings of touch in the clinical encounter. *Journal of Alternative and Complementary Medicine*, *14*(3), 321–327.
3. Ruffin PT. (2011). A history of massage in nurse training school curricular (1860–1945). *Journal of Holistic Nursing*, *29*(1), 61–67.
4. Quinn JF. (1992). Holding sacred space: The nurse as healing environment. *Holistic Nursing Practice*, *6*(4), 26–36.

5. Bruhn JG. (1978). The doctor's touch: Tactile communication in the doctor-patient relationship. *Southern Medical Jounal, 71*(12), 1469–1473.

6. Institute of Medicine of the National Academies. (2010). *Integrative medicine and the health of the public: A summary of the February 2009 summit.* Washington, DC: National Academies Press.

7. Kemper KJ & Shaltout HA. (2011). Non-verbal communication of compassion: Measuring psychophysiologic effects. *BMC Complementary Alternative Medicine, 11*, 132.

8. Varney H, Kriebs JM, & Gegor C. (2004). *Varney's midwifery*, 4th ed. Burlington, MA: Jones & Bartlett.

9. American College of Nurse-Midwives. (2004). Philosophy of the American College of Nurse-Midwives. Retrieved from: http://www.midwife.org/index.asp?bid=59&cat=2&button=Search&rec=49. Accessed August 20, 2012.

10. American College of Nurse-Midwives. (2012). Core competencies for basic midwifery practice. Retrieved from: http://www.midwife.org/ACNM/files/ACNMLibraryData/UPLOADFILENAME/000000000050/Core%20Comptencies%20Dec%202012.pdf. Accessed August 20, 2012.

11. American College of Nurse-Midwives. (2003). Position statement: Appropriate use of technology in childbirth. Retrieved from: http://www.midwife.org/ACNM/files/ACNMLibraryData/UPLOADFILENAME/000000000054/Approp%20Use%20of%20Tech%2005.pdf. Accessed August 20, 2012.

12. Hodnett ED, Gates S, Hofmeyr GJ, Sakala C, & Westin J. (2011). Continuous labour support for women during childbirth. *Cochrane Database of Systematic Reviews*, issue 3. Art. No.: CD003766. DOI:10.1002/14651858.CD003766.pub2.

13. American Holistic Nurses Association. (ND). Position on the role of nurses in the practice of complementary therapies. Retrieved from: http://www.ahna.org/Resources/Publications/PositionStatements/tabid/1926/Default.aspx. Accessed August 18, 2012.

14. Wardell DW & Engebretson J. (2001). Ethical principles applied to complementary healing. *Journal of Holistic Nursing, 19*(4), 318–334.

15. Snyder M, Kreitzer M, & Loen M. (2001). Complementary and healing practices in nursing. In NL Chaska, ed., *The nursing profession: Tomorrow and beyond*, pp. 527–535. Thousand Oaks, CA: Sage.

16. Hellstrom A & Willman A. (2011). Promoting sleep by nursing interventions in healthcare settings: A systematic review. *Worldview's Evidence Based Nursing, 8*(3), 128–142.

17. Fortney L, Rakel D, Rindfleisch JA, & Mallory J. (2010). Introduction to integrative primary care: The health-oriented clinic. *Primary Care Clinical Office Practice, 37*, 1–12.

18. Maizes V, Rakel D, & Niemiec C. (2009). Integrative medicine and patient-centered care. *Explore, 5*(5), 277–289.

19. Watson J. (1985). *Nursing: The philosophy and science of caring.* Boulder: University Press of Colorado.

20. Engebretson J & Wardell D. (2002). Experience of a Reiki session. *Alternative Therapies in Health and Medicine, 8*(2), 48–53.

21. Brathovde A. (2006). A pilot study: Reiki for self-care of nurses and healthcare providers. *Holistic Nursing Practice, 20*(2), 95–101.

22. Benson H. (1975). *The relaxation response.* New York: William Morrow.

23. Tiran D & Chummun H. (2004). Complementary therapies to reduce physiological stress in pregnancy. *Complementary Therapies in Nursing and Midwifery, 10*(3), 162–167.

24. Simkin P & Ancheta R. (2011). *The labor progress handbook: Early interventions to prevent and treat dystocia*, 3rd ed. San Fransciso: Wiley-Blackwell.

25. Dickinson HO, Beyer FR, Ford GA, Nicolson D, Campbell F, Cook JV, & Mason J. (2008). Relaxation therapies for the management of primary hypertension in adults. *Cochrane Database of Systematic Reviews* CD004935. DOI: 10.1002/14651858.pub2.

26. Jorm AF, Morgan AJ, & Hetrick SE. (2008). Relaxation for depression. *Cochrane Database of Systematic Reviews* CD007142. DOI: 10.1002/14651858.pub2.

27. Proctor M, Murphy PA, Pattison HM, Suckling JA, & Farquhar C. (207). Behavioral interventions for dysmenorrhea. *Cochrane Database of Systematic Reviews* CD002248. DOI: 10.1002/14651858.

28. Krisanaprakorkit W, Sriaj W, Piyavhatkul N, & Laopaiboon M. (2006). Meditation therapy for anxiety disorders. *Cochrane Database of Systematic Reviews* CD004998. DOI: 10.1002/14651858.pub2.

29. Rada G, Capurro D, Patnoja T, Corbalan J, Moreno G, Letelier LM, & Vera C. (2010). Non-hormonal interventions for hot flushes in women with a history of breast cancer. *Cochrane Database of Systematic Reviews* CD004923. DOI: 10.1002/14651858.pub2.

30. Ramaratnam S, Baker GA, & Goldstein LH. (2008). Psychological treatments for epilepsy. *Cochrane Database of Systematic Reviews* CD002029. DOI: 10.1002/14651858.pub3.

31. Izquierdo de Santiago I & Khan M. (2007). Hypnosis for schizophrenia. *Cochrane Database of Systematic Reviews* CD004160. DOI:10.1002/14651858.pub3.

32. Yorke J, Fleming SL, & Shuldham C. (2009). Psychological interventions for adults with asthma. *Cochrane Database of Systematic Reviews* CD002982. DOI: 10.1002/14651858.pub3.

33. Ersser SJ, Latter S, Sibley A, Satherley PA, & Welbourne S. (2007). Psychological and educational interventions for atopic eczema in children. *Cochrane Database of Systematic Reviews* CD004054. DOI: 10.1002/14651858.pub2.

34. Zijdenbos IL, de wit NJ, van der Heijden GJ, Rubin G, & Quartero AO. (2009). Psychological interventions for the management of irritable bowel syndrome. *Cochrane Database of Systematic Reviews* CD006442. DOI: 10.1002/14651858.pub2.

35. Henschke N, Ostelo RWJG, van Tulder MW, Vlaeyan JWS, Morley S, Assendelft WJ, et al. (2010). Behavioural treatment for chronic low-back pain. *Cochrane Database of Systematic Reviews, 7*, CD002014.

36. Jones L, Othman M, Dowswell T, Alfirevic Z, Gates S, Newborn M, Jordan S, Lavendar T, & Neilson JP. (2012). Pain management for women in labour: An overview of systematic reviews. *Cochrane Database of Systematic Reviews* CD009234. DOI: 10.1002/14651858.pub2.

37. Khunpadit S, Tavender E, Lumbiganon P, Laopaiboon M, Wasiak J, & Gruen R. (2011). Non-clinical interventions for reducing unnecessary caesarean section. *Cochrane Database of Systematic Reviews* CD005528. DOI: 10.1002/14651858.pub2.

38. Becker GE, Cooney F, & Smith HA. (2011). Methods of milk expression for lactating women. *Cochrane Database of Systematic Reviews* CD006170. DOI: 10.1002/14651858.pub3.

39. Henricson M, Ersson A, Maatta S, Segesten K, & Berglund AL. (2008). The outcome of tactile touch on stress parameters in intensive care: A randomized controlled trial. *Complementary Therapies in Clinical Practice, 14*(4), 244–254.

40. Harris M & Richards KC. (2010). The physiological and psychological effects of slow-stroke back massage and hand massage on relaxation in older adults. *Journal of Clinical Nursing, 19*(7–8), 917–926.

41. Lindgren L, Rundgren S, Winso O, Lehtipalo S, Widlund U, Karlsson M, Stenlund H, Jacobsen C, & Brulin C. (2010). Physiologic responses to touch massage in healthy volunteers. *Autonomic Neuroscience, 158*(1–2), 105–110.

42. Weze C, Leathard HL, Grange J, Tiplady P, & Stevens G. (2007). Healing by gentle touch ameliorates stress and other symptoms in people suffering with mental health disorders or psychological stress. *Evidence Based Complementary Alternative Medicine, 4*(1), 115–123.

43. Anderson JG & Taylor AG. (2011). Effects of Healing Touch in clinical practice: A systematic review of randomized clinical trials. *Journal of Holistic Nursing, 29*(3), 221–228.

44. Birocco N, Guillame C, Storto S, Ritorto G, Catino C, et al. (2012). The effects of Reiki therapy on pain and anxiety in patients attending a day oncology and infusion services unit. *American Journal of Hospice and Palliative Care, 29*(4), 290–294.

45. Bowden D, Goddard L, & Gruzelier J. (2010). A randomized controlled single-blind trial of the effects of Reiki and positive imagery on well-being and salivary cortisol. *Brain Research Bulletin, 81*(1), 66–72.

46. Caitlin A & Taylor-Ford RL. (2011). Investigation of standard care versus sham Reiki placebo versus actual Reiki therapy to enhance comfort and well-being in a chemotherapy infusion center. *Oncology Nursing Forum, 38*(3), E212–E220.

47. Collinge W, Wentworth R, & Sabo S. (2005). Integrating complementary therapies into community mental health practice: An exploration. *Journal of Alternative and Complementary Medicine, 11*(3), 569–574.

48. Diaz-Rodriquez L, Arroyo-Morales M, Fernandez-de-las-Penas C, Garcia-Lafuente F, Garcia-Royo C, & Tomas-Rojas I (2011). Immediate effects of Reiki on heart rate variability, cortisol levels, and body temperature in health care professionals with burnout. *Biological Research in Nursing, 13*(4), 376–382.

49. Friedman RSC, Burg NM, Miles P, Lee F, & Lampert R. (2010). Effects of Reiki on autonomic activity after acute coronary syndrome. *Journal of the American College of Cardiology, 56*(2), 995–996.

50. Mackay N, Hansen S, & McFarlane O. (2004). Autonomic nervous system changes during Reiki treatment: A preliminary study. *Journal of Alternative and Complementary Medicine, 10*(6), 1077–1081.

51. Park J, McCaffrey R, Dunn D, & Goodman R. (2011). Managing osteoarthritis: Comparisons of chair yoga, Reiki, and education (pilot study). *Holistic Nursing Practice, 25*(6), 316–326.

52. Potter P. (2003). What are the distinctions between Reiki and Therapeutic Touch? *Clinical Journal of Oncology Nursing, 7*(1), 89–91.

53. Richeson N, Spross J, Lutz K, & Peng C. (2010). Effects of Reiki on anxiety, depression, pain, and physiological factors in community-dwelling older adults. *Research in Gerontological Nursing, 3*(3), 187–199.

54. Ring ME. (2009). Reiki and changes in pattern manifestations. *Nursing Science Quarterly, 22*(3), 250–258.

55. Shore A. (2004). Long-term effects of energetic healing on symptoms of psychological depression and self-perceived stress. *Alternative Therapies in Health and Medicine, 10*(3), 42–48.

56. Toms R. (2011). Reiki therapy: A nursing intervention for critical care. *Critical Care Nursing Quarterly, 34*(3), 213–217.

57. Vitale AT & O'Connor PC. (2006). The effect of Reiki on pain and anxiety in women with abdominal hysterectomies: A quasi-experimental pilot study. *Holistic Nursing Practice, 20*(6), 263–274.

58. Wardell D & Engebretson J. (2001). Biological correlates of Reiki touch healing. *Journal of Advanced Nursing, 33*(4), 439–445.

59. Witte D & Dundes L. (2001). Harnessing life energy or wishful thinking? *Alternative and Complementary Therapies, 7*(5), 304–309.

60. Burr JP. (2005). Jayne's story: Healing touch as a complementary treatment for trauma recovery. *Journal of Holistic Nursing Practice, 19*(5), 211–216.

61. Cook C, Guerrerio J, & Slater VE. (2004). Healing touch and quality of life in women receiving radiation treatment for cancer: A randomized controlled trial. *Alternative Therapies in Health and Medicine, 10*(3), 34–44.

62. Dauhauer S, Tooze J, Holder P, Miller C, & Jesse M. (2008). Healing touch as a supportive intervention for adult acute leukemia patients: A pilot investigation of effects on distress and treatment-related symptoms. *Journal for the Society of Integrative Oncology, 6*(3), 89–97.

63. Dowd T, Kolcaba K, Steiner R, & Fashingpaur D. (2007). Comparison of Healing Touch, coaching, and a combined intervention on comfort and stress in younger college students. *Holistic Nursing Practice, 21*(4), 194–202.
64. Hart LK, Freel MI, Haylock PJ, & Lutgendorf SK. (2011). The use of Healing Touch in integrative oncology. *Clinical Journal of Oncology Nursing, 15*(5), 519–525.
65. MacIntyre B, Hamilton J, Fricke T, Ma W, Mehle S, & Michel M. (2008). The efficacy of Healing Touch in coronary artery bypass surgery recovery: A randomized clinical trial. *Alternative Therapies in Health and Medicine, 14*(4), 24–32.
66. Maville J, Bowen J, & Benham G. (2008). Effect of Healing Touch on stress perception and biological correlates. *Holistic Nursing Practice, 22*(2), 103–110.
67. Post-White J, Kinney ME, Savik K, Gau JB, Wilcox C, & Lerner I. (2003). Therapeutic massage and Healing Touch improve symptoms in cancer. *Integrative Cancer Therapies, 2*(4), 332–344.
68. Schnepper LL. (2004). Healing touch and health-related quality of life in women with breast cancer receiving radiation therapy. *Journal of Society for Integrative Oncology, 7*, 178.
69. Seskevich JE, Crater SW, Lane JD, & Krucoff MW. (2004). Beneficial effects of noetic therapies on mood before percutaneous intervention for unstable coronary syndromes. *Nursing Research, 53*(2), 116–121.
70. Sneed NV, Olson M, Bubolz B, & Finch N. (2001). Influences of a relaxation intervention on perceived stress and power spectral analysis of heart rate variability. *Progressive Cardiovascular Nursing, 16*(2), 57–64, 79.
71. Tang R, Tegeler C, Larrimore D, Cowgill S, & Kemper KJ. (2010). Improving well-being of nursing leaders through Healing Touch training. *Journal of Alternative and Complementary Medicine, 16*(8), 837–841.
72. Wardell DW, Decker SA, & Engebretson JC. (2012). Healing touch for older adults with persistent pain. *Holistic Nursing Practice, 26*(4), 194–202.
73. Wilkinson D, Knox P, Chatman J, Johnson T, Barbour N, Myles Y, & Reel A. (2002). The clinical effectiveness of Healing Touch. *Journal of Alternative and Complementary Medicine, 8*(1), 33–47.
74. Wong J, Ghiassuddin A, Kimata C, Patelesio B, & Siu A. (2013). The impact of Healing Touch on pediatric oncology patients. *Integrative Cancer Therapies, 12*(1), 25–30.
75. Coakley AB & Duffy ME. (2010). The effect of Therapeutic Touch on postoperative patients. *Journal of Holistic Nursing, 28*(3), 193–200.
76. Cox C & Hayes J. (1999). Physiologic and psychodynamic responses in the administration of Therapeutic Touch in critical care. *Complementary Therapies in Nurse Midwifery, 5*(3), 87–92.
77. Heidt P. (1981). Effect of Therapeutic Touch on the anxiety level of hospitalized patients. *Nursing Research, 30*(1), 32–37.
78. Fenton M. (2003). Therapeutic touch: A nursing practice. *Alternative Therapies in Health and Medicine, 9*(1), 34–36.
79. Gagne D & Toye RC. (1994). The effects of Therapeutic Touch and relaxation therapy in reducing anxiety. *Archives of Psychiatric Nursing, 8*(3), 184–189.
80. Giasson M & Bouchard L. (1998). Effect of Therapeutic Touch on the well-being of persons with terminal cancer. *Journal of Holistic Nursing, 16*(3), 383–398.
81. Kramer N. (1990). Comparison of Therapeutic Touch and casual touch in stress reduction of hospitalized children. *Pediatric Nursing, 16*(5), 483–485.
82. Lothian JA. (1993). A modern version of the laying on of hands can aid in relaxation during labor—and beyond: Therapeutic Touch. *Childbirth Instructor, 32*, 34–36.

83. Krieger D, Peper E, & Ancoli S. (1979). Therapeutic Touch: Searching for evidence of physiologic change. *American Journal of Nursing, 79*(4), 660–662.

84. Quinn JF. (1988). Therapeutic touch as energy exchange: Replication and extension. *Nursing Science Quarterly, 2*(2), 79–87.

85. Smith DW & Broida JP. (2007). Pandimensional field pattern changes in healers and healees: Experiencing Therapeutic Touch. *Journal of Holistic Nursing, 25*(4), 217–225.

86. Turner J, Clark A, Gauthier D, & Williams M. (1998). The effect of Therapeutic Touch on pain and anxiety in burn patients. *Journal of Advanced Nursing, 28*(1), 10–20.

87. Zolfaghari M, Eybpoosh S, & Hazrati M. (2012). Effects of therapeutic touch on anxiety, vital signs, and cardiac dysrhythmia in a sample of Iranian women undergoing cardiac catheterization: A quasi-experimental study. *Journal of Holistic Nursing, 30*(4), 225–234.

88. Baldwin AL & Schwartz GE. (2006). Personal interaction with a Reiki practitioner decreases noise-induced microvascular damage in an animal model. *Journal of Alternative and Complementary Medicine, 12*(1), 15–22.

89. Baldwin AL, Wagers C, & Schwartz GE. (2008). Reiki improves heart rate homeostasis in laboratory rats. *Journal of Alternative and Complementary Medicine, 14*(4), 417–422.

90. Vanitallie TB. (2002). Stress: A risk factor for serious illness. *Metabolism, 51*(6 Suppl 1), 40–45.

91. Field T, Diego M, & Hernandez-Reif M (2010). Prenatal depression effects and interventions: A review. *Infant Behavioral Development, 33*(4), 409–418.

92. Field T. (2010). Pregnancy and labor massage. *Expert Review in Obstetrics and Gynecology, 5*(2), 177–181.

93. Field T, Hernandez-Reif M, Hart S., Theakson H, Schanberg S, & Kuhn C. (1999). Pregnant women benefit from massage therapy. *Journal of Psychosomatic Obstetrics and Gynecology, 20*(1), 31–38.

94. Field T, Diego M, Hernandez-Reif M, Schanberg S, & Kuhn C. (2004). Massage therapy effects on depressed pregnant women. *Journal of Psychosomatic Obstetrics and Gynecology, 25*(2), 115–122.

95. Field T, Diego M, Hernandez-Reif M, Deeds O, & Fiqueiredo B. (2009). Pregnancy massage reduces prematurity, low birthweight and postpartum depression. *Infant Behavioral Development, 32*(4), 454–460.

96. Chang MY, Wang SY, & Chen CH. (2002). Effects of massage on pain and anxiety during labour: A randomized controlled trial in Taiwan. *Journal of Advanced Nursing, 38*(1), 68–73.

97. Keenan P. (2000). Benefits of massage therapy and use of doula during labor and childbirth. *Alternative Therapies in Health and Medicine, 6*(1), 66–74.

98. Simkin P. (2012). Comfort in labor: How you can help yourself to a normal satisfying childbirth. Retrieved from: www.childbirthconnection.org. Accessed May 29, 2012.

99. Moyer CA, Seefeldt L, Mann ES, & Jackley LM. (2011). Does massage therapy reduce cortical? A comprehensive quantitative review. *Journal of Bodywork Movement Therapy, 15*(1), 3–14.

100. Kerr CE, Wasserman RH, & Moore CI. (2007). Cortical dynamics as a therapeutic mechanism for touch healing. *Journal of Alternative Complementary Medicine, 13*(1), 59–66.

101. National Center for Complementary and Alternative Medicine. (2008). What is complementary and alternative medicine? Retrieved from: http://nccam.nih.gov/heatlh/whatiscam. Accessed August 18, 2012.

102. Eisenberg DM, Cohen MH, Hrbek A, Grayzel J, Van Rompay MI, & Cooper RA. (2002). Credentialing complementary and alternative medical providers. *Annals of Internal Medicine, 137*(12), 965–973.

103. Minnesota Board of Nursing. (2003). Statement of accountability for utilization of integrative therapies in nursing practice. Retrieved from: mn.gov/health-licensing-boards/nursing. Accessed August 18, 2012.
104. Ananth S. (2011). 2010 Complementary and Alternative Medicine Survey of Hospitals. Samueli Institute. Retrieved from: http://www.samueliinstitute.org/File%20Library/Our%20 Research/OHE/CAM_Survey_2010_oct6.pdf. Accessed August 20, 2012.
105. American Massage Therapy Association. (2010). Code of Ethics. Retrieved from: www. amtamassage.org/About-AMTA/Core-Documents/Code-of-Ethics.html. Accessed August 20, 2012.
106. Burgan B. (2012). Taking charge of your health: Massage therapy. Retrieved from: www. takingcharge.csh.umn.edu/explore-healing-practices/massage-therapy. Accessed August 19, 2012.
107. Snyder M & Taniguki S, (2010). Massage therapy. In M Snyder & R Lindquist, eds., *Complementary and alternative therapies in nursing*, 6th ed., pp. 337–348. New York: Springer.
108. Massage: Bottom line monograph. (2012). Retrieved from: www.naturalstandard.com. Accessed July 25, 2012.
109. American Massage Therapy Association. (2012). 2012 massage therapy industry fact sheet. Retrieved from: www.amtamassage.org/articles/2/PressRelaease/detail/2545. Accessed August 19, 2012.
110. Touch Research Institute. (2012). History of Touch Research Institute. Retrieved from: www6. miami.edu/touch-research/About.html. Accessed August 20, 2012.
111. Moyer CA, Rounds J, & Hannum JW. (2004). A meta-analysis of massage therapy research. *Psychological Bulletin*, *130*(1), 13–18.
112. Ernst E. (1999). Abdominal massage therapy for chronic constipation: A systematic review of controlled clinical trials. *Forsch Komplementarmed*, *6*(3), 149–151.
113. Furlan AD, Imamura M, Dryden T, & Irvin E. (2009). Massage for low back pain: An updated systematic review within the framework of the Cochrane Back Review Group. *Spine*, *34*(16), 1669–1684.
114. Ezzo J, Donner T, Nickols D, & Cox M. (2001). Is massage useful in the management of diabetes: A systematic review. *Diabetes Spectrum*, *14*(4), 218–225.
115. Corbin L. (2005). Safety and efficacy of massage therapy for patients with cancer. *Cancer Control*, *12*(3), 158–164.
116. Ernst E. (2012). Massage therapy for cancer palliation and supportive care: A systematic review of randomized clinical trials. *Supportive Care in Cancer*, *17*(4), 333–337.
117. Jane SW, Wilkie D, Galluci BB, & Beaton RD. (2008). Systematic review of massage intervention for adult patients with cancer: A methodological perspective. *Cancer Nursing*, *31*(6), E24–E35.
118. Lee MS, Lee E-N, & Ernst E. (2011). Massage therapy for breast cancer patients: A systematic review. *Annals of Oncology*, *22*(6), 1459–1461.
119. Coelho HF, Boddy K, & Ernst E. (2008). Massage therapy for the treatment of depression: A systematic review. *International Journal of Clinical Practice*, *62*(2), 325–333.
120. Chaibi A, Tuchin PJ, & Russell MB. (2011). Manual therapies for migraine: A systematic review. *Journal of Headache Pain*, *12*(2), 127–133.
121. Sarris J & Byrne GJ. (2011). A systematic review of insomnia and complementary medicine. *Sleep Medicine Review*, *15*(2), 99–106.
122. Furlan AD, Imamura M, Dryden T, & Irvin E. (2008). Massage for low-back pain. *Cochrane Database of Systematic Reviews*, issue 4. Art. No.: CD001929. DOI: 10.1002/14651858.
123. Haraldson B, Gross A, Myers CD, Ezzo J, Morien A, Goldsmith CH, Peloso MJ, Bronfort G, & Cervical Overview Group. (2006). Massage for mechanical neck disorders. *Cochrane Database of Systematic Reviews*, issue 3. Art. No.: CD004871. DOI: 10.1002/14651858.

124. Smith CA, Collins CT, Cyna AM, & Crowther CA. (2006). Complementary and alternative therapies for pain management in labour. *Cochrane Database of Systematic Reviews* CD003521. DOI: 10.1002/14651858.

125. Smith CA, Levett KM, Collins CT, & Crowther CA. (2011). Relaxation techniques for pain management in labour. *Cochrane Database of Systematic Reviews*, issue 12. Art. No.: CD009514. DOI: 10.1002/14651858.

126. Smith CA, Levett KM, Collins CT, & Jones J. (2012). Massage, reflexology, and other manual methods for pain management in labor. *Cochrane Database of Systematic Reviews*, issue 2. Art. No.: CD009290. DOI: 10.1002/14651858.

127. Dennis CL & Allen K. (2008). Interventions (other than pharmacological, psychosocial or psychological) for treating antenatal depression. *Cochrane Database of Systematic Reviews*, issue 4. Art. No.: CD006795. DOI: 10.1002/14651858.

128. Hillier SL, Louw Q, Morris L, Uwimana J, & Statham S. (2010). Massage therapy for people with HIV/AIDS. *Cochrane Database of Systematic Reviews* CD007502. DOI: 10.1002/14651858.

129. Viggo Hansen N, Jorgensen T, & Ortenblad L. (2006). Massage and touch therapy for dementia. *Cochrane Database of Systematic Reviews* CD004989. DOI: 10.1002/14651858.

130. Ezzo J. (2007). What can be learned from Cochrane systematic reviews of massage that can guide future research? *Journal of Alternative and Complementary Medicine*, *13*(2), 291–295.

131. Goldstone LA. (2000). Massage as an orthodox medical treatment past and future. *Complementary Therapies in Nursing and Midwifery*, *6*(4), 169–175.

132. Miles P & True G. (2003). Reiki—review of a biofield therapy history, theory, practice, and research. *Alternative Therapies in Health and Medicine*, *9*(2), 62–72.

133. Jain S & Mills PJ. (2010). Biofield therapies: Helpful or full of hype? A best evidence synthesis. *International Journal of Behavioral Medicine*, *17*(1), 1–16.

134. Hover-Kramer D. (1996). *Healing touch: A resource for health care professionals.* New York: Delmar.

135. Macrae J. (1988). *Therapeutic Touch: A practical guide.* New York: Knopf.

136. Ringdahl D. (2010). Reiki. In M. Snyder & R. Lindquist (Ed). *Complementary and alternative therapies in nursing*, 6th ed., pp. 271–286. New York: Springer.

137. Engebretson J & Wardell D. (2007). Energy-based modalities. *Nursing Clinics of North America*, *42*(2), 243–259.

138. Anderson JG & Taylor AG. (2011). Biofield therapies in cardiovascular disease management: A brief review. *Holistic Nurisng Practice*, *25*(4), 199–204.

139. Davies E. (2001). My journey into the literature of Therapeutic Touch and Healing Touch: Part 1. *Australian Journal of Holistic Nursing*, *7*(2), 20–28.

140. Anderson JG & Taylor AG. (2012). Biofield therapies and cancer pain. *Clinical Journal of Oncology Nursing*, *16*(1), 43–48.

141. Eschiti VS. (2007). Healing touch: A low-tech intervention in high-tech settings. *Dimensions in Critical Care Nursing*, *26*(1), 9–14.

142. Fischer S & Johnson P. (1999). Therapeutic touch: A viable link to midwifery practice. *Journal of Nurse-Midwifery*, *44*(3), 300–309.

143. Todaro-Franceschi V. (2001). Energy: A bridging concept for nursing science. *Nursing Science Quarterly*, *14*(2), 132–140.

144. Rogers ME. (1970). *An introduction to the theoretical basis of nursing.* Philadelphia: Davis.

145. Herdtner S. (2000). Using Therapeutic Touch in nursing practice. *Orthopedic Nursing*, *19*(5), 77–82.

146. Kryak E & Vitale A. (2011). Reiki and its journey into a hospital setting. *Holistic Nursing Practice*, *25*(5), 238–245.

147. Meeham TC. (1993). Therapeutic touch and postoperative pain: A Rogerian research study. *Nursing Science Quarterly, 6*(2), 69–78.

148. Quinn JF & Strelkauskas AJ. (1993). Psychoimmunologic effects of Therapeutic Touch on practitioners and recently bereaved recipients: A pilot study. *ANS Advances in Nursing Science, 15*(4), 13–26.

149. Smith DW. (2000). Pattern changes in people experiencing Therapeutic Touch, phase 1. *Rogerian Nursing Science News, 12*(3), 3–4.

150. Thornton L. (1996). A study of Reiki using Rogers' science: Part II. *Rogerian Nursing Science News, 8*(4), 13–14.

151. Vitale AT. (2007). An integrative review of Reiki touch therapy research. *Holistic Nursing Practice, 21*(4), 167–179.

152. Nurse Healers—Professional Associates International. (2012). Definition of therapeutic touch. Retrieved from: therapeutic-touch.org. Accessed September 17, 2012.

153. Krieger D. (1979). *The Therapeutic Touch.* New York: Prentice Hall.

154. Krieger D. (1976). Healing by "laying-on" of hands as a facilitator of bioenergetic change: The response of in-vivo human hemoglobin. *Psychoenergetic Systems, 1,* 121–129.

155. Lin Y & Taylor AG. (1998). Effects of Therapeutic Touch in reducing pain and anxiety in an elderly population. *Integrative Medicine, 1*(4), 155–162.

156. Simington J & Laing G. (1993). Effects of Therapeutic Touch on anxiety in the institutionalized elderly. *Clinical Nursing Research, 2*(4), 438–451.

157. Gordon A, Merenstein JH, D'Amico F, & Hudgens D. (1998). The effects of Therapeutic Touch on patients with osteoarthritis of the knee. *Journal of Family Practice, 47*(4), 271–277.

158. Keller E & Bzdek VM. (1986). Effects of Therapeutic Touch on tension headache pain. *Nursing Research, 35*(2), 101–106.

159. Newshan G. (1989). Therapeutic Touch for symptom control for persons with AIDS. *Holistic Nursing Practice, 5*(4), 45–51.

160. Peck SD. (1998). The efficacy of Therapeutic Touch for improving functional ability in elders with degenerative arthritis. *Nursing Science Quarterly, 11*(3), 123–132.

161. Olson M, Sneed N, Bonadonna R, Ratliff J, & Dias J. (1992). Therapeutic Touch and post-Hugo stress. *Journal of Holistic Nursing, 10*(2), 120–136.

162. Peters RM. (1999). The effectiveness of Therapeutic Touch: A meta-analytic review. *Nursing Science Quarterly, 12*(1), 52–61.

163. Winstead-Frye P & Kijek J. (1999). An integrative review and meta-analysis of Therapeutic Touch research. *Alternative Therapies in Health and Medicine, 5*(6), 58–67.

164. Newshan G & Schuller-Civitella D. (2003). Large clinical study shows value of Therapeutic Touch program. *Holistic Nursing Practice, 17*(4), 189–192.

165. Aghabati N, Mohammadi E, & Pour EZ. (2010). The effect of Therapeutic Touch on pain and fatigue of cancer patients undergoing chemotherapy. *Evidence Based Complementary Alternative Medicine, 7*(3), 375–381.

166. Coakley AB & Barron AM. (2012). Energy therapies in oncology nursing. *Seminars in Oncology Nursing, 28*(1), 55–63.

167. Jackson E, Kelley M, McNeil P, Meyer E, Schlegel L, & Eaton M. (2008). Does Therapeutic Touch help reduce pain and anxiety in patients with cancer? *Clinical Journal of Oncology Nursing, 12*(1), 113–120.

168. Madrid MM, Barrett EA, & Winstead-Fry P. (2010). A study of the feasibility of introducing Therapeutic Touch into the operative environment with patients undergoing cerebral angiography. *Journal of Holistic Nursing, 28*(3), 168–174.

169. McCormick GL. (2009). Using non-contact Therapeutic Touch to manage post-surgical pain in the elderly. *Occupational Therapies International, 16*(1), 44–56.

170. Smyth PE. (2001). Therapeutic touch for a patient after a Whipple procedure. *Critical Care Nursing North America, 13*(3), 357–363.

171. Zare Z, Shahsavari H, & Moeini M. (2006). Effects of Therapeutic Touch on the vital signs of patients before coronary artery bypass graft surgery. *Iran Journal of Nurse Midwifery Research, 15*(1), 37–42.

172. O'Mathuna DP & Ashford RA. (2003). Therapeutic Touch for healing acute wounds. *Cochrane Database of Systematic Reviews*, issue 4. Art. No.: CD002766. DOI: 10.1002/14651858.

173. Robinson J, Biley FC, & Dolk H. (2007). Therapeutic touch for anxiety disorders. *Cochrane Database of Systematic Reviews*, issue 3. Art. No.: CD006240. DOI: 10.1002/14651858.

174. So P, Jiange Y, & Qin Y. (2008). Touch therapies for pain relief in adults. *Cochrane Database of Systematic Reviews*, issue 3. CD006535.

175. Bronfort G, Nilsson N, Haas M, Evans R, Goldsmith CH, Assendelft WJ, & Bouter LM. (2004). Non-invasive physical treatments for chronic-recurrent headache. *Cochrane Database of Systematic Reviews* CD001878. DOI: 10.1002/14651858.

176. Hutchison CP. (1999). Healing touch: An energetic approach. *American Journal of Nursing, 99*(4), 43–48.

177. Mentgen JL. (2001). Healing touch. *Nursing Clinics of North America, 36*(1), 143–158.

178. Taylor B & Lo R. (2001). The effects of Healing Touch on the coping ability, self esteem and general health of undergraduate nursing students. *Complementary Therapies in Nurse Midwifery, 7*(2), 122.

179. Wardell DW, Rintala DH, Duan Z, & Tan G. (2006). A pilot study of Healing Touch and progressive relaxation for chronic neuropathic pain in persons with spinal cord injury. *Journal of Holistic Nursing, 24*(4), 231–240.

180. Wardell DW & Weymouth KF. (2004). Review of studies of Healing Touch. *Journal of Nursing Scholarship, 36*(2), 147–154.

181. Krucoff MW, Crater SW, Green CL, Maas AC, Seskevich JE, Lane JD, Loeffler KA, Morris K, Bashore TM, & Koenig HG. (2001). Integrative noetic therapies as adjuncts to percutaneous intervention during unstable coronary syndrome: The monitoring and acutualization of noetic training (MANTRA) feasibility project. *American Heart Journal, 142*, 760–769.

182. Miles P & Ringdahl D. (2012). Taking charge of your health, Reiki. Retrieved from: www. takingcharge.csh.umn.edu/explore-healing-practices/reiki. Accessed August 19, 2012.

183. Assefi N, Bogart A, Goldberg J, & Buchwald D. (2008). Reiki for the treatment of fibromyalgia: A randomized controlled trial. *Journal of Alternative and Complementary Medicine, 14*(9), 1115–1122.

184. Bossi LM, Ott MJ, & DeCristofaro S. (2007). Reiki as a clinical intervention in oncology nursing practice. *Clinical Journal of Oncology Nursing, 12*(3), 489–494.

185. Burden B, Herron-Marx S, & Clifford C. (2005). The increasing use of Reiki as a complementary therapy in specialist palliative care. *International Journal of Palliative Care Nursing, 11*(5), 248–253.

186. Crawford SE, Leaver VW, & Mahoney SD. (2006). Using Reiki to decrease memory and behavior problems in cognitive impairment and mild Alzheimer's disease. *Journal of Alternative and Complementary Medicine, 12*(9), 911–913.

187. Dressen LJ & Singg S. (1998). Effects of Reiki on pain and selected affective and personality variables of chronically ill patients. *Subtle Energy and Energy Medicine, 9*, 51–82.

188. Gillipsie E, Gillipsie B, & Stevens M. (2007). Painful diabetic neuropathy: Impact of an alternative approach. *Diabetes Care, 30*(4), 999–1001.

189. Kennedy P. (2001). Working with survivors of torture in Sarajevo with Reiki. *Complementary Therapies in Nurse Midwifery, 7*(1), 4–7.

190. Lee MS. (2008). Is Reiki beneficial for pain management? *Focus on Alternative and Complementary Therapies*, *13*(2), 78–81.

191. Meland B. (2009). Effects of Reiki on pain and anxiety in the elderly diagnosed with dementia: A series of case reports. *Alternative Therapies in Health and Medicine*, *15*(4), 56–57.

192. Olson K, Hanson J, & Michaud M. (2003). A phase II trial of Reiki for the management of pain in advanced cancer patients. *Journal of Pain and Symptom Management*, *26*(5), 990–997.

193. Pocotte SL & Salvador D. (2008). Reiki as a rehabilitative nursing intervention for pain management: A case study. *Rehabilitation Nursing*, *33*(6), 231–232.

194. Shiftlett S, Nayak S, Bid S, Miles P, & Agostinelli M. (2002). Effect of Reiki treatments on functional recovery in patients in poststroke rehabilitation: A pilot study. *Journal of Alternative and Complementary Medicine*, *8*(6), 755–763.

195. Tsang K, Carlson L, & Olson K. (2007). Pilot crossover of Reiki versus rest for treating cancer-related fatigue. *Journal of Pain Symptom Management*, *6*(1), 25–35.

196. Herron-Marx S, Price-Knol F, Burden B, & Hicks C. (2008). A systematic review of the use of Reiki in health care. *Alternative and Complementary Therapies*, *14*(1), 37–42.

197. Lee MS, Pittler MH, & Ernst E. (2008). Effects of Reiki in clinical practice: A systematic review of randomized clinical trials. *International Journal of Clinical Practice*, *62*(6), 947–954.

198. vanderVaart S, Gijsen VM, de Wildt SN, & Koren G. (2009). A systematic review of the therapeutic effects of Reiki. *Journal of Alternative and Complementary Medicine*, *15*(11), 1157–1169.

199. Mansour A, Beuche M, Laing Leis A, & Nurse J. (1999). A study to test the effectiveness of placebo /Reiki standardization procedures developed for a planned Reiki efficacy study. *Journal of Alternative and Complementary Therapies*, *5*(2), 153–164.

200. Samarel N. (1992). The experience of receiving Therapeutic Touch. *Journal of Advanced Nursing*, *17*(6), 651–657.

201. Cuneo C, Cooper M, Drew C, Naoum-Heffernan C, Sherman T, & Walz K. (2011). The effect of Reiki on work-related stress of the registered nurse. *Journal of Holistic Nursing*, *29*(1), 33–43.

202. Diaz-Rodriquez L, Arroyo-Morales M, Cantarero-Villanueva I, Fernandez-Lao C, Polley M, & Fernandez-de-las-Penas C. (2011). The application of Reiki in nurses diagnosed with burnout syndrome has beneficial effects on concentration of salivary IgA and blood pressure. *Latin American Journal of Nursing*, *19*(5), 1132–1138.

203. Raingruber B & Robinson C. (2007). The effectiveness of Tai Chi, Yoga, meditation, and Reiki healing sessions in promoting health and enhancing problem solving abilities of registered nurses. *Issues in Mental Health Nursing*, *28*(10), 1141–1155.

204. Whelan KM & Wishnia GS. (2003). Reiki therapy: The benefits to a nurse/Reiki practitioner. *Holistic Nursing Practice*, *17*(4), 209–217.

205. Vitale A. (2009). Nurses' lived experiences of Reiki for self-care. *Holistic Nursing Practice*, *23*(3), 129–145.

206. Kemper K, Bulla S, Krueger D, Ott MJ, McCool JA, & Gardiner P. (2011). Nurses' experiences, expectations, and preferences for mind-body practices to reduce stress. *BMC Complementary Alternative Medicine*, *11*, 26.

207. Shang C. (2001). Emerging paradigms in mind-body medicine. *Journal of Alternative and Complementary Medicine*, *7*(1), 83–91.

208. Judith A. (1997). *Wheels of life: A users guide to the chakra system*. Woodbury, MN: Llewellyn Publications.

209. Maslow A. (1954). *Motivation and personality*. New York: Harper & Row.

210. Slater VE. (1995). Toward an understanding of energetic healing. Part 1: Energetic structures. *Journal of Holistic Nursing, 13*(3), 209–224.

211. American Medical Association. (2007). AMA code of medical ethics. Retrieved from: www. ama-assn.org/ama/pub/physician-resources/medical-ethics/code-medical-ethics.page. Accessed August 20, 2012.

212. American Nurses Association. (2001). Code of ethics for nurses with interpretive statements. Retrieved from: nursingworld.org/MainMenuCategories/EthicsStandards/CodeofEthicsforNurses/Code-of-Ethics.pdf. Accessed August 20, 2012.

213. DONA International. (2012). Code of ethics for birth doulas. Retrieved from: www.dona.org/aboutus/code_of_ethics_birth.php. Accessed August 20, 2012.

214. International Confederation of Midwives. (2008). International code of ethics for midwives. Retrieved from: www.internationalmidwives.org/Portals/5/2011/International%20of%20 Ethics%20for%20Midwives%20jt%202011rev.pdf. Accessed August 20, 2010.

215. Midwives Alliance of North America. (2010). MANA statement of values and ethics. Retrieved from: mana.org/valuesethics.html. Accessed August 20, 2012.

216. Healing Touch International. (2006). Code of ethics and standards of practice for Healing Touch. Retrieved from: www.healingtouchinternational.org/?option=com_content&task=view&id=26&Itemid=58. Accessed August 20, 2012.

217. International Association of Reiki Professionals. (2010). Code of ethics for Reiki practitioners and Reiki master teachers. Retrieved from: www.iarp.org/IARPReikiCodeofEthics.html.

218. International Center for Reiki Training. (2012). ICRT Reiki membership code of ethics. Retrieved from: www.reikimembership.com/Code_of_Ethics.aspx. Accessed August 20, 2012.

219. Nurse Healers—Professional Associates International. (2007). Unified code of ethics for healers. Retrieved from: 222.councilforhealing.org/Ethics.html. Accessed August 20, 2012.

220. Hover-Kramer D. (2011). *Creating healing relationships: Professional standards for energy therapy practitioners.* Santa Rosa, CA: Energy Psychology Press. http://mn.gov/health-licensing-boards/images/Integrative_Therapies_statement.pdf.

221. Sawyer J. (1998). The first Reiki practitioner in our OR. *AORN Journal, 67*(3), 679–677.

222. Schiff E, Ben-Arye E, Shilo M, Levy M, Schachter L, Weitchner N, Golan O, & Stone J. (2010). Development of ethical rules for boundaries of touch in complementary medicine—outcomes of a Delphi process. *Complementary Therapies in Clinical Practice, 16*(4), 194–197.

223. Simkin PP & O'Hara M. (2002). Nonpharmocologic relief of pain during labor: Systematic reviews of five methods. *American Journal of Obstetrics and Gynecology, 186*(5 Suppl. Nature), S131–159.

224. Birch ER. (1986). The experience of touch received during labor: Postpartum perceptions of therapeutic value. *Journal of Nurse-Midwifery, 31*(6), 270–276.

225. Penny KS. (1979). Postpartum perceptions of touch received during labor. *Research in Nursing Health, 2*(1), 9–16.

226. Leslile MS, Romano A, & Wooley D. (2007). Step 7: Educates staff in nondrug methods of pain relief and does not promote use of analgesic, anesthetic drugs. *Journal of Perinatal Education, Suppl, 16*(1), 65S–73S.

227. Huntley AL, Coon JT, & Ernst E. (2004). Complementary and alternative medicine for labor pain: A systematic review. *American Journal of Obstetrics and Gynecology, 191*(1), 36–44.

228. Field T, Hernandez-Reif M, Taylor S, Quintino O, & Burman I. (1997). Labor pain is reduced by massage therapy. *Journal of Psychosomatic Obstetrics and Gynecology, 18*(4), 286–291.

229. Chang MY, Chen CH, & Huang KF. (2006). A comparison of massage effects on labor pain using the McGill Pain Questionaire. *Journal of Nursing Research, 14*(3), 190–197.

230. Mortazavi SH, Khaki S, Moradi R, Heidari K, & Vasegh Rahimparvar SF. (2012). Effects of massage and presence of attendant on pain, anxiety, and satisfaction during labor. *Archives of Gynecology and Obstetrics*, *286*(1), 19–23.

231. Kimber L, McNabb M, McCourt C, Haines A, & Brocklevorst P. (2008). Massage or music for pain relief in labour: A pilot randomized placebo controlled trial. *European Journal of Pain*, *12*(8), 961–969.

232. Marsh-Prelesnik J. (2009). Calming the tumultuous storm: Alleviating stress and pain with gentle touch. *Midwifery Today International Midwife*, *92*, 24–25.

233. Mills J. (2003). Reiki in hospitals: How I introduced Reiki treatments into my obstetrics and gynecologic practice. *Reiki News*, *2*(2), 16–21.

234. Rakestraw T. (2009). Reiki: The energy doula. *Midwifery Today International Midwife*, *92*, 16–17.

235. Peck S. (2008). Integrating CAM therapies into NP practice. *American Journal for Nurse Practitioners*, *12*(5), 10–18.

236. Bishop JL, Northstone K, Green JR, & Thompson EA. (2011). The use of complementary and alternative medicine in pregnancy: Data from the Avon Longitudinal Study of Parents and Children (ALSPAC). *Complementary Therapies in Medicine*, *19*, 303–310.

237. Gaffney L & Smith C. (2004). The views of pregnant women towards the use of complementary therapies and medicines. *Birth Issues*, *13*, 43–50.

238. Adams J, Liu C-W, Sibbritt D, Broom A, Wardle J, & Homer C. (2010). Attitudes and referral practices of maternity care professionals with regard to complementary and alternative medicine: An integrative review. *Journal of Advanced Nursing*, *67*(3), 472–483.

239. Hall HG, Griffiths DL, & McKenna LG. (2011). The use of complementary and alternative medicine by pregnant women: A literature review. *Midwifery*, *27*(6), 817–824.

240. Bishop F & Lewith G. (2010). Who uses CAM? A narrative review of demographic characteristics and health factors associated with CAM use. *Evidence-Based Complementary and Alternative Medicine*, *7*(1), 11–28.

241. Skouteris H, Wetheim E, Rallis S, Paxton S, Kelly L, & Milgrom J. (2008). Use of complementary and alternative medicines by a sample of Australian women during pregnancy. *Australian and New Zealand Journal of Obstetrics and Gynecology*, *48*(4), 384–390.

242. Wang S, Dezinno P, Fermo L, William K, Caldwell-Andrews, AA, Braveman F, & Kain ZN. (2005). Complementary and alternative medicine for low-back pain in pregnancy: A cross-sectional survey. *Journal of Alternative and Complementary Medicine*, *11*(3), 459–464.

243. Collinge W, Kahn J, Yarnold P, Bauer-Wu S, & McCorkle R. (2007). Couples and cancer: Feasibility of brief instruction in massage and touch therapy to build caregiver efficacy. *Journal of Social Integrative Oncology*, *5*(4), 147–154.

244. Raisler J. (1999). Complementary and alternative healing in midwifery care. *Journal of Nurse-Midwifery*, *44*(3), 189–191.

245. Larden CN, Palmer ML, & Janssen P. (2004). Efficacy of Therapeutic Touch in treating pregnant inpatients who have a chemical dependency. *Journal of Holistic Nursing*, *22*(4), 320–332.

246. Kiernan J. (2002). The experience of Therapeutic Touch in the lives of five postpartum women. *American Journal of Maternal Child Nursing*, *27*(1), 47–53.

247. Alandydy P & Alandydy K. (1999). Using Reiki to support surgical patients. *Journal of Nursing Care Quality*, *13*(4), 89–91.

248. Frank LS, Frank JL, March D, Makari-Judson G, Barham RB, & Mertens WC. (2007). Does Therapeutic Touch ease the discomfort or distress of patients undergoing sterotactic core breast biopsy? A randomized clinical trial. *Pain Medicine*, *8*(5), 419–424.

249. Hardwick ME, Pulido PA, & Adelson WS. (2012). Nursing intervention using Healing Touch in bilateral total knee arthroplasty. *Orthopedic Nursing, 31*(1), 5–11.

250. Hulse RS, Stuart-Shor EM, & Russo J. (2010). Endoscopic procedure with a modified Reiki intervention. *Gastroenterology Nursing, 33*(1), 20–26.

251. Potter P. (2007). Breast biopsy and distress: Feasibility of testing a Reiki intervention. *Journal of Holistic Nursing, 25*(4), 238–248.

252. Simmons D, Chabal C, Griffith J, Rausch M, & Steele B. (2004). A clinical trial of distraction techniques for pain and anxiety control during cataract surgery. *Insight, 29*(4), 13–16.

253. Wang HL & Keck JF. (2004). Foot and hand massage as an intervention for postoperative pain. *Pain Management Nursing, 5*(2), 59–65.

254. Wirth DP, Brenlan DR, Levine RJ, & Rodriguez CM. (1993). The effect of complementary healing therapy on postoperative pain after surgical removal of impacted third molar teeth. *Complementary Therapies in Medicine, 1*(3), 133–138.

255. Becker NB. (2000). Healing journey spans high-tech, high-touch at Hawaiian hospital. *Alternative Therapies in Health and Medicine, 6*(2), 99–100.

256. Dooley M. (2006). Complementary therapy and obstetrics and gynecology: A time to integrate. *Current Opinions in Obstetrics and Gynecology, 18*(6), 648–652.

257. Fortney L, Rakel D, Rindfleisch JA, & Mallory J. (2010). Introduction to integrative primary care: The health-oriented clinic. *Primary Care, 37*(1), 1–12.

258. Hemphill L & Kemp J. (2000). Implementing a therapeutic massage program in a tertiary and ambulatory care VA setting: The healing power of touch. *Nursing Clinics in North America, 35*(2), 489–497.

259. Ernst LS & Ferrer L. (2012). Reflection of a 7-year patient care program: Implementing and sustaining an integrative hospital program. *Journal of Holistic Nursing, 27*(4), 276–281.

260. Newshan G & Schuller-Civitella D. (2003). Large clinical study shows value of Therapeutic Touch program. *Holistic Nursing Practice, 17*(4), 189–192.

261. Knutson L & Weiss P. (2009). Exploring integrative medicine: The story of a large, urban, tertiary care hospital. In B Dossey & L Keegan, ed., *Holistic nursing: A Handbook for Practice*, 6th ed., pp. 523–529. Sudbury, MA: Jones & Bartlett.

262. Engebretson J. (2002). Hands-on: The persistent metaphor in nursing. *Holistic Nursing Practice, 16*(4), 20–35.

Chapter 9

Water immersion for labor and birth

Michelle R. Collins and Dawn M. Dahlgren-Roemmich

Key points

- Water immersion is therapeutic and can help relieve discomfort during pregnancy, labor, and birth.
- There is no evidence of an increase in adverse effects of water immersion in labor or water birth for newborns or mothers.
- Women experience increased relaxation using water immersion during labor and report increased satisfaction with the labor and birth experience.
- When planning to add water immersion and water birth to clinical practice, involve all labor unit staff in the process.
- Women with a singleton pregnancy, at least 37 weeks gestation, spontaneous labor, Category 1 fetal heart rate tracing, and normal maternal vital signs are good candidates for water immersion.
- Women requiring continuous EFM may be candidates for water labor/birth if telemetric monitoring is available.

Water . . . this is where he came from, and what he's known all his life. It's gentle, it's familiar. It is the very familiarity that in the end will completely calm him. It will be like meeting an old friend when one is far from home.

Frederick Leboyer

Introduction

The use of warm water is a common comfort measure employed in many situations, whether a warm compress for a sore muscle or a luxurious soak in a hot tub after a long hike or day of skiing. Water immersion for labor and birth was first used in the United States in the 1980s and continues to increase in popularity among women and clinicians. In this chapter we provide a brief history of water birth, review the research evidence to support its use, and provide practical guidance and suggestions for those who wish to begin offering this choice to women in their birthing units.

Supporting a Physiologic Approach to Pregnancy and Birth: A Practical Guide, First Edition.
Edited by Melissa D. Avery.
© 2013 John Wiley & Sons, Inc. Published 2013 by John Wiley & Sons, Inc.

History

The first documented water birth occurred in 1805 in Haut Languedoc, France. The story goes that a young woman had been laboring for 48 hours when her obstetrician consulted midwives who recommended she try the bath to help with the strength of her contractions and aid her slow progress. Upon being immersed in the water, she quickly began pushing and birthed her baby, who let out a hearty cry [1]!

Modern-day pioneers of water birth were drawn to the practice for a variety of reasons. Igor Charkovsky, a Russian swim coach and scientist, was attracted to water birth primarily for the effect on the baby. Charkovsky gained a somewhat notorious reputation for assisting women giving birth in such water environments as the frigid Crimean Sea. Film footage of Charkovsky encouraging submersion of infants into freezing lake water did not help his credibility, though his contribution to the introduction of water immersion for labor and birth cannot be understated [2]. At the same time as Charkovsky was introducing water birth in Russia, Frederick Leboyer was introducing the concept of a warm bath for the baby after the birth. His supposition was that newborns required warm water to support the transition from intrauterine to extrauterine life, and that any birth trauma would be diminished by the effects of water and massage. Leboyer is best known for his 1975 book *Birth without Violence* [1,3].

Michel Odent, considered the French pioneer of water birth, came to the idea of using water for labor after reading Leboyer's book. Odent arrived at the Centre Hospitalier General de Pithiviers in 1962 to direct a surgical unit and was consistently called upon by the midwives to perform cesarean sections or forceps deliveries. At Pithiviers, he redecorated the birth unit with warm colors and installed birth pools in each room. Intending to use the tubs only for labor, he quickly discovered that women laboring in the tub did not want to leave the water to give birth and eventually acknowledged the benefit of actually giving birth in the water. As a result, women began to be encouraged by staff to not only labor but also give birth in the water [3].

A champion of water birth in the United States was obstetrician Michael Rosenthal, who founded the Family Birthing Center in Upland, California, in 1985, the first institutional setting in the United States to offer water birth [2]. Barbara Harper, registered nurse, certified doula, and childbirth educator, has also been an American pioneer of water birth, having been instrumental in assisting birth centers and hospitals throughout the United States to initiate water birth programs. Harper has been invaluable in establishing guidelines for water birth that have been used nationwide as the basis for many institutions' water birth programs.

Research

Pregnant women are drawn to warm water throughout their pregnancies. Water can be helpful in relieving many common discomforts of pregnancy [4]. Modern women seek out birth environments that offer choices they want including warm water immersion with the option to give birth in water [5–7]. The Cochrane review of immersion in water in labor and birth [8] included twelve trials (3,243 women): eight trials evaluated the use of water in first stage of labor only, one examined early versus late immersion in the first stage of labor, two examined the use of immersion in the first and second stages, and another involved the use of water for second stage labor only. No studies evaluated the issue of variance between types of baths/pools, nor the management of third stage of labor in water. Few studies have examined the physiologic benefits of warm water immersion.

Evaluating existing research and designing new studies examining water immersion and water birth can be difficult. First, much of the existing literature does not clearly delineate the activity of laboring in water versus actually giving birth in the water. Second, there are no regulations that require institutions offering water immersion and/or birth to keep or report statistics related to water immersion and/or birth.

Infant outcomes

The recent Cochrane review concluded that "there is no evidence of increased adverse effects to the fetus/neonate or woman from laboring in water or water birth." The review further acknowledged that those studies exploring the safety of neonates during water immersion and birth were variable in design and outcome measures, increasing the difficulty of drawing valid conclusions. Additional research is needed to more accurately assess the effect of immersion in water on neonatal morbidity.

Individual papers have demonstrated beneficial outcomes for infants born in water. A descriptive report from England reported that of 343 babies born in water, 94% had Apgar scores of 7 or greater at 1 minute and 99.7% had Apgar scores of 7 or greater at 5 minutes [9,10]. Anecdotally, the Family Birth Center in Upland, California, reported that of 1,400 women who labored in water, and 679 who gave birth in water, none of the infants had an Apgar score of less than 5 at 1 minute and none had a score less than 7 at 5 minutes [9]. A recent report from New Zealand described four infants with poor neonatal outcomes related to freshwater aspiration after water births. Little documentation was provided about the mother's prenatal care, labor/birth history, or the type of neonatal care unit available to the infants; important information when interpreting the results in such case reports [11]. Infant Apgar scores, infection rates, and NICU admission rates have been shown to be similar in studies comparing water birth and conventional birth [6,12–14].

Maternal outcomes

Women report multiple benefits of giving birth in water, including a high level of satisfaction with their birth, enhanced ability to achieve relaxation during labor, a feeling of being sheltered or protected by the surrounding water, and an improved ability to move about freely while in the water, compared to being out of the water [15]. Other women describe that water immersion gives them a greater sense of control over their birth experience, possibly contributing to greater emotional well-being in the postpartum period [4]. The Cochrane review outcomes for water immersion in first stage of labor include significant reduction in the use of epidural/spinal/paracervical analgesia/

anesthesia; reduction in duration of the first stage of labor (~32 minutes); no difference in assisted vaginal deliveries, cesarean section, use of oxytocin, perineal trauma, or maternal infection; and no differences for Apgar score less than 7 at 5 minutes, NICU admissions, or neonatal infection rates [16]. Of three trials included in the review that compared water immersion during second stage labor with no immersion at all, one showed a significantly higher level of satisfaction with the birth experience.

The gate theory of pain and water immersion

The gate control theory of pain is helpful in understanding how hydrotherapy may relieve the pain of labor. Warm water stimulates large, high-velocity afferent nerve fibers, blocking smaller, slower pain fiber impulses, thus reducing the amount of painful stimuli reaching the reticular activating system in the cerebral cortex through the "gate" [17,18]. Water immersion has been hypothesized to reduce the use of recumbent labor positions, encouraging uterine perfusion, muscle relaxation, and pain relief, and consequently decreasing catecholamine levels, maternal anxiety, and fatigue [9,19].

Therapeutic effects of water

Five basic principles described below underlie the positive physiologic effects of immersion in warm water.

Buoyancy

An individual immersed in water is essentially buoyed by a counterforce that supports the submerged body against the downward pull of gravity. A direct result of buoyancy is that the body immersed in water "appears" to weigh less, and in fact, the greater the depth that the body is immersed in water, the greater the apparent weight loss. For example, a woman submerged to hip height in water weighs 50% of her weight on land, whereas a woman submerged to her neck weighs 90% less under water than what she weighs on land. Body fat is more buoyant than lean body tissue, thus women have a greater buoyant effect than their male counterparts [20]. This buoyant effect undoubtedly accounts for women's feelings of weightlessness, contributing to greater freedom of movement in the water.

Specific gravity and density

Water has a specific gravity of 1.0, and anything with a lower specific gravity will float when placed into water. A specific gravity greater than 1.0 will cause an object to sink. The average human body has a specific gravity of 0.974, indicating that most individuals will float when submerged in water [1,20]. Persons with a very lean body mass will not float as readily as those with more adipose tissue. Adipose stores are increased in pregnancy, contributing to a pregnant woman's tendency to float. Floating enhances a woman's ability to relax, removing much of the weight burden of her limbs and organs off the muscles and body frame.

Hydrostatic pressure

When a body is submerged in water, the force exerted to all submerged body surfaces equalizes to the density of the water in which those surfaces are submerged. As a result, the physiologic response to the hydrostatic force is to remobilize the blood to direct it to the body's surface [21]. Therapeutically, this translates to the sensation of support of all of the body surfaces and a decrease in muscular tension.

Specific heat

Water has the capacity to both hold and transfer heat. The specific heat of water is higher than most substances; thus water has great capability to hold and maintain its temperature, as well as to transfer that heat. A high specific heat also means there will be less alteration in water temperature, compared to other substances, and water will remain at a more constant temperature, making it an ideal medium for transfer of heat to skin and body tissues [21].

Thermal effect

This *thermal effect* of warm water causes peripheral vasodilation and resultant decreased vascular resistance. Because of these hemodynamic changes, the submerged woman may exhibit a slight increase in blood pressure soon after getting into the tub or pool. However, the body adapts to the water environment with a resulting overall reduction in blood pressure [21,22]. Hypothesized as a result of the synergistic effect of these five principles, water immersion in labor has been shown to result in reduced use of epidural analgesia and intravenous pain medication [1,6,8,12,23].

Theoretical risks to mother during water immersion and/or water birth

Infection, hemorrhage, emboli, and reduced strength of uterine contractions are considered theoretical risks because quality research has not demonstrated their occurrence as a result of water immersion and/or water birth.

Infection

Maternal infection during water labor and birth is a complication that occurs infrequently [9,10,14,24,25]. Few case reports of infection after water birth have been published. In a classic descriptive study published in 1960, tampons were placed per vagina in pregnant and laboring women who then bathed in an iodine bath. On postbath measurement, no iodine was found in the tampons of women in either group, demonstrating that bath water did not enter the vagina [26]. A study comparing infection rates among women birthing in water compared to those birthing out of water demonstrated that chorioamnionitis and endometritis were related to length of time of rupture of membranes, the number of vaginal examinations, the length of labor, and incidence of operative birth, and not to water immersion during labor [27].

Hemorrhage

Rates of hemorrhage have actually been shown to be lower for water births than for births occurring out of water; however, further research is needed [28,29]. Postpartum hemorrhage is of particular interest because third stage following water birth is typically managed expectantly rather than using an active approach.

Emboli

Suggested as a potential risk of water birth, where bath water could potentially enter the circulatory system from inside the uterus at the moment of placental separation and become an embolus, there has never been a documented case reported. Studies that have demonstrated that bath water does not enter the vagina strengthen the argument that an embolism caused by water immersion is highly improbable [30].

Reduction in uterine contractile activity

Some early papers reported that women entering the water at less than 5 centimeters cervical dilatation or those who remain in the water for longer than 2 hours may experience a reduction in uterine activity [25,28]. Cluett et al. [8] conducted the first trial evaluating the impact of water immersion in labor for nulliparous women with dystocia. The authors found that compared with the women who underwent standard labor augmentation (defined as artificial rupture of membranes and oxytocin), the women treated with water immersion had lower rates of epidural anesthesia use, decreased pain scores, and increased satisfaction rates. Operative birth rates were similar between the two groups, and the overall length of labor was not significantly different. Cluett hypothesized that immersing a woman in water may actually have the opposite effect of diminishing labor efficacy. Endorphin release resulting from physical relaxation in the water is a possible mechanism. Theoretically, decreased catecholamine production following relaxation may actually enhance rather than diminish uterine activity.

Risks to baby

The risks listed for the newborn are not considered theoretical, similar to those proposed for mothers immersed in water. Many of the fetal/neonatal risks that will be discussed have been documented in case reports or studies. Those that have been hypothesized, but not substantiated, will be highlighted.

Fetal hyperthermia

Intrauterine fetal temperature is 0.5–1.0°C higher than the average body temperature of 37°C. A woman immersed in water can easily cool down if she becomes overheated by getting out of the tub. Given the surface area of the skin, standing up out of the tub will allow evaporation to occur and quickly cool the mother. The fetus, however, must decrease its temperature via its own circulatory system, which takes markedly longer than the process of cooling the mother. Fetal tachycardia is typically observed in cases of fetal hyperthermia; fetal deaths and cases of fetal encephalopathy resulting from fetal hyperthermia have been reported in the literature [31,32].

Infection

Cases of neonatal pseudomonas, with the identical strain cultured from the birth tub, have been reported [33]. One case of lethal *Legionella* infection following home water birth in a spa-type tub has been reported from Japan [34]. Spa-type tubs, where water actually circulates through the tub jets, are much more difficult to clean thoroughly and may harbor reservoirs of bacteria. Therefore, spa-type tubs are not recommended for water labor or birth. Zanetti-Dallenbach and colleagues [35] evaluated colonization rates of infants born in water to group B streptococcus (GBS)-positive mothers. Although the water was cultured with high rates of GBS, those infants born in the water were less frequently colonized with GBS than those born to GBS-positive mothers out of the water. The researchers proposed a possible "wash out" effect of the water over the fetus as the baby was born and was brought from the uterus to the mother's arms.

Polycythemia

One recorded case of polycythemia occurring after water birth has been published in the literature [28]. There is no further evidence that neonatal polycythemia is a common occurrence, or that it is problematic for the baby if it does occur, following birth in water.

Water aspiration, drowning

Arguably the most frequently verbalized concern about water birth is the potential for neonatal drowning. Understanding the normal physiologic process of neonatal respiratory adaptation is imperative to comprehending why drowning is not a realistic concern for the low-risk, uncompromised neonate. First, many physiologic factors inhibit fetal breathing efforts during labor. Prostaglandin E2 production increases sharply approximately 48 hours prior to the onset of labor. Coupled with the increase in production, the placental release of E2 and adenosine hinder fetal breathing efforts [36].

The neonatal dive reflex is another important factor to consider when discussing the potential for neonatal drowning. Harding, Johnson, and McClelland [37] investigated the fetal and newborn breathing response using fetal lambs. The researchers isolated chemoreceptors on the laryngeal mucosa of the fetal sheep that analyze and interpret the content of any fluid passing over them. When a nonphysiologic fluid was detected, the dive reflex was enabled, in other words the glottis closed and the fetus swallowed. Physiologic fluids (species-specific milk, isotonic glucose solutions, gastric solutions, and species saliva) did not trigger the dive reflex, while water, non-species-specific milk, progressively dilute sodium chloride solutions, isotonic alkalis, and ammonia triggered the dive reflex. It is crucial to note, however, that the dive reflex can be overridden by fetal hypoxia, thus allowing fetal aspiration of nonphysiologic substances [1,32,36].

Finally, neonatal breathing is initiated after birth when the neonate's temperature cools as little as 1–2°C. Therefore, birth into water with the temperature comparable to body temperature actually contributes to the inhibition of infant breathing. Healthy neonates begin breathing when they are brought to the surface of the water and exposed to the cooler air temperature [36].

Cord avulsion or snapping of the umbilical cord

Although the phenomenon of cord snapping at various sites has been documented to have occurred during water birth in case reports [38], careful attention to slow and deliberate lifting of the neonate from the water should eliminate accidental separation of an umbilical cord that may be unusually short. As with birth occurring out of water, movement of neonate too rapidly from vagina to mother's arms, without attention to a potentially short umbilical cord, could result in cord breakage.

Incorporating water birth into practice

Staff involvement

A critical step in incorporating water birth into clinical practice is to begin with discussions among other key care providers involved with one's clientele, that is, obstetricians, pediatricians, infection control specialists, nursing staff, administration, housekeeping, and maintenance staff. It is crucial that all of those involved in caring for clients choosing water birth have the opportunity to verbalize any concerns or questions. Another helpful step is to complete a needs assessment of one's clientele including women's thoughts, opinions, and requests related to their preferences within the birth environment. Water birth may not be a familiar practice to many clinicians or administrative or support staff. Providing some key resources (Cochrane review, individual good-quality research reports) can help staff understand potential benefits of water birth.

Nursing staff may be concerned that offering water birth may impact their workload. Time to fill, empty, and clean tubs as well as management of birth complications in the tub will likely top their list of concerns. Assure nursing staff that although there are subtle differences in caring for women choosing water birth, they will still employ the same core labor and delivery basic nursing skills utilized while caring for women birthing outside of the water. Having staff "buy in" prior to initiation of a water birth program will help ensure success.

Equipment

Birthing unit staff have the option of choosing from free-standing permanent tubs or tubs that can be moved from room to room. Permanently placed tubs connected into the room's plumbing have the advantage of not having to be filled or drained with hoses. Movable tubs on wheels, however, may allow greater access, as they can be shifted to a room with a women desiring to use the tub. Nonpermanent tubs made of plastic or like materials that can be set up and taken down multiple times are another option.

An advantage of nonpermanent tubs is that they are much less expensive than the permanent tubs or those on wheels. This can be an ideal starting point if the labor unit staff is unsure of consumer response to water birth. Purchase of a less expensive model allows the unit to "dip their toe" into water birth slowly, as well as have a tub that can be taken down and stored on the unit inconspicuously when not in use. A disadvantage of plastic pools is that there is a risk of puncture to the tub, and hence a greater risk of a leak causing a safety hazard. Portable tubs can be a short-term solution until either the bathrooms or the birthing rooms can be remodeled with permanent tubs.

Other necessary equipment includes a waterproof Doppler device, waterproof personal protective equipment, preferably shoulder-length gloves (like those used by veterinary professionals), aquarium nets to skim debris from the water, single-use floating water thermometers, and preferably a blanket warmer nearby for supplying women with warmed blankets once they step out of the tub after their birth.

Infection control

Infection control policies should be meticulously designed and followed closely. If hoses are utilized for filling and draining the tub, separate hoses must be used for filling than those that are used for draining, to prevent contamination. A protocol for regular culturing of tubs and hoses must also be included in the unit policy. A very methodical cleaning process must be detailed in the policy, and monitoring must be in place to ensure that the process is followed meticulously after every water birth. The policy should delineate clearly which tasks fall to nursing personnel and which to housekeeping staff, so there is no confusion about one's role in tub cleaning, with all infection control procedures completed according to guidelines.

Candidate selection for water immersion/water birth

Sample criteria

While there is no national or international standard of agreement on the appropriate candidate, we propose sample criteria for selection of women that may be included in the unit policy. These include singleton pregnancy, 37 or greater weeks gestation, established Category I electronic fetal monitor (EFM) tracing, maternal vital signs in normal range, and spontaneous versus augmented or induced labor. If there is the ability to monitor contractions continuously then Pitocin may be considered for the woman using the tub.

Contraindications

Again, a single standard does not exist; institutions will want to examine the protocols of several established water birth units and determine guidelines for the individual unit. Contraindications may include gestation less than 37 weeks, multifetal gestation, prior cesarean birth, maternal fever (defined as temperature greater than 38°C) or signs of infection, Category II or III EFM tracing, epidural or spinal anesthesia, or vaginal bleeding that is heavier than a normal bloody show in labor. Evidence of a communicable vaginal, blood, or skin infection, keeping in mind that GBS-positive status is not a contraindication, may also be included. Herpes simplex, human immunodeficiency virus, or hepatitis B should be considered contraindications to water immersion or birth. Thick meconium stained amniotic fluid (MSAF) has also been proposed as a contraindication, primarily because MSAF may be the indicator for fetal distress. High body mass index (BMI) has been considered a contraindication for water immersion/water birth. Advocates cite a risk of complication at birth for women with a high BMI, purporting that being in the tub may prevent necessary emergency access or delay in emergency treatment if removal from the tub takes some time. Another reason high BMI has been cited as a contraindication is the possible risk of injury to staff attempting to lift the woman from the tub in the event of emergency. Proponents of women with a high BMI considered as candidates for water immersion/water birth cite the ease of movement in the water experienced by women who essentially become weightless during submersion. Units can consider having emergency lift equipment (i.e., Hoyer or similar lifts) available tubside to assist the woman who needs a quick exit.

Some conditions proposed as contraindications reflect situations that require EFM. Waterproof telemetric monitoring systems are available. A labor unit with a system to continually monitor women in the tub may consider offering water immersion for women with pitocin augmentation or a trial of labor after cesarean. The availability of a telemetric fetal monitoring system on the unit should be considered when determining contraindications to water immersion.

Considerations when developing water immersion guidelines

The topics below are helpful to review and keep in mind when first developing water immersion/water birth guidelines.

Consent for water immersion and/or water birth

Some labor units offering hydrotherapy for labor and/or birth require a written formal consent signed by the woman prior to entering the water. While this practice is not widespread, an alternate perspective is that water immersion is a nonpharmacologic mode of pain relief similar to ambulating, getting into the shower, sitting on the commode or birth ball, using aromatherapy or music, or having a doula present. Written consent is not obtained prior to use of those nonpharmacologic pain relief methods and therefore most likely unnecessary when water is employed as the therapeutic modality. Some unit policies require written consent for water birth and not for water immersion during labor, acknowledging that a woman's written consent serves as documentation that her provider has discussed both the benefits and risks associated with water birth.

Parameters for water temperature

There is no agreement in the literature of the exact preferred water temperature. However, most unit guidelines suggest somewhere in the range of 35–38°C, close to maternal body temperature [32,39]. The rationale for maintaining the water temperature within such a strict range is that the core temperature of the fetus is 0.5–1°C higher than the maternal temperature. As discussed previously, a woman who gets overheated in the water can quickly decrease her core temperature simply by getting out of the water while the fetus must cool down slowly via the mechanism of the circulatory system. For the overheated fetus, fetal hyperthermia can ensue and the fetus with limited reserve may exhibit signs of distress [1]. Water that is too cool will likely be uncomfortable for the laboring woman; water too warm may result in fetal hyperthermia.

Parameters for monitoring water and maternal temperature

Timing for checking water and maternal temperature varies in the literature from monitoring every 30 minutes to every 2 hours. The rationale for close attention to maternal and water temperature allows that mild temperature elevations in the laboring woman will be detected early enough to cool her before the fetus can become hyperthermic.

Method of fetal surveillance

Women who are candidates for water immersion and birth are generally also candidates for intermittent auscultation according to Association of Women's Health, Obstetric and Neonatal Nurses (AWHONN) and American Congress of Obstetricians and Gynecologists (ACOG) guidelines. Exclusions would be those women with a prior cesarean section desiring a planned vaginal birth, or in the case of pitocin augmentation wherein telemetric EFM is unavailable.

Vaginal examinations

The policy will address the method for performing vaginal examinations of the laboring woman. There is no reason that the examination cannot be done in the tub; asking the woman to get out of the tub for vaginal examinations represents an unnecessary annoyance for her.

Intravenous access

Submersion in water, with its resulting mobilization of blood to internal organs, causes a resultant diuresis. Thus it is imperative that women are encouraged to take oral fluids generously. Water immersion in and of itself is not a requisite for IV access. If a woman requires IV access for other reasons (antibiotic treatment of GBS, for example), the site can be easily covered to maintain dryness while in the tub.

Analgesic use in the tub

Individual units will decide how the topic of analgesia with the use of water immersion is approached. There is no existing rationale describing why IV narcotics cannot be used while the patient is in the water, provided that there is a family member tubside to assist if the woman desires to stand or get out of the tub. Nitrous oxide, widely used in Europe and gaining popularity in the United States, may also be used by the laboring woman while in the tub. As has been widely anecdotally noted, often the synergistic effects of combining warm water and another modality results in very effective and safe pain relief.

Timing of entry into the water

Unit staff will need to decide if they wish to designate specific timing of entry into the water according to progress in labor. Some unit policies require that the woman must be dilated to 4 cm. We suggest caution in including restrictive criteria for water immersion in unit policies and procedures. A woman who is not dilated to 4 cm, for example, yet is very anxious at admission and does not progress in the first hour or 2 after admission may be an excellent candidate to immerse in water. Providing her with this method will assist her to relax and decrease her catecholamine production and may be exactly the remedy to promote her progress. As with many aspects of clinical care of laboring women, clinical judgment is critical in determining the course of management.

Consideration of time limitation of water use

As with timing of entry into the water, some unit policies have limited a woman's immersion in the water to 2 consecutive hours. Again, we advise prudence in incorporating rigid time frames into a formal policy without evidence to support the practice. The scenario wherein a woman is immersed in water for 3 hours and makes no labor progress is a very different situation than a woman sitting in water for several hours who does make steady progress. Individualized care for the specific situation considering the woman's preferences is an appropriate approach when considering time limits in the water. Composing unit guidelines allowing for individual differences will best serve the women using water immersion for labor or birth.

Managing complications at birth

Management of specific possible birth complications is described below.

Shoulder dystocia

The management of shoulder dystocia while in the water requires slight variation from common maneuvers practiced in a bed. Because the woman cannot assume a position where her hips are over the edge of a firm surface (similar to moving her to the edge of the bed), she should first be asked to squat in the tub. McRobert's maneuver and suprapubic pressure may be attempted prior to assisting her to the squatting position. The squatting position is achieved easily enough, as the woman can support herself by holding onto the sides of the tub. An alternative to the squatting position is the hands and knees position in the tub. If the fetus is not born utilizing these positions, the woman must be assisted from the tub to the bed for further attempted maneuvers. It is very helpful to "rehearse" the scenario of having to leave the tub quickly with the woman and her support persons prior to the onset of second stage labor so that everyone is clear about required actions should the situation occur.

Nuchal cord management

The newborn should be assisted slowly and deliberately from the water, watching the nuchal cord carefully and unwrapping while bringing the baby up if possible. This will help ensure that the umbilical cord is not accidentally torn or snapped. If cord avulsion does occur for some reason, the neonate should be swiftly moved to the warmer and the cord clamped to minimize blood loss. Nuchal cord management is the same in and out of the water. The somersault maneuver, described as a technique to successfully manage nuchal cord during birth [40], can easily be utilized during birth in the water.

Postpartum hemorrhage

Accurate assessment of blood loss at birth (whether in or out of water) has long been proven to be an enigma to birth attendants. The added complexity of blood loss occurring in water, and the difficulty estimating that amount, adds to the issue of accurate measurement. One misconception about water birth is that the tub water automatically becomes bloody once the birth occurs. However, because of the dilution of blood by the water, it may be surprising to many how very little the water actually does discolor. When greater than expected blood loss occurs, the water does become heavily blood stained and no longer translucent. In this case, the woman should be removed from the tub for closer evaluation of blood loss.

Conclusion

Water immersion and water birth are options that labor units can initiate with a fairly low degree of expense and workload to make the option available to low-risk pregnant women. The therapeutic effects of water are undisputed, and although more research is needed, there is no evidence of increased adverse effects to the fetus/neonate or laboring woman from experiencing water immersion or water birth. While many laboring women will want epidural anesthesia for their labor, a significant number of women prefer nonpharmacologic methods to promote comfort in labor and relieve labor pain. For those women, water immersion and water birth are safe options that clinicians can offer. (See Box 9.1 and Case Study 9.1.)

Box 9.1   Considerations in water immersion/water birth guidelines

- Determination of desire for signed consent.
- Water temperature guidelines, including parameters for regular measurement.
- Instructions for when maternal temperature is evaluated.
- Method of fetal surveillance.
- How vaginal examinations will be accomplished.
- IV access and necessity, as well as measures to keep area dry if IV in place.
- Supplemental use of either narcotics or nitrous oxide while in tub.
- Entry point into water (whether the unit will want a designated point or not).
- Time parameters for duration of immersion (whether none, or based on the individual clinical situation).

Case Study 9.1

Water birth

DJ is a 34-year-old G4P3 at 40 1/7 weeks gestation in spontaneous labor who requests to utilize hydrotherapy for comfort during labor. Her pregnancy has been uncomplicated and all prenatal lab work rules out any blood-borne infection. Written informed consent is not required on this unit; the prenatal record documents a thorough discussion about water immersion/water birth between DJ and her primary midwife. The EFM tracing is Category I. Contractions are every 3–6 minutes, palpate of moderate intensity, and she has a slight amount of bloody show. Her cervix is 5 cm dilated, 70% effaced, the fetus is at −1 station, with amniotic sac intact. DJ enters the tub and within 10 minutes reports that she feels as though her contractions have ceased. Uterine palpation for contraction strength reveals a continued pattern of contractions every 4–5 minutes, palpating moderate. Fetal heart rate surveillance per Doppler continues to be reassuring. The midwife continues to observe DJ in the tub, while DJ dozes between contractions. Within 20 minutes she reports a "popping sensation" and the midwife notes the fetal head beginning to emerge from the vaginal introitus. DJ continues to bear down through the contraction to birth her baby. The infant is brought to the surface within seconds and handed to her mother to place skin to skin. After the cord is noted to have stopped pulsating, it is clamped, and the father of the baby cuts. The baby is then wrapped in prewarmed blankets and handed to the waiting father. DJ is helped out of the tub and back to bed where she is also wrapped in prewarmed blankets. Third stage of labor is managed in the bed, with the placenta delivering intact via Schultze mechanism. When questioned about her birth experience on postpartum day 1, DJ reports a very different birth experience as compared to her previous births. "I felt an overwhelming sense of calm when I entered the water. It was like the contractions just disappeared. I actually thought that the tub had made my labor stop! When the midwife confirmed that contractions were still coming regularly I thought to myself, then rest! I also was surprised at how comfortable pushing was, I was not feeling the burning sensation that I remember with my previous births."

References

1. Mackey MM. (2001). Use of water in labor and birth. *Clinical Obstetrics and Gynecology*, 44(4), 733–749.
2. Cassidy T. (2006). *Birth: The surprising history of how we are born*. New York: Atlantic Monthly Press.
3. Balaskas J. (1992). *Active birth: The new approach to giving birth naturally*, 2nd ed. Boston: Harvard Common Press.
4. Katz VL, Ryder RM, Cefalo RC, Carmichael SC, & Goolsby R. (1990). A comparison of bed rest and immersion for treating the edema of pregnancy. *Obstetrics & Gynecology*, 75, 147–151.
5. Hawkins S. (1995). Water vs. conventional births: Infection rates compared. *Nursing Times*, 91(11), 38–40.
6. Geissbuhler V & Eberhard J. (2000). Waterbirths: A comparative study. *Fetal Diagnosis and Therapy*, 15, 291–300.
7. Jessiman W & Bryers H. (2000). The highland experience: Immersion in water in labor. *British Journal of Midwifery*, 8, 357–361.
8. Cluett ER, Pickering RM, Getliffe KG, & St George Saunders NJ. (2004). Randomized controlled trial of labouring in water compared with standard augmentation for management of dystocia in first stage of labour. *British Medical Journal*, 328, 314–319.

9. Rosenthal MJ. (1991). Warm-water immersion in labor and birth. *Female Patient*, 16, 44–50.

10. Brown L. (1998). The tide has turned: Audit of water birth. *British Journal of Midwifery*, 6, 236–243.

11. Nguyen S, Kuschel C, Teele R, & Spooner C. (2002). Water birth—a near-drowning experience. *Pediatrics*, 110(2 Pt 1), 411–413.

12. Burke E & Kifoyle A. (1995). A comparative study: Waterbirth and bedbirth. *Midwives*, 3–7.

13. Gilbert RE & Tookey PA. (1999). Perinatal mortality and morbidity among babies delivered in water: Surveillance study and postal survey. *British Medical Journal*, 319, 483–486.

14. Fehervary P, Lauinger-Lorsch E, Hof H, Melchert F, Bauer L, & Zieger W. (2004). Water birth: Microbiological colonization of the newborn, neonatal and maternal infection rate in comparison to conventional bed deliveries. *Archives of Gynecology and Obstetrics*, 270, 6–9.

15. Duffin C. (2004). Water birth findings reveal high levels of satisfaction. *Nursing Standard*, 18(37), 8.

16. Cluett ER & Burns E. (2011). Immersion in labour and birth. *Cochrane Database of Systematic Reviews, issue* 2. DOI: 10.1002/14651858.CD000111.pub3.

17. Gentz BA. (2001). Alternative therapies for the management of pain in laborand delivery. *Clinical Obstetrics and Gynecology*, 44, 704–732.

18. Teschendorf ME & Evans CP. (2000). Hydrotherapy during labor: An example of developing a practice policy. *American Journal of Maternal/Child Nursing*, 25, 198–203.

19. Benfield RD, Herman J, Katz VL, Wilson SP, & Davis JM. (2001). Hydrotherapy in labor. *Research in Nursing & Health*, 24, 57–67.

20. Edlich R, Towler M, Goitz R, Wilder R, Buschbacher L, Morgan ER, & Goitz R. (1987). Bioengineering principles of hydrotherapy. *Journal of Burn Care and Rehabilitation*, 8(6), 580–584.

21. Brown C. (1982). Therapeutic effects of bathing during labor. *Journal of Nurse-Midwifery*, 27(1), 13–16.

22. Griffin J & Karselis T. (1978). *Physical agents for physical therapists*. Springfield, IL: Charles C. Thomas.

23. Burns E & Greenish K. (1993). Pooling information. *Nursing Times*, 89(8), 47–49.

24. Church LK. (1989). Water birth: One birthing center's observations. *Joournal of Nurse-Midwifery*, 34, 165–170.

25. Eriksson M, Mattsson LA, & Ladfors L. (1997). Early or late bath during the first stage of labour: A randomized study of 200 women. *Midwifery*, 13, 146–148.

26. Siegel P. (1960). Does bath water enter the vagina? *Obstetrics & Gynecology*, 15, 660–661.

27. Robertson PA, Huang LJ, Croughan-Minihane MS, & Kilpatrick SJ. (1998). Is there an association between water baths during labor and the development of chorioamnionitis or endometritis? *American Journal of Obstetrics and Gynecology*, 178, 1215–1221.

28. Odent M. (1998). Use of water during labour—updated recommendations. *Midwifery Digest*, 8(1), 68–69.

29. Garland D. (2006). On the crest of a wave; completion of a collaborative audit MIDIRS. *Midwifery Digest*, 16(1), 81–85.

30. Garland D. (2011). Revisiting waterbirth: An attitude to care. New York: Palgrave Macmillan.

31. Rosevear S, Fox R, Marlow N, & Stirrat G. (1993). Birthing pools and the fetus. *Lancet*, 342, 1048–1049.

32. Chapman V & Charles C, eds. (2009). *The midwife's labour and birth handbook*, 2nd ed. Southern Gate, UK: Blackwell.

33. Byard RW & Zuccollo JM. (2010). Forensic issues in cases of water birth fatalities. *American Journal of Forensic Medicine & Pathology*, 31(3), 258–260. DOI: 10.1097/PAF.0b013e3181e12eb8.

34. Nagai T, Sobajima H, Iwasa M, Tsuzuki T, Kura F, Amemura J, & Watanabe H. (1993). Neonatal sudden death due to Legionella pneumonia associated with water birth in a domestic spa bath. *Journal of Clinical Microbiology*, 41(5), 2227–2229. DOI: 10.1128/JCM.41.5.2227-2229.2003.
35. Zanetti-Dallenbach RA, Holzgreve W, & Hosli I. (2007). Neonatal group B streptococcus colonization in water births. *International Journal of Gynecology & Obstetrics*, 98(1), 54–55. Retrieved from: http://www.rcog.org.uk/womens-health/clinical-guidance/group-b-strep-and-water-birth-query-bank.
36. Johnson P. (1996). Birth underwater; to breathe or not to breathe. *American Journal of Obstetrics and Gynecology*, 103, 202–208.
37. Harding R, Johnson P, & McClelland ME. (1978). Liquid-sensitive laryngeal receptors in the developing sheep, cat and monkey. *Journal of Physiology*, 277, 409–422.
38. Crow S & Preston J. (2002). Cord snapping at a waterbirth delivery. *British Journal of Midwifery*, 10(8), 494–497.
39. National Institute for Health and Clinical Excellence. (2007). *Clinical guideline 55: Intrapartum care*. London: National Institute for Health and Clinical Evidence.
40. Mercer JS, Scovgaard RL, Peareara-Eaves J, & Bowman TA. (2005). Nuchal cord management and nurse-midwifery practice. *Journal of Midwifery & Women's Health*, 50, 373–379.

Chapter 10

Aromatherapy in pregnancy and childbirth

Linda L. Halcón

Key points

- Aromatherapy is the intentional use of plant essential oils for preventive or therapeutic purposes.
- Essential oil from a single plant contains multiple chemical constituents and can have therapeutic effects.
- Essential oils are usually applied to humans by inhalation or topical applications.
- While essential oils are generally regarded as safe, most experts recommend *avoiding* their use in the first trimester of pregnancy and with newborns.
- Aromatherapy can be considered for use in maternity care for conditions such as anxiety, pain relief in labor, perineal care, and postpartum blues.
- Current high-quality evidence to support aromatherapy practice in maternity care is limited and more research is needed.

Smell is a potent wizard that transports you across thousands of miles and all the years you have lived.

Helen Keller

Introduction

Aromatherapy is rapidly being integrated into health care settings such as acute care, long-term care, home care, and maternity care. In the UK, some National Health Service midwifery practices have included aromatherapy during birthing and the postnatal period for decades, while in the United States and Canada it is a more recent addition in many regions. Exposure to essential oils is not new; they are common ingredients in foods, perfumes, cosmetics, and hygiene and aesthetic products. Because essential oils are natural products from plants, many people incorrectly assume that they are all harmless. For this reason and in light of growing evidence of their therapeutic potential in maternity

---

Supporting a Physiologic Approach to Pregnancy and Birth: A Practical Guide, First Edition.
Edited by Melissa D. Avery.
© 2013 John Wiley & Sons, Inc. Published 2013 by John Wiley & Sons, Inc.

services, it is critical that clinicians have a basic knowledge of essential oils and aromatherapy. This chapter is not a substitute for good texts that can provide detailed information on the chemistry, actions, and cautions for individual essential oils, nor is it a substitute for a course of study to practice aromatherapy. It is an introduction and overview that aims to highlight aspects of aromatherapy that are most relevant to pregnancy, childbirth, patient education, and maternity care practice.

Brief history and definitions

History

Aromatherapy is part of plant medicines. It would be difficult to imagine a time in which humans did not appreciate the mind- and mood-altering effects of plant aromatics, the "ahhh" that comes with smelling a rose blossom or the zest from a lemon peel. The earliest plant distillation evidence is thought to be about 5,000 years old. Early civilizations in the Middle Eastern region, Asia, and North Africa used essential oils for disease prevention, healing, hygiene, esthetics, embalming, and spiritual purposes. In Europe during the Middle Ages, essential oils were used in certain industries such as glove making and perfumery. Herbal remedies in medical books of the day in the eighteenth and nineteenth centuries sometimes recommended essential oils for healing a variety of common ailments and infectious diseases.

The modern history of aromatherapy began in the early 1900s when a French chemist named René-Maurice Gattefossé sustained a serious injury in a laboratory accident. Gattefossé applied lavender essential oil when the wound infection appeared gangrenous and reportedly was amazed at his rapid and full recovery. Following this incident, he devoted his scientific career to essential oils research and coined the term "aromatherapie" [1]. Important promoters of aromatherapy in Europe during the early twentieth century were Marguerite Maury, a nurse, who brought essential oils to health care in the UK, and Jean Valnet, a French physician, who wrote extensively about his clinical applications of essential oils for chronic and infectious diseases [2] and popularized aromatherapy in France. At about that same time, papers about the healing and antiseptic properties of essential oils appeared in Australian medical journals [3] during a period of scientific interest and investigation. However, when pharmaceuticals and especially antibiotics came into widespread use, plant medicines were largely forgotten by allopathic medicine.

Definition of clinical aromatherapy

Aromatherapy can be defined as *the intentional, evidence-based application of plant essential oils for preventive or therapeutic purposes*. This definition contains several key concepts. First, application is intentional and for a specific purpose. The purpose may be either preventive or therapeutic or both. In other words, neither the chosen essential oils nor the application methods are haphazard or accidental. Second, application is evidence-based. For some essential oils there is little published empirical research evidence. There may, however, be other types of evidence that are acceptable in some situations, for example, where there is an abundance of qualitative or subjective data over time. Third, applications involve plant essential oils rather than other botanical substances, such as flower essences or plant tinctures.

Other definitions may be useful and some have limitations. The National Institutes of Health National Center for Complementary and Alternative Medicine [4] defines aromatherapy as "a therapy in which the scent of essential oils from flowers, herbs and trees is inhaled to promote health and well being." This definition limits aromatherapy applications to inhalation, when in practice topical applications are very common. The National Cancer Institute [5] definition is more inclusive, describing aromatherapy as the "therapeutic use of essential oils from flowers, herbs, and trees for the improvement of physical, emotional and spiritual well being."

Context of aromatherapy

Aromatherapy and NIH CAM domains

The National Center for Complementary and Alternative Medicine (NCCAM), an established center of the National Institutes of Health, uses the term "complementary and alternative medicine" or "CAM" to describe what many others, refer to as "integrative health and healing." NCCAM [6] defines CAM as "a group of diverse medical and health care systems, practices, and products that are not generally considered part of conventional medicine (also called Western or allopathic medicine)." NCCAM categorizes integrative practices as natural products, manipulative and body-based practices, whole medical systems, mind and body medicine, and energy medicine. A particular modality may not always fit clearly in one category, and some modalities may fit in more than one. Essential oils, as botanical substances, most clearly fit into the category of natural products along with other forms of botanical medicines. Aromatherapists and others who use essential oils, however, recognize the mind/body and energetic aspects of essential oils as well.

Aromatherapy within a botanical medicine continuum

In order to use essential oils competently in clinical practice, it is necessary to understand aromatherapy within the field of botanical medicines. Essential oils are volatile secondary metabolites of plants. Only a small percentage of plants produce essential oils, but many plant species have not yet been assessed for the presence of essential oils. Known essential oils come from all of the major plant groups but are often restricted to particular plant families within an order. They may be found in any plant part, such as flowers, leaves, stems, seeds, and roots, and some plants produce different essential oils in different anatomical locations, for example, angelica root and angelica seed. Essential oils perform a variety of known functions for plants, including attracting pollinators, retaining moisture, healing wounds, and repelling predators. Essential oils are responsible for the odors of many aromatic plants, and about half of the orders of flowering plants contain families with species that produce essential oils [7].

Botanical medicines can be visualized as a continuum of plant substances (Figure 10.1). *Whole herbs* or completely unprocessed plants lie on one end of the continuum (far right box). Using a whole plant or plant part is the oldest and most common form of botanical medicine worldwide. Chemical or medicinal substances existing in the plant also exist in the whole herb. Keep in mind that even when the whole plant is used, physical and chemical

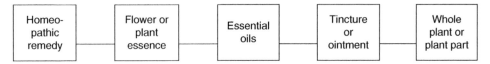

Figure 10.1   A simple continuum of plant medicines.

changes may occur with drying and packaging. The selected plant material might also include only part of the plant, for example, ginger roots, dogwood bark, lavender flowers, or basil leaves. For any form of botanical medicine, it is important to know what part of the plant was used because the chemicals present and the therapeutic effects vary accordingly.

Tinctures and ointments

Tinctures and ointments are found next on the continuum (Figure 10.1, second box from right). These are not chemically identical to the whole plant. Many people confuse tinctures and essential oils, thus it is extremely important that health care providers understand the difference so that they can provide credible advice about safety. The tincturing process extracts chemicals from plant material using alcohol as a solvent. To make a tincture, one would (a) pack small pieces of the desired plant material in a jar; (b) cover the plant material with 100 proof alcohol and seal the jar; (c) remove the plant material after 6–8 weeks; and (d) bottle the remaining liquid. One hundred proof alcohol (often vodka) is half water and half alcohol, thus it absorbs both water-soluble and oil-soluble chemicals from the plant material. The final product is concentrated and is usually ingested in amounts of 1–10 drops at a time, orally or sublingually, from one to several times a day for a specified number of days depending on the practitioner and the purpose.

Ointments are made in a similar manner using vegetable oil (e.g., olive oil) rather than alcohol as the solvent. After removing the plant material from the oil, melted beeswax is often added to produce a semi-solid product that can be applied topically. Plant-derived ointments often are used for first aid (e.g., calendula or arnica). Tinctures and ointments are readily available in natural foods markets and health food stores, and they are easy to make at home. Specific directions are found in many widely available herbal medicine texts. Locally produced tinctures of local plants are often obtainable; a regional or local herbalist guild can provide names of reputable herbalists.

Flower or plant essences

Flower or plant essences (Figure 10.1, second box from left) also are frequently confused with essential oils. A simple essence can be made by placing flowers or other plant material in a bowl of pure water and exposing the water to sunlight for a specified number of hours. After removing the plant material from the water, the water is thought to have absorbed some of the medicinal properties or "essence" of the plant. Flower essences often are applied as several drops sublingually. With understanding of how essences are made, it becomes clear that the oil-soluble chemicals in the plant material are likely to be absent because water molecules would attract only water-soluble substances. Essences used medicinally are believed to incorporate the vibrations or frequencies of the plants from which they are made. This frequency, then, is considered a major source of their therapeutic action rather than physical chemistry.

Homeopathy

Homeopathy (Figure 10.1, far left box) was developed in Europe in the 1800s as a complete system of health care. It was very popular in the United States around the turn of the twentieth century but declined in popularity as allopathic medicine expanded. There is a renaissance of public interest in homeopathy today, and classically trained homeopaths can be found in many parts of the country and most large cities. Homeopathic remedies are produced from plants and other materials but contain no molecules of the materials they are produced from. Thus they are farthest from the whole plant in their physical chemistry. The remedies are produced using water and plant material that undergoes multiple and successive dilutions along with sucussion, or shaking. When the appropriate dilution or concentration is reached, the liquid is removed. The final product is tiny tablets. The more dilute the remedy, the stronger it is considered in homeopathic theory [8]. The tablets are taken as prescribed by a homeopathic physician or, if the remedies are obtained over the counter, as directed on the bottle. Homeopathic remedies may not have the same therapeutic properties as those an herbalist would identify for the same plant. They are thought to contain the vibration or frequency of the plant or substance and to work subtly on that level to promote balance and healing.

Essential oils: Production and constituents

Processing of essential oils

Essential oils (Figure 10.1, middle box) are obtained from plant material using distillation, expression, or carbon dioxide extraction. Most essential oils in common use are distilled or expressed, but CO_2-extracted oils are not rare today. The processing method affects the chemistry and properties of essential oils, thus it is important to have basic understanding of the main extraction methods and their implications. When essential oils are distilled, the plant material is subjected to steam or boiling water. The steam passes through the plant, material rises and moves through cooling coils, after which it condenses into liquid form in a separate receptacle. When aromatic plant material is distilled, this final receptacle contains two products. First, it contains a *hydrosol* or *hydrolat*, an aqueous solution containing the lighter water-soluble chemicals present in the plant material. This is by far the major portion by volume. Second, it contains a film of essential oil floating on top of the hydrosol (the specific gravity of essential oils is lower than that of water). Essential oils obtained by distillation contain the lighter oil-soluble molecules that were present in the original plant material.

Expression is the process used for obtaining essential oils from citrus fruit peels. It involves scraping or grating the peels of citrus fruits to rupture the essential oil sacs and then removing other substances to leave only the essential oil. Because these essential oils have not been subjected to heat and steam, expressed citrus oils differ chemically from distilled oils extracted from the same plant material. They may contain a broader molecular weight range of chemicals than distilled oils. Expressed oils (only citrus oils are expressed) tend to oxidize faster than distilled oils, thus they do not retain their original chemistry as long, which has implications for shelf life.

Carbon dioxide extraction is a third common processing method. Although it is a form of solvent extraction, the CO_2 residue does not remain in the essential oil, as often occurs when other solvents are used. Like expression, CO_2 extraction can capture a broader range of chemical constituents than distillation, thus it may be closer to the original plant material in odor and color [9]. CO_2 extraction is also a more expensive process than distillation or extraction.

In summary, different extraction methods may be selected based on the plant material, desired qualities, and economic factors. It is helpful for clinicians to understand that different extraction methods yield essential oils with different chemical constituencies and, therefore, different therapeutic and toxicity profiles. Reference books and essential oil bottles should specify the processing method used so that clinicians can match the information appropriately and safely.

Chemistry and its impact on physiologic effects

Essential oils are complex substances. Each essential oil from a single plant source contains many (over a hundred) separate chemical molecules, largely terpenes and oxygenated terpenoid compounds, functional groups such as alcohols, aldehydes, esters, ketones, and oxides. Different essential oils, when compared, often contain some of the same and some different molecules and classes of molecules (functional groups). This contributes to the therapeutic complexity and sometimes confusion when several essential oils are purported to have some of the same therapeutic effects. For example, true lavender essential oil (*Lavandula angustifolia*) contains a large proportion of esters and a large proportion of alcohols. Roman chamomile (*Chamaemelum nobile*) contains an even higher proportion of esters and a very low proportion of alcohols. Both contain many other terpenoid compounds in small amounts. Esters are antispasmodic and calming, while alcohols are antiseptic. Thus, aromatherapy texts list both true lavender and Roman chamomile as calming essential oils, but of these two essential oils it is likely that only lavender will be mentioned for its antiseptic properties. This example is an oversimplification because of the many separate chemical constituents in each essential oil, but it illustrates why a number of essential oils might have overlapping or similar properties. Botanicals contain the complexity of nature, in contrast to single chemical pharmaceutical products, and using essential oils appropriately in clinical practice requires understanding and working with that complexity. (See Table 10.1.)

Essential oils are terpenoid molecules and as such have a number of physical characteristics in common. They are volatile, thus they vaporize or evaporate quickly if released into the air. They are flammable, and as such should be stored in a cool place and never exposed to flame or high heat (such as being dripped onto a light bulb). Essential oils are less dense than water (lower specific gravity), and most are fragrant. Most are nonpolar, meaning that they are not soluble and do not disperse well in water. Other chemical behaviors depend on the polarity, solubility, and other properties of the constituents in individual essential oils.

Table 10.1   Major chemical constituents of essential oils, examples of stated health effects, and representative essential oils containing more than 25% of constituent.

Chemical component or functional group	Examples of generalized health effects*	Essential oil Example (*Latin names* and common names)	Molecule comprising the largest % of this functional group in this essential oil
Monoterpenes	Analgesic, antiseptic, tonics and stimulants	*Citrus sinensis* Sweet orange	Limonene
Sesquiterpenes	Anti-inflammatory	*Matricaria recutita* German chamomile	Chamazulene
Monoterpene alcohols	Anti-infectious, uplifting or stimulating	*Lavandula angustifolia* True lavender	Linalool
Sesquiterpene alcohols	Anti-inflammatory	*Santalum album* Sandalwood	Beta-santanol
Phenols	Immune stimulant, antibacterial, nervous system stimulant	*Thymus vulgaris* Thyme	Thymol
Aldehydes	Sedative, calming, anti-infectious	*Melissa officinalis* Lemon balm	Geranial
Esters	Antispasmodic, sedative, calming	*Chamamaelum nobile* Roman chamomile	Isobutyl angelate
Ketones	Mucolytic, cicatrizant	*Mentha spicata* Spearmint	Carvone
Oxides	Expectorant	*Eucalyptus globulus* Blue gum eucalyptus	1,8 cineole
Lactones	Mucolytic	*Nepeta cataria* Catnip	Nepetalactone

*There are always exceptions to the generalized properties of the functional groups. Generalized health effects listed here were noted in at least three of four aromatherapy texts consulted. Each text also listed additional health effects of the functional groups [24,52,79,80]; those other effects are not included here.

Methods of application

Essential oils are applied to humans in three main ways: inhalation, topical applications, and internal applications. The method of application chosen depends on the therapeutic objective(s), characteristics of the essential oil(s) chosen, and characteristics of the person or population being treated. With inhalation, essential oil molecules enter the body via the olfactory system and the respiratory system. Topical applications allow essential oils to enter the body through the integumentary system. Because essential oils are volatile they are also likely to enter the body through inhalation when applied to the skin. With internal applications (oral, rectal, or vaginal) absorption is through mucous membranes or through the gastrointestinal tract with oral applications. In the United States, it is uncommon to encounter internal aromatherapy applications in allopathic health care settings. Internal use of essential oils requires considerable knowledge about dose and toxicity and is never recommended for pregnant women or infants.

Inhalation is one of the most common aromatherapy application methods in home and health care settings. Inhalation requires little equipment; it may be as simple as putting a couple of drops of essential oil on a tissue or cotton ball and placing it within a few feet of the nose. Many people enjoy using a diffuser that sends the odor out to a farther range and automatically turns on and off at intervals. A variety of diffusers are readily available online or in shops that sell essential oils. Electric burners and candle/water burners are also available at lower cost but may require more attention in order to remain safe from fire. Steam inhalation with or without essential oils has been long popular for helping to improve cold symptoms. Two or three drops of an essential oil such as *Eucalyptus smithii* or *Eucalyptus radiata* added to a bowl of steaming water and then inhaled (with eyes closed) can help open stuffy nasal passages. In pregnancy, especially early pregnancy, steam alone is preferred. Simple spritzers made by placing a few drops of an essential oil in a spray bottle of water can be effective for short-term room diffusion and air freshening, similar to commercial room freshener products.

Essential oils often are applied topically with massage. Massage has the added benefits associated with touch; however, for that reason it may be difficult to determine how much of the therapeutic effects are attributable to the essential oils. For massage, essential oils generally must be diluted in a carrier oil (unscented massage oil or vegetable oil), for example, at 1–3% for an adult and 1–2% or 10–20 drops in an ounce of carrier for pregnant women. Topical application of tea tree oil results in little skin penetration, possibly 10% at most [10,11]. In early pregnancy, massage without essential oils is recommended [12].

Aromatherapy baths are another often used topical application of essential oils. It is very important to mix essential oils with a dispersant prior to adding them to bath water because essential oils are physically nonpolar, meaning that they do not dissolve in water. Without a dispersant, the skin can be exposed to full-strength essential oils, many of which are very irritating. Common dispersants include bath salts, full fat milk, or lecithin. Bath salts can be easily made at home by mixing one part baking soda, two parts Epsom salts, and three parts sea salt. About 3–6 drops of an essential oil can be mixed with a half cup of the above mixture and added to the bath just before entering the water. Baths with or without essential oils may be helpful with symptoms of insomnia, nervous tension, or muscular aches. Footbaths or handbaths can be used for arthritis symptoms or dermatitis. Similarly, warm or cold compresses can be made by soaking a cloth in water to which essential oils have been added, applying to the affected area, and covering with plastic and a source of heat or cold for pain, swelling, or inflammation. Principles of common sense always apply in choosing essential oils and application methods.

Toxicity, sensitization, and irritation

Toxicity

Integrative therapies are often included in maternity services in response to patient demand, and health care providers may not be aware of the potential risks involved in aromatherapy [13]. Despite the very real risks, it is widely acknowledged that the risks are small when essential oils are used properly. Generally, proper use means using safe essential oils for appropriate reasons at low dilutions of 2% or less topically, and avoiding use in early pregnancy. The greatest potential risk is fetal toxicity [14–16]. Nearly all sources recommend not using essential oils in early infancy, with rare possible exceptions when the mother and infant are under the care of a very knowledgeable aromatherapist.

Despite some lack of toxicity data, essential oils are known to be very concentrated substances, and some essential oils or components are known to have caused harm [17]. In a controlled study of the effects of menthol on the risk of jaundice in G6PD-deficient newborns, those whose umbilical cords were dressed daily with a mentholated powder developed significantly more jaundice than controls [18]. Although the product was not an essential oil, peppermint oil also contains menthol. The study underscores the importance of asking patients about the use of natural products. Numerous reports in the literature describe essential oil toxicity after accidental ingestion or inappropriate use in infants and small children. A toddler and a newborn accidentally exposed to sage essential oil experienced generalized tonic-clonic seizures. Sage oil contains substances that may be convulsant, such as thujone, camphor, and cineole [19].

Increasing in vitro and animal evidence suggests that some essential oils and chemical components may be teratogenic. Results of a study in mice suggested that nerolidol, a component of neroli essential oil that is used as a flavor and aroma enhancer and previously considered nontoxic, may be weakly genotoxic [20]. Another study of fetal mice suggested that citral, an ingredient in many essential oils, can block tooth and cranial bone formation by inhibiting retinoic acid synthesis when used in high concentrations [21,22]. Extrapolation from these animal studies to humans is difficult, and thus it is unclear whether small therapeutic doses may be teratogenic in human fetuses. Citral, the chemical studied, is used extensively in the food and flavor industry and is present in citrus fruits. Thus, it would be difficult to avoid; however, it is prudent to expose mother and fetus to as few potentially harmful substances as possible once pregnancy is suspected [23].

Some essential oils should never be used during pregnancy, and many others used only with caution. The most toxic essential oils include those that contain the chemicals apiole, sabinyl acetate, or pulegone (dill seed, parsley leaf and seed, sage, savin, wormwood, yarrow, and pennyroyal) [10]. Price and Price [24] noted that essential oils are often contraindicated for general reasons that have nothing directly to do with pregnancy, such as those with danger of phototoxicity (many citrus oils) or hepatotoxicity. Cautions in pregnancy largely are aimed at protecting the vulnerable fetus. It must also be noted that many of the case reports of essential oil toxicity involved ingestion of much larger quantities than therapeutic doses. For example, there are historical case reports of women ingesting large amounts of pennyroyal essential oil to induce abortion, with resultant adverse effects to other organ systems [24, p. 69].

All essential oils most likely cross the placenta to some degree, and the fetus is especially sensitive to toxicity up to the latter part of pregnancy [10]. Although authors do not always agree about which essential oils should be avoided altogether or used only cautiously, clinicians are advised to use similar caution with essential oils in pregnancy and birth as they would with pharmaceutical or other products, including minimizing chemical exposures to the extent possible in early pregnancy.

Dose is an important factor even for nonpregnant adults, although adult bodies are accustomed to small exposures to essential oils and their constituents because they are so commonly used as food and flavoring additives [10], as well as in soaps, lotions, and cosmetics.

In some cases, toxicity may not be caused by essential oils themselves but associated with impurities and adulterants in poor-quality essential oils, or to synergistic relationships with other products or drugs. In vitro studies have found interactions between essential oils and drugs. Synergistic, additive, or antagonistic effects were found when essential oils such as peppermint and rosemary were combined with standard antibiotics in cultures of a variety of bacteria [25]. Pesticides and plasticizer residues have also been found in citrus essential oils from different countries [26], underscoring the importance of obtaining organic and pure essential oils. This brief introduction to toxicity with a few examples is not meant to provide a complete discussion of toxicity. Clinicians who use essential oils in practice should remain up to date on the literature or consult a text or aromatherapist that can provide current toxicity information.

Skin sensitivity and irritation

Contact allergy is not uncommon with topical applications, affecting more than 1% of large populations tested. Patch testing should be done if individuals have a strong history of sensitivity to plants or multiple other skin sensitivities [27]. Skin sensitization is a relatively infrequent issue with topical applications; however, there have been a number of reports of skin sensitivity to essential oils [28,29]. Women should be cautioned to discontinue topical application if skin irritation or sensitivity occurs. Essential oils obtained through CO_2 extraction may be more sensitizing because they contain water-soluble chemicals such as alkaloids, chlorophylls, and carotenoids [19]. For this reason and because essential oil references and texts most often refer to distilled or expressed (for citrus oils) essential oils when listing their chemistries and properties, it may be best to avoid CO_2 extracted essential oils in pregnancy.

General safety

Clinical safety with essential oils has many aspects. First, it is important to obtain good-quality essential oils. The plant source should be clearly identified by its botanical name, the part of the plant used, the extraction method, the country of origin, and chemical specificity (chemotype, etc.) when applicable. Second, essential oils should be packaged in dark glass containers with an integral dropper that releases only 1 drop at a time. The concentration should be noted on the container, and generally only pure, undiluted oils should be purchased if the clinician plans to mix the product for the patient. In some cases, premixed essential oils may be purchased from a trusted aromatherapist. Third, essential oils should be stored in a cool, dark location to slow the oxidation process, as chemical changes may result in increased risk of skin sensitivity or irritation [30]. In clinical settings, the date the bottle was opened should be recorded, and old essential oils should be discarded in an environmentally safe manner that includes evaporation of the substance. Individuals using essential oils in home settings should be advised to keep essential oils out of reach of children, not to ingest essential oils, to use less rather than more, and to avoid applying undiluted essential oils to mucous membranes. Phototoxicity precautions must be taken with citrus oils because severe burns can result from sun exposure after applying even diluted citrus oils to the skin.

Aromatherapy in maternity care

Current practice

Positive public opinion about the contribution of complementary therapies such as aromatherapy to improved health is one of the major influences on their spread within health care systems. Maternity care is no exception. Like the public, health care providers also favor the use of integrative therapies. Aromatherapy is one of the most popular complementary therapies currently used in maternity care and midwifery, along with massage, reflexology, acupuncture, imagery, and herbal therapies [31–34].

Essential oils generally regarded as safe in pregnancy

Aromatherapy self-help books list a number of essential oils as safe to use sparingly during pregnancy and for particular purposes, such as anxiety, backache, constipation, hemorrhoids, indigestion, insomnia, nausea and vomiting, pain relief in labor, perineal care, fatigue, and postpartum blues [12,35]. Some of these applications are not supported by research evidence, as most human studies are not specific to pregnant women. However, oils have been used over time with no observed adverse effects. These books generally include advice to avoid essential oils in the first trimester and for newborns. Authors seem to generally agree on which essential oils are helpful and safe, but aromatherapists and clinicians also use their own clinical experience as a guide, resulting in inconsistent recommendations. Clinicians who wish to use essential oils in practice will need a good understanding of essential oils and the best reference books available. When clinicians recommend essential oils to women, it is important to consider the available evidence as well as the chemistry, toxic potential, dose, administration route, and therapeutic objective when determining whether aromatherapy is the right approach for a particular woman and condition. Helpful considerations are highlighted in Box 10.1.

Evidence for therapeutic effects

Mood, stress, and anxiety

Many studies in animals and humans have examined the effects of essential oils on stress, mood, and anxiety. Although some studies have found no effect [36,37], others have shown positive findings. Few of these studies have included pregnant women [38].

A number of studies have examined the effects of essential oils on measures of sympathetic and parasympathetic activity. One randomized, controlled trial found that after a stressor, based on self-report and unobtrusive mood measures, lemon oil increased

---

Box 10.1   Sample maternity care essential oil applications and cautions

- Oil-soluble substances such as essential oils cross the placental barrier.
- Avoidance of exposure in the first trimester is prudent due to rapid fetal development and higher risk of spontaneous abortion during this time.
- As with any chemical or pharmacologic substance, the lowest possible therapeutic doses of essential oils are recommended in pregnancy [64,77].

A few examples of commonly recommended applications are:

- Cypress (*Cupressus sempervirens*) essential oil in a dilute mixture for hemorrhoids. A compress can be applied or a couple of drops can be added to a sitz bath [35].
- Clary sage (*Salvia sclarea*) for stress and anxiety during labor and to ease pain (contraindicated prior to labor) [12].
- Lavender (*Lavandula angustifolia*) for its analgesic, antiseptic, and anxiolytic properties [12,78].
- Rose (*Rosa damascena*) for its regulating, toning, uplifting, and hormone balancing qualities [35,78].

---

positive mood. Immune function was not affected by the odors, nor were salivary cortisol, pulse, blood pressure, or pain ratings. Lavender performed no better than water in this study [39]. Another study [40] found that a blend of lemon, lavender, and ylang ylang essential oils noticeably decreased systolic blood pressure and sympathetic nervous system activity in hypertensive adults compared to controls receiving an artificial fragrance mixture. Similarly, the effects of inhaled lavender and rosemary essential oils were measured on EKG results, blood pressure, fingertip blood flow, galvanic skin conductance, and heart rate variability [41]. Lavender was better than rosemary at producing calm and relaxation as measured by increased blood flow, decreased skin conductance, and decreased systolic blood pressure. Rosemary was found to decrease blood flow and increase systolic blood pressure immediately after inhalation. Other researchers examined the effects of inhaled essential oils on sympathetic activity in normal adults and found pepper oil to increase plasma adrenaline, while fennel and grapefruit oils increased sympathetic activity, and rose oil and patchouli oil decreased relative sympathetic activity. Rose oil was found to decrease adrenaline concentration by 30% in healthy adults [42].

Both inhaled lavender and rosemary were found to lower cortisol levels in saliva in twenty-two healthy volunteers [43]. A clinical trial testing inhaled lavender and rosemary on perceived stress of nursing students (measured by test anxiety, pulse rates, and personal statements) found they perceived less stress with the essential oils [44]. Ambient odors of orange and lavender have been found to reduce anxiety and improve mood when tested among adult dental patients waiting for their appointments [45,46]. Lee and others [47] reviewed published research on the anxiolytic effects of aromatherapy among individuals with anxiety symptoms. Of sixteen randomized controlled trials, most reported positive effects and no adverse effects. Methodological problems such as small sample size and lack of a control group were identified in some of the reviewed studies. The effects of essential oils on stress and anxiety during pregnancy have not been well studied; however, aromatherapy may be a viable stress- and anxiety-reducing strategy when other nonpharmacologic approaches have not been successful.

Pain

Lavender (*L. angustifolia*) has been studied most frequently for its effect on pain. When applied to a face mask, lavender was shown to reduce the use of opioids following anesthesia in morbidly obese patients undergoing surgery [48]. Lavender applied with a face mask for five minutes prior to needle insertion resulted in decreased stress and significantly reduced perceived pain among healthy adults [49]. Although the mechanism of action for the effect of essential oils on pain is unknown and the results are mixed, some research evidence supports the use of essential oils for pain relief [50].

Hormonal effects

Animal studies have suggested that some essential oil–producing plants can affect hormones, and it has been hypothesized that the essential oils themselves may affect certain hormone levels. For example, a rat study found that fennel seed extract taken orally stimulated the estrus cycle and increased the weight of mammary glands and genitalia [51]. Fennel and anise plants have been used by herbalists to increase milk production, promote menstruation, facilitate birth, and increase libido. Most aromatherapists recommend not using essential oils that may have estrogenic effects during pregnancy, childbirth, and lactation, as the evidence for safety or harm is scant [52].

Topical applications of lavender and tea tree oils in shampoos or lotions have been linked to gynecomastia in boys [53]. Although the evidence was not high quality, it raises questions about hormonal effects of essential oils and if perceived safety in adults extends to children and even pregnant women.

Lavender

Lavender is often recommended for relaxation, pain relief, and stress reduction, and its use in pregnancy has been controversial. Many aromatherapy textbooks recommend caution, suggesting that it may be a uterine stimulant. Dr. Robert Tisserand, author of the most widely used text on the safety of essential oils, reviewed the literature and concluded that there is no evidence of toxicity or uterine stimulation with lavender essential oil or its major chemical constituents [54]. One double-blind, placebo-controlled trial of an oral preparation of lavender oil found it to be beneficial for quality and duration of sleep and improved physical/mental health without unwanted sedative or other adverse effects. The product is considered safe and efficacious for relief of anxiety [55]; however, ingestion of essential oils is not recommended in pregnancy because of a lack of evidence supporting safety.

A body of research suggests that lavender may have positive effects that can be helpful in maternity care practice, but the evidence is not clear. Several studies have examined the effect of lavender on anxiety, mood, outlook, blood pressure, and pulse with mixed results

[56–58]. Most of this research has not included pregnant women. Few studies have reported adverse effects when lavender is used properly.

Evidence for essential oils in pregnancy and postpartum

Labor and birth

A well-known and frequently cited study of aromatherapy in midwifery practice was conducted in a large UK teaching hospital between 1990 and 1998 [59]. Ten different essential oils (rose, jasmine, Roman chamomile, eucalyptus, lemon, mandarin, clary sage, frankincense, lavender, and peppermint) were included. Essential oils were administered to a nonrandom sample of over eight thousand women during labor and birth to reduce anxiety, pain, and nausea and/or vomiting and to strengthen contractions. Oils were selected by the midwife based on symptoms of her patient and the qualities of the essential oils. Administration included inhalation, massage, or baths. Outcomes were compared with those of women in the same facility who had not used essential oils during labor and birth. Most mothers rated the essential oil treatments as helpful. The midwives reported that the oils were helpful for pain, that adverse effects were minor and there were few side effects, and that the use of pethidine had declined over the study period from 6% to 0.2%. In concluding that aromatherapy is helpful in addressing anxiety, pain, nausea, or poor contractions during labor and childbirth, the authors noted that fewer women receiving aromatherapy needed epidural analgesia. Although this study did not meet criteria for the highest quality of evidence, it is important research because of its size and effort to evaluate an aromatherapy program offered in a real-life scenario where essential oils and administration methods were chosen based on the individual woman's needs. Additional studies should place more emphasis on objective measures and ensuring a control group comparable to the treatment group.

Subsequently, in a pilot study (N = 513) conducted in Italy [60], researchers assessed the feasibility of conducting a true randomized controlled trial on the use of aromatherapy in labor. Again, the decision about which essential oil to use was made by the midwife and the mother utilizing a smaller number of essential oils: Roman chamomile, clary sage, frankincense, lavender, and mandarin. Aromatherapy treatment was used for reducing fear, anxiety, or pain or for augmenting contractions. There were no differences in the rates of caesarean section, ventouse, Kristeller maneuver, spontaneous vaginal delivery, or first or second stage augmentation between treated and nontreated groups. Pain perception was lower for nulliparas in the aromatherapy group, but not statistically significant. Significantly more infants in the control group required NICU services. A study funded by NCCAM is currently under way in the UK to assess whether aromatherapy (peppermint, lavender, clary sage, or frankincense) can lower anxiety, decrease analgesia use, or increase perceived satisfaction of women in labor [61].

A Cochrane review of aromatherapy for pain management in labor examined two randomized controlled trials that assessed essential oils compared to placebo, no treatment, or other nonpharmacologic pain management strategies. One study was summarized above [60]. The authors of the review determined that the data were inconclusive. Neither trial found differences in pain intensity, length of labor, or use of pharmacologic pain relief. Methodologic issues were identified for both studies [60,62].

Perineal healing

In addition to labor and birth, essential oils have been used for perineal healing following birth, also with mixed results. One review article found scant evidence for the efficacy of lavender oil on perineal trauma itself; however, the authors concluded that there is some evidence that it may be helpful for anxiety and pain [63]. Nearly all studies of lavender oil refer to *Lavandula angustifolia*, one of three major species of lavender. However, a different species of lavender oil (*Lavendula stoechas*) was assessed in a trial of its effect on episiotomy healing. Sixty women were assigned to receive sitz baths with 5–7 drops of *L. stoechas* essential oil twice daily for 10 days, while the control group received treatment with povodine-iodine. There were no significant differences between the treatment and control groups, although less erythema was found in the lavender group. Because of its camphor content of 15–30%, *L. stoechas* may have small risk of neurotoxicity and is contraindicated during pregnancy [64, p. 145]. The importance of knowing both the genera and species of essential oils along with their differential chemical properties and safety profiles is highlighted [65].

Dale and Cornwell [66] examined the effect of natural lavender essential oil baths on perineal discomfort following childbirth, compared to both synthetic lavender oil and an inert substance, among 635 women who gave birth vaginally to healthy infants. It can be assumed contextually that *L. angustifolia* was the essential oil used, although this was not stated explicitly. Randomly assigned participants were asked to add 6 drops of their assigned product to a daily bath for ten days postpartum. Data were gathered on discomfort level, mood, and perineal healing. Mothers using the lavender product had lower mean discomfort scores, although the difference was not statistically significant. No side effects from any treatment were observed. One possible confounder was the presence of linalyl acetate, a principal constituent of both natural and synthetic lavender, which may have affected the results.

Postpartum well-being

Aromatherapy has also been used to promote postpartum well-being. Researchers used a quasi-experimental, between-groups design to compare a 20-minute aromatherapy massage on the second postpartum day between first-time mothers with healthy infants and a control group. Pre-/postmeasures were: Maternity Blues Scale (MBS), State-Trait Anxiety Inventory (STAI), Profile of Mood States (POMS), and Feeling Toward Baby Scale (FTBS). The massage group had significantly decreased scores on the MBS and STAI, and higher scores on the POMS and FTBS. The researchers concluded that aromatherapy massage might be a good intervention for postpartum mothers to improve physical and mental status and facilitate mother-infant interaction [67]. Similarly, Conrad & Adams [68] conducted a pilot study showing that aromatherapy improved anxiety and depression in postpartum women.

Incorporating aromatherapy in practice

Findings from established aromatherapy practices

A few evaluations of aromatherapy services in midwifery practice have been published. Researchers obtained qualitative data from six nurses and two midwives with a credential in aromatherapy. They were asked to describe how they had subsequently changed their clinical practices, if at all, after completing aromatherapy coursework. All of the participants were employees of the UK National Health Service. Although some of the nurses and midwives stated they had not intended it, all said they felt their practice was more holistic and that they felt more confident of their skills. Those who used aromatherapy massage focused primarily on the effects of the massage rather than the therapeutic effects of the essential oils in their discussion, illustrating the difficulty of separating the therapeutic effects of essential oils from those of massage when both are used together. Neither of the two midwives worked in an environment where there was a policy or protocol for essential oils, thus they did not yet use them at work. Generally, they were frustrated that they had not been able to incorporate aromatherapy into their work, stating that they saw much potential benefit [69].

An audit was conducted in the UK to assess clinical effectiveness of the aromatherapy service, maternal satisfaction, and staff training needs 2 years after starting an aromatherapy service in a maternity unit. Eighty mothers and 24 midwives participated in the evaluation of the aromatherapy service initiated by the midwives. Results of the audit suggested that the service was well accepted after 2 years, although it was used more by primigravidas than by multigravidas. Women were able to choose from ten essential oils, with lavender and frankincense being most popular. Participants reported that aromatherapy helped with relaxation and somewhat for pain. After this audit was completed, an interdisciplinary Holistic Midwifery Group was formed at the facility. In addition to aromatherapy, the group intended to add shiatsu, reflexology, and baby massage to their range of available therapies. Further staff workshops were planned to continue to raise skill and confidence levels [70].

Examples of aromatherapy in maternity care

Example 1

At Woodwinds Health Campus in Woodbury, Minnesota, the use of clinical essential oils has been included in maternity care for over 10 years as part of nursing practice. A 4% specially made blend of essential oils may be offered to women in labor. Also, in the third trimester a lavender blend may be used for headache, insomnia, anxiety, or pain, and a mandarin blend may be offered for general well-being, digestive problems, fluid elimination, and general circulation, or for its calming and uplifting properties. Nursing staff at this facility are provided essential oil education and protocols that include the goals of clinical treatment, safety and storage guidelines, best practices, cautions and contraindications, specific procedures, and documentation requirements. Because holistic healing is part of the institutional philosophy of Woodwinds, it is considered routine that patients may be offered a variety of integrative modalities. In addition to the use of essential oils, Woodwinds holistic nursing model of care includes energy healing, therapeutic presence, acupressure, use of guided imagery and healing music to address pain, stress/anxiety, nausea, or other symptoms. Symptoms, treatments, and responses are documented in the electronic health record, providing a record over time of aromatherapy practice and results [71].

Example 2

Pam Conrad, RN, BSN, PGd, CCAP, a nurse and qualified aromatherapist, developed a program called Aromatic Childbirth. Conrad teaches complementary therapies and clinical aromatherapy at Purdue University in Indiana and is a consultant in an outpatient hospital pharmacy. In 2008, she conducted an aromatherapy pilot program in a large, suburban Indianapolis hospital. The purpose of the project was to "explore the impact of aromatherapy in reducing anxiety, pain, nausea, and in enhancing the childbirth experience" [72]. In this project, Conrad educated nurses on the maternity unit, developed and implemented guidelines, policies, and protocols for nurses who had participated in the education, and implemented the aromatherapy program. Data were obtained on aromatherapy treatments using pre- and posttreatment ratings by patients and nurses. Almost half of patients included were in labor, about a third postpartum. The major reasons for using aromatherapy were anxiety (42%), pain (38%), contractions (8%), nausea (8%), and sleep (4%). Application methods included massage/skin (51%), inhalation (34%), spritzer (14%), and compress (1%). For skin applications and spritzers, the essential oils were diluted to 1–2% concentration. The ten essential oils included were identical to those in the Burns [59] study in the UK. The most frequently used oils were lavender (27%), mandarin (22%), and rose (13%). Results of this pilot project were positive, with both nurses and patients reporting effectiveness of the intervention. There were no negative effects other than rare dislike of the scent. Aromatic Childbirth nursing and midwifery programs continue at this hospital and have expanded to nine Indiana hospitals. Development in Arizona and California is in process. At this point, data exist on over eight hundred labor and postpartum aromatherapy interventions. Private consultations are available to women throughout the United States. The aromatherapy postpartum anxiety and depression pilot study completed in 2011 indicated positive responses [68]. A new pilot study of aromatherapy and postpartum anxiety and depression has begun [72,73].

Example 3

North Hawaii Regional Community Hospital, Kamuela, Hawaii, has had an aromatherapy program for several years. In the labor and delivery unit, 3–5 drops of a lavender (*Lavandula angustifolia*) and grapefruit (*Citrus paradisi*) blend is often used in the labor tub to promote comfort and well-being. Anecdotal results have been positive from the mothers, and staff has conjectured that this aromatherapy practice may speed the labor process in some cases; however, these perceptions have not been systematically evaluated. In addition to labor and birth, peppermint (*Mentha piperita*) is used for postnatal urinary retention by placing a couple of drops of peppermint essential oil in the toilet or bedpan. Again, anecdotal results have been positive [74].

Guidelines for aromatherapy services

Clinicians wishing to incorporate aromatherapy services in practice will find it helpful to first evaluate the environment and obtain support from key individuals or departments. Initial assessment should include information about the level of support and interest from patient groups and from staff. A brief survey or focus groups can help gauge the knowledge level and current use of essential oils in these two groups. Although aromatherapy supplies are not expensive relative to many other services, it will be important to obtain intellectual and financial support from management prior to beginning. Other key relationships for success include other providers, pharmacists, safety personnel, an essential oil supplier, and an aromatherapist if there is none within the staff group.

Clinicians may want to consider a variety of integrative therapies to include in their practices, aromatherapy being one option. Discussion should also include which integrative modalities would be provided by which type of provider. Sharing of information is important when implementing any new integrative service, and protocols developed by those with special aromatherapy training may be adapted or adopted by others. In most health care settings, persons who will be administering essential oils will employ protocols that specify the conditions or symptoms that can be treated, which essential oils can be used, what application methods are acceptable, any contraindications, and documentation requirements. Protocols also may include literature searches and evidence summaries [75].

Education of aromatherapy service providers is needed to ensure safety and adherence to practice standards. In addition to the basics of essential oils and aromatherapy, staff training should include review of the rationale and evidence base for the program and the integrative therapies scope of practice for each discipline involved. Documentation needs vary depending on the facility but generally include:

- Indication for using essential oils (e.g., anxiety, insomnia, pain, digestive complaint, wound healing, relaxation).
- Goal(s) of treatment.
- Treatment plan.
- Relevant flow sheets or checklists.
- Patient education provided.
- Patient response to the treatment.

Both the education process and content should be evaluated periodically. After initiation, program expansion should go forward slowly based on documented results and any new evidence. There is a need for basic, applied, and program evaluation research in this field to answer such questions as:

- Is there an effect?
- What is the mechanism for the effect?
- How can the effect be improved?
- Which of two treatments is more effective? [76]

Nurses, midwives, and physicians are in an excellent position to conduct this research, having an understanding of the complexities of holistic practice and the importance of both subjective and objective measurement.

Credentialing issues

There is no licensure of aromatherapists in the United States at this time. A variety of certification programs are available. Most of these follow education guidelines of the Alliance for International Aromatherapists (http://www.alliance-aromatherapists.org) or the National Association for Holistic Aromatherapy (http://www.naha.org) and are designed to meet the requirements for the Aromatherapy Registration Council's registration exam (http://www.aromatherapycouncil.org). Clinical-level aromatherapy education offerings include at least 400 hours of training, as well as safety standards, standards of practice, and codes of ethics. Information about recommended programs can be found on the websites of these organizations.

Conclusion

By design, this chapter focused on the safety aspects of aromatherapy and the limitations of current evidence. The intent is to encourage provision of aromatherapy services in maternity care practice in a prudent and safe manner, using the experience of others and the available evidence. Essential oils currently are used in maternity services and other health care settings to the benefit of patients. A body of anecdotal and historical evidence has accumulated, and there is a great need for more clinical research to provide scientific evidence. The relative paucity of research evidence at this time may reflect the multiple barriers for clinicians to conduct research rather than the clinical effectiveness or ineffectiveness of essential oils. Collaborations between practitioners and researchers may help to address this lack of evidence in the future.

References

1. Gattefossé R. (1937; English translation 1993). *Gattefossé's aromatherapy*. Essex, UK: C.W. Daniels.
2. Valnet J. (1980; English translation 1982). *The practice of aromatherapy: A classic compendium of plant medicines and their healing properties*. R Tisserand, ed. Rochester, VT: Healing Arts Press.
3. Humphrey E. (1930). A new Australian germicide. *Medical Journal of Australia*, *1*, 417–418.
4. National Center for Complementary and Alternative Medicine. (2012). Aromatherapy. Retrieved from: http://nccam.nih.gov/health/aromatherapy. Accessed January 24, 2012.
5. National Cancer Institutes at the National Institutes of Health. (2011). Retrieved from: Aromatherapy and essential oils. http://www.cancer.gov/cancertopic/pdq/cam/aromatherapy/HealthProfessionals/page2 and http://www.cancer.gov/cancertopics/pdq/cam/aromatherapy/patient. Accessed February 2012.

6. National Center for Complementary and Alternative Medicine. (2011). What is complementary and alternative medicine? NCCAM publication No. D347. Retrieved from: http://nccam.nih.gov/health/whatiscam/. Accessed January 15, 2012.

7. Shawe K. (2001). *Taxonomy and distribution of essential oil bearing plants.* Oral presentation, Essential Oils: Advanced Studies, Rutgers University, August 6–16.

8. Dooley TR. (2002). *Homeopathy: Beyond flat earth medicine: An introduction for students and patients: A family physician explains this holistic medical science.* San Diego: Timing Publications.

9. Kerr J. (2002). Carbon dioxide extraction. *Aromatherapy Today, 22,* 28–29.

10. Tisserand R. (2010). *Essential oil therapeutics.* Workshop for Plant Extracts International, Hopkins, MN, May 22–23.

11. Cross S, Russell M, Southwell I, & Roberts M. (2008). Human skin penetration of the major components of Australian tea tree oil applied in its pure form and as a 20% solution *in vitro. European Journal of Pharmaceutics & Biopharmaceutics, 69*(1), 214–222.

12. Tiran D. (2000). Massage and aromatherapy. In D Tiran & S Mack, eds., *Complementary therapies for pregnancy and childbirth,* 2nd ed. pp. 129–167. Edinburgh: Ballière Tindall.

13. Tiran D. (2006). Complementary therapies in pregnancy: Midwives and obstetricians' appreciation of risk. *Complementary Therapies in Clinical Practice, 12*(2), 126–131.

14. Field T. (2008). Pregnancy and labor alternative therapy research. *Alternative Therapies, 14*(5), 28–34.

15. Duddridge E. (2002). Using complementary therapies during the childbearing process. *British Journal of Midwifery, 10*(11), 699–704.

16. Maddox-Jennings W & Wilkinson J. (2004). Aromatherapy practice in nursing: Literature review. *Journal of Advanced Nursing, 48*(1), 93–103.

17. Lis-Balchin M. (1999). Possible health and safety problems in the use of novel plant essential oils and extracts in aromatherapy. *Journal of the Royal Society for the Promotion of Health, 119,* 240–243.

18. Olowe S & Ransome-Kuti O. (1980). The risk of jaundice in Glucose-6-phosphate dehydrogenase deficient babies exposed to menthol. *Acta Paediatrica Scandinavica, 69,* 341–345.

19. Halicioglu O, Astarcioglu G, Yaprak I, & Aydinlioglu H. (2011). Toxicity of *Salvia officinalis* in a newborn and a child: An alarming report. *Pediatric Neurology, 45*(4), 259–260.

20. Piculo F, Macedo G, de Andrade S, & Maistro L. (2011). *In vivo* genotoxicity assessment of nerolidol. *Journal of Applied Toxicology, 31*(7), 633–639.

21. Koussoulakou D, Margaritis L, & Doussoulakos S. (2011). Antagonists of retinoic acid and BMP4 affect fetal mouse osteogenesis and odontoblast differentiation. *Pathophysiology, 18,* 103–109.

22. Kronmiller J, Beeman C, Nyugen T, & Berndt W. (1995). Blockade of the initiation of murine odontogenesis in vitro by citral, in inhibitor of endogenous retinoic acid synthesis. *Archives of Oral Biology, 40*(7), 645–652.

23. Tisserand R. Personal communication, February 1, 2012.

24. Price S & Price L. (2007). *Aromatherapy for health professionals,* 3rd ed. Philadelphia: Churchill Livingstone.

25. Toroglu S. (2011). *In-vitro* antimicrobial activity and synergistic/antagonistic effect of interactions between antibiotics and some spice essential oils. *Journal of Environmental Biology, 32*(1), 23–29.

26. Di Bella G, Lo Turco V, Rando R, Arena G, Pollicino D, & Luppino R. (2010). Pesticide and plasticizer residues in citrus essential oils from different countries. *Natural Product Communications, 5*(8), 1325–1328.

27. Uter W, Schmidt E, Geier J, Lessmann H, Schnuch A, & Frosch P. (2010). Contact allergy to essential oils: Current patch test results (2000–2008) from the Information Network of Departments of Dermatology (IVDK). *Contact Dermatitis, 63*(5), 277–283.

28. Brandao F. (1986). Occupational allergy to lavender oil. *Contact Dermatitis*, 249–250.
29. Sugiura M, Hayakawa R, Kato T, Sugiura K, & Hashimoto R. (2000). Results of patch testing with lavender oil in Japan. *Contact Dermatitis*, *43*, 157–160.
30. Hammer K, Carson C, Riley T, & Nielsen J. (2006). A review of the toxicity of Melaleuca alternifolia (tea tree) oil. *Food & Chemical Toxicology*, *44*(5), 616–625.
31. Allaire A, Moos M, & Wells S. (2000). Complementary and alternative medicine in pregnancy: A survey of North Carolina certified nurse-midwives. *Obstetrics & Gynecology*, *95*(1), 19–23.
32. Gaffney L & Smith C. (2004). Use of complementary therapies in pregnancy: The perceptions of obstetricians and midwives in South Australia. *Australian & New Zealand Journal of Obstetrics and Gynaecology*, *44*(1), 24–29.
33. Mitchell M, Williams J, Hobbs E, & Pollard K. (2006). The use of complementary therapies in maternity services: A survey. *British Journal of Midwifery*, *14*(10), 576–582.
34. Skouteris H, Wertheim E, Rallis S, Paxton S, Kelly L, & Milgrom J. (2008). Use of complementary and alternative medicines by a sample of Australian women during pregnancy. *Australian and New Zealand Journal of Obstetrics and Gynaecology*, *48*, 384–390.
35. England A. (2000). *Aromatherapy and massage for mother and baby*. Rochester, VT: Healing Arts Press.
36. Muzzarelli L, Force M, & Sebold M. (2006). Aromatherapy and reducing preprocedural anxiety: A controlled prospective study. *Gastroenterology Nursing*, *29*(6), 466–471.
37. Graham P, Browne L, Cox H, & Graham J. (2003). Inhalation aromatherapy during radiotherapy: Results of a placebo-controlled double-blind randomized trial. *Journal of Clinical Oncology*, *21*(12), 2372–2376.
38. Bastard J & Tiran D. (2006). Aromatherapy and massage for antenatal anxiety: Its effect on the fetus. *Complementary Therapies in Clinical Practice*, *15*(4), 230–233.
39. Kiecolt-Glaser J, Graham J, Malarkey W, Porter K, Lemeshow S, & Glaser R. (2007). Olfactory influences on mood and autonomic, endocrine, and immune function. *Psychoneuronendocrinology*. DOI: 10.1016/j.psyneuen.2007.11.015.
40. Cha J, Lee S, & Yoo Y. (2010). Effects of aromatherapy on changes in the autonomic nervous system, aortic pulse wave velocity and aortic augmentation index in patients with essential hypertension. *Journal of Korean Academy of Nursing*, *40*(5), 705–713.
41. Saeki Y & Shiohara M. (2001). Physiological effects of inhaling fragrances. *International Journal of Aromatherapy*, *11*(3), 118–125.
42. Haze S, Sakai K, & Gozu Y. (2002). Effects of fragrance inhalation on sympathetic activity in normal adults. *Japanese Journal of Pharmacology*, *90*, 247–253.
43. Atsumi T & Tonosaki K. (2007). Smelling lavender and rosemary increases free radical scavenging activity and decreases cortisol level in saliva. *Psychiatry Research*, *150*(1), 89–96.
44. McCaffrey R, Thomas D, & Kinzelman A. (2009). The effects of lavender and rosemary essential oils on test-taking anxiety among graduate nursing students. *Holistic Nursing Practice*, *23*(2), 88–93.
45. Lehrner J, Marwinski G, Lehr S, Johren P, & Deeke L. (2005). Ambient odors of orange and lavender reduce anxiety and improve mood in a dental office. *Physiology & Behavior*, *86*(1–2), 92–95.
46. Kritsidima M, Newton T, & Asimakopoulou K. (2010). The effects of lavender scent on dental patient anxiety levels: A cluster randomized-controlled trial. *Community Dentistry & Oral Epidemiology*, *38*(1), 83–87.
47. Lee Y, Wu Y, Tsang H, Leung A, & Cheung W. (2011). A systematic review on the anxiolytic effects of aromatherapy in people with anxiety symptoms. *Journal of Alternative & Complementary Medicine*, *17*(2), 101–108.

48. Kim J, Ren C, Fielding G, Pitti A, Kasumi T, Wajda M, Lebovits A, & Bekker A. (2007). Treatment with lavender aromatherapy in the post-anesthesia care unit reduces opioid requirements of morbidly obese patients undergoing laparoscopic adjustable gastric banding. *Obesity Surgery, 17*(7), 920–925.

49. Kane F, Brodie E, Couli A, Coyne L, Howd A, Milne A, Niven C, & Robbins R. (2004). The analgesic effect of odour and music upon dressing change. *British Journal of Nursing, 13*(19), S4–S12.

50. Kim S, Kim J, Yeo J, Hong S, Lee J, & Jeon Y. (2011). The effect of lavender oil on stress, bispectral index values, and needle insertion pain in volunteers. *Journal of Alternative & Complementary Medicine, 17*(9), 823–826.

51. Malini T, Vanithakumari G, Megala N, Anusya S, Devi K, & Elango V. (1985). Effect of *Foeniculum vulgare* mill seed extract on the genital organs of male and female rats. *Indian Journal of Physiology and Pharmacology, 29*(1), 21–26.

52. Battaglia S. (2003). *The complete guide to aromatherapy*, 2nd ed. Brisbane, Australia: International Centre of Holistic Aromatherapy.

53. Henley D, Lipson N, Korach K, & Bloch C. (2007). Prepubertal gynecomastia linked to lavender and tea tree oils. *New England Journal of Medicine, 365*(5), 479–485.

54. Tisserand R. (2011). http://roberttisserand.com/2011/07/lavender-oil-and-pregnancy/. Accessed July 23, 2011.

55. Kasper S, Gastpar M, Muller W, Volz H, Moller H, Dienel A, & Schlafke S. (2010). Silexan, an orally administered Lavandula oil preparation, is effective in the treatment of "subsyndromal" anxiety disorder: A randomized, double-blind, placebo controlled trial. *International Clinical Psychopharmacology, 25*(5), 277–287.

56. Morris N. (2002). The effects of lavender (*Lavendula angustifolium*) baths on psychological well-being: Two exploratory randomized control trials. *Complementary Therapies in Medicine, 10*, 223–228.

57. Howard S & Hughes M. (2008). Expectancies, not aroma, explain impact of lavender aromatherapy on psychophysiolical indices of relaxation in young healthy women. *British Journal of Health Psychology, 13*(4), 603–617.

58. Grunbaum T, Murdock J, Castenedo-Tardan M, Baumann L. (2011). Effects of lavender olfactory input on cosmetic procedures. *Journal of Cosmetic Dermatology, 10*(2), 89–93.

59. Burns E, Blamey C, Ersser S, Barnetson M, & Lloyd A. (2000). An investigation into the use of aromatherapy in intrapartum midwifery practice. *Journal of Alternative and Complementary Therapies, 6*(2), 141–147.

60. Burns E, Zobbi V, Panzeri D, Okrochi R, & Regalia A. (2007). Aromatherapy in childbirth: A pilot randomized controlled trial. *BJOG, 114*(7), 838–844.

61. Walker D. (2010). Effects of aromatheraphy on childbirth. www.ClinicalTrials.gov. Study ID number NCT01051726.

62. Smith C, Collins C, & Crowther C. (2011). Aromatherapy for pain management in labor. *Cochrane Database of Systematic Reviews, 7*, Art. No.: CD009215.

63. Jones C. (2011). The efficacy of lavender oil on perineal trauma: A review of the evidence. *Complementary Therapies in Clinical Practice, 17*, 215–220.

64. Tisserand R & Balacs T. (1998). *Essential oil safety: A guide for health professionals*. Edinburgh: Churchill Livingstone.

65. Vakilian K, Atarha M, Bekhradi R, & Chaman R. (2011). Healing advantages of lavender essential oil during episiotomy recovery: A clinical trial. *Complementary Therapies in Clinical Practice, 17*, 50–53.

66. Dale A & Cornwell S. (1994). The role of lavender oil in relieving perineal discomfort following childbirth: A blind randomized clinical trial. *Journal of Advanced Nursing, 19*, 89–96.

67. Imura M, Misao H, & Ushijima H. (2006). The psychological effects of aromatherapy-massage in healthy postpartum mothers. *Journal of Midwifery & Women's Health*, *51*(2), e21–e27.
68. Conrad P & Adams C. (2012). The effects of clinical aromatherapy for anxiety and depression in the high risk postpartum woman: A pilot study. *Complementary Therapies in Clinical Practice*, *18*, 164–168.
69. Rawlings F & Meerabeau L. (2003). Implementing aromatherapy in nursing and midwifery practice. *Journal of Clinical Nursing*, *12*, 405–411.
70. Mousley S. (2011). Audit of an aromatherapy service in a maternity unit. *Complementary Therapies in Clinical Practice*, *11*(3), 205–210.
71. Nowak E & Lincoln V, Integrative Services, Woodwinds Health Campus. Personal communication, March 2, 2012.
72. Conrad P. (2010). A new approach to American maternity care. *In Essence*, *9*(2), 18–20.
73. Conrad P. Personal communication, April 5, 2012.
74. Myers K, FBU Director. Personal communication, March 15, 2012.
75. Tiran D. (2003). Implementing complementary therapies into midwifery practice. *Complementary Therapies in Nursing and Midwifery*, *9*(1), 10–13.
76. Kirk-Smith M. (1996). Clinical evaluation: Deciding what questions to ask. *Nursing Times*, *92*(19), 34–35.
77. Tillett J & Ames D. (2010). The uses of aromatherapy in women's health. *Journal of Perinatal and Neonatal Nursing*, *24*(3), 238–245.
78. Fawcett M. (1993). *Aromatherapy for pregnancy and childbirth*. Shaftesbury Dorset, UK: Element.
79. Buckle J. (2003). *Clinical aromatherapy: Essential oils in practice*, 2nd ed. Philadelphia: Churchill Livingstone.
80. Bowles EJ. (2003). *The chemistry of aromatherapeutic oils*, 3rd ed. NSW, Australia: Allen & Unwin.

Chapter 11

Acupressure and acupuncture in pregnancy and childbirth

Katie Moriarty and Kennedy Sharp

Key points

- "Acupuncture" is derived from the Latin words "acus" (needle) and "punctura" (penetration). Acupressure is the use of pressure to the acupoint rather than sterile needle insertion.
- Acupuncture has been practiced in China and throughout Asia for thousands of years.
- A family of procedures are used to stimulate acupoints such as acupuncture, electro-acupuncture, moxibustion, TENS to acupoints, and acupressure.
- Traditional Chinese medicine (TCM) involves the concepts of qi, yin and yang, five-elements theory, and the Eight Principle patterns.
- Western proposed mechanism of action has several physiologic models to explain acupuncture effects.
- Acupuncture is very safe when given by appropriately trained licensed and certified practitioners utilizing appropriate sterile techniques.
- Pregnancy is well suited for the incorporation of this integrative modality.

A pregnant woman carries within her the finest piece of jade. She should enjoy all things, look at fine pictures and be attended by handsome servants.
The Chinese Classic—Admonitions to the Ladies, c. 500 B.C.

Introduction

Acupuncture and acupressure are two modalities included in the holistic medical system Traditional Chinese Medicine (TCM). This chapter will present information about the use of acupuncture and acupressure within the maternity care cycle. A review of the historical background, basic principles, theories, and philosophical framework of TCM will be presented, as well as Western theories about the mechanism of action. While the Chinese practice of acupuncture and acupressure is thousands of years old, the incorporation of its

---

Supporting a Physiologic Approach to Pregnancy and Birth: A Practical Guide, First Edition.
Edited by Melissa D. Avery.
© 2013 John Wiley & Sons, Inc. Published 2013 by John Wiley & Sons, Inc.

use in Western obstetric and midwifery care is a modern development. Current evidence related to the application of acupuncture and acupressure in maternity care will be presented, as well as information related to licensure and certification of acupuncturists to guide clinician referral or women's selection of a practitioner.

Definition of acupuncture and acupressure

Acupuncture is the insertion of single-use, sterilized needles into the skin and underlying tissue at specific points in the body (Figure 11.1). The actual word is derived from the Latin words "acus," meaning needle, and "punctura," to prick or puncture. The depth of the insertion is reliant upon the anatomy of the patient and the "de qi" sensation (dull ache, numbness, or tingling sensation) felt under the needle by the patient while the practitioner feels a "grabbing" of the needle. There are different styles of acupuncture practiced throughout the world, and some examples include TCM, Japanese, Korean, Tibetan, Vietnamese, French, British, and now Western. There is also five-element acupuncture (a subset of TCM), electro-acupuncture, scalp, hand, and auricular (ear) acupuncture.

Acupressure is a variation of acupuncture whereby fingers, instead of needles, are used to apply manual pressure to an acupoint. Applications of acupressure can be in the form of firm stationary pressure, slow-motion kneading, brisk rubbing, quick tapping, pushing and pulling strokes, gentle stretching, and rubbing or squeezing [1–3]. In TCM, it is called "tuina," which literally means "pushing-pulling," and the Japanese have an equivalent called "anma." Many

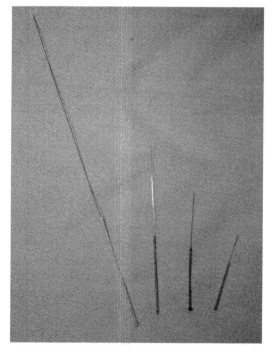

Figure 11.1   Acupuncture needles.

people have heard of "shiatsu," which is Japanese for "finger pressure." In both acupressure and acupuncture, the locations of the points (acupoints) lie along meridians or channels that traverse the human body and they are used to restore the body to balance and health.

Brief history

The history of Chinese medicine dates back thousands of years. There is evidence of "stone needle acupuncture" as early as the Neolithic period, where sharpened, polished stones were used to treat illnesses by pricking the body [4]. During the Bronze and Iron Ages, the transition from stone to needles made of silver, gold, bronze, and iron occurred. Alongside the use of acupuncture in records from the Warring States Period, 475 B.C. to 221 B.C., is moxibustion. Moxibustion is the burning of the herb mugwort (*Artemisia vulgaris*) while placed on or near an acupuncture point, used to warm the body energetically. The *Huang Di Nei Jing* (Yellow Emperor's Internal Classic), one of the oldest medical texts still in use today, references both stone and metal needles in acupuncture as well as moxibustion [5]. There is conflicting opinion as to when the text was compiled by scholars and physicians but dates ranging from the fifth to the first century B.C. are commonly referenced [4]. Acupuncture as a medical therapy emerged during the same period as Confucianism and Taoism. The philosophical influence is seen within the underpinnings of the concepts central to TCM theory.

With the introduction of Western medicine in China in the mid-seventeenth–nineteenth centuries, TCM experienced a decline, as it was associated with the lower classes. Yet in the 1950s, Mao Tse-tung, Communist Party chairman, advocated the revival of acupuncture. In 1958, the Chinese began experimenting with electro-acupuncture as a method of surgical anesthesia. Electro-acupuncture uses low-voltage electrical current via small clips that are connected to the needles.

American physicians first learned about acupuncture for acute back pain from Sir William Osler [6], often considered the father of modern medicine. However, it wasn't until the summer of 1971, when *New York Times* reporter James Reston covered President Nixon's historic trip to China, that acupuncture received widespread notice in the Western world. Reston had an emergency appendectomy and experienced a postoperative paralytic ileus that was successfully treated with acupuncture and moxibustion. He returned to the United States and wrote his seminal front-page article [7]. Interest and the use of acupuncture have continued to grow. In 1997, the U.S. National Institutes of Health issued a consensus development conference statement whereby they recognized acupuncture as a mainstream medicine healing option, documenting acupuncture's safety and efficacy for a range of health conditions [8].

Mechanism of action: Eastern theories

Concept of qi

According to the TCM perspective, the mechanism of action involved in acupuncture and acupressure is reliant upon the existence of qi (pronounced as "chee") and its dynamic dual energies of yin qi and yang qi. Qi has numerous translations, including energy, vital force, breath, and life force. Qi is the primal, motive force underlying all functions, states, and patterns of being within the human body and the larger universe.

Yin yang theory

From both a traditional Chinese medical and philosophical standpoint, yin and yang are created out of the chaos of qi. They are two opposite yet mutually related aspects existing in the same and one thing, qi. The original meaning of yin is "the side of a mountain turning away from the sun," and the original meaning of yang is "the side of a mountain facing the sun." Yin exhibits the properties of being in the shade, turned away from the sun. Yin is cool, dark, still, moves inward, and is symbolic of water and the moon. Yang exhibits the properties of being in the sun. Yang is warm, bright, active, moves upward, and is symbolic of fire and the sun. Further, yang is light and moves upward to create heaven. Yin is heavy and turbid and condenses to create earth [9].

In TCM, yin and yang relate to each other in four different ways: (1) mutual opposition, (2) interdependence, (3) wane and wax and equilibrium, and (4) transformation. Mutual opposition means that yin and yang are opposite to each other in nature and struggle against each other. It is this struggle that promotes the movement of qi. The interdependence of yin and yang means that yin and yang generate and create each other, for example, without cold there is no heat and without heat there is no cold. The waning, waxing, and equilibrium of yin and yang describe the balance that is maintained between the two essences. Similar to the waxing and waning of the moon, yin rises while yang declines followed by yang rising while yin declines. Transformation can occur in extreme cases whereby yin completely turns into yang or yang completely turns into yin.

The Tao symbol (Figure 11.2) exhibits the relationships between yin and yang. It is black and white, demonstrating mutual opposition. It is round and in the shape of a circle, demonstrating the cyclical process and movement of nature and interdependence. The small black dot within the larger white space and the small white dot within the larger black space represent equilibrium; there is a little yin within yang and yang within yin. At the top and bottom of the symbols, the tails of white and black meet the largest spaces of the opposing colors, representing transformation; at the extreme of one it turns into the other.

In short, health and homeostasis exist when the natural movement of qi is maintained and flowing smoothly. Disease in the body occurs when the movement of qi is out of

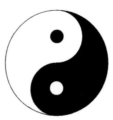

Figure 11.2   The Tao symbol.

Table 11.1   The five elements and associations.

Element	Zang-Fu Meridians	Emotion	Developmental Phase	Season	Color	Direction
Wood	Liver Gall-bladder	Anger	Birth	Spring	Green	East
Fire	Heart Small intestine	Joy	Growth	Summer	Red	South
Earth	Spleen Stomach	Worry	Transition	Late summer	Yellow	Center
Metal	Lung Large intestine	Grief	Fruition	Autumn	White	West
Water	Kidney Urinary bladder	Fear	Decline	Winter	Black or blue	North

order, disorganized, blocked, or deficient. Acupuncture and acupressure can help the body restore the natural movement, flow, and balance of qi, thereby strengthening the body's defensive ability to resist pathogenic factors.

Five-elements theory

The Taoist Chinese philosophers concluded that wood, fire, earth, metal, and water were the five basic materials or elements for life. They expanded their principles to the human body and associated seasons, tastes, orientations, colors, environmental factors, and emotions to the five elements (Table 11.1). Within the five-elements theory, there are four main relationships of interaction among the elements. The four relationships are (a) generating or interpromoting (Shen cycle), (b) controlling or interrestraining (Ko cycle), (c) overacting (Cheng cycle), and (d) counteracting (Wu cycle). The cycles explain both the normal physiology and pathology experienced by the human body. The normal physiologic cycles are the generating and controlling cycles while the cycles overacting and counteracting are seen within pathological conditions.

Zang Fu organ theory

In the body, the five elements are manifested through five yin organs (Zang) and five yang organs (Fu). Along with these five yin and yang organs are the pericardium and triple warmer, which are considered special physiologic organs. Each organ system has a yin and yang aspect, yet overall, the Zang organs are considered yin, as they store the body's essence and are solid in shape. The Fu organs are considered yang, as they are hollow and their functions are transformative in nature. The Zang or yin organs are the liver, heart, spleen, lungs, kidneys, and pericardium. The Fu or yang organs are the gall-bladder, small intestine, stomach, large intestine, urinary bladder, and triple warmer. The introduction of philosophical concepts and theories heavily influenced the formation of the Zang Fu theory. These Chinese conceptualizations are based on thousands of years of clinical observation and on a physiologic aspect of the body systems.

Meridians/collaterals/acupuncture points

The Chinese use the words "jing luo" to refer to the meridians and collaterals of the body in which qi flows. Jing is used to describe the main channels or meridians. Luo is the term used for collaterals that branch from the main meridians to circulate qi.

Jing is composed of Twelve Regular Meridians with six yin channels (Heart, Lungs, Kidneys, Liver, Spleen, and Pericardium) and the six yang channels (Large Intestine, Small intestine, Stomach, Gallbladder, Urinary Bladder, and Triple Warmer). Of the Eight Extraordinary Meridians, two are commonly used in practice. The two commonly used Extra Meridians are the Du or Governing Vessel (GV) and the Ren or Conception Vessel (CV) channels. The meridians and collaterals connect all aspects of the body: superior to inferior, anterior to posterior, right to left, interior to exterior, and the internal Zang-Fu with the limbs of the body.

Located along these meridians are the acupuncture points (acupoints). Classical acupuncturists describe 361 acupoints on the Twelve Regular Meridians with 50 more points located along the Du (Governing Vessel/GV) and Ren (Conception Vessel/CV) meridians [10]. The points serve as entry points into the meridians, allowing the practitioner to manipulate the qi of the human body.

Diagnosis and the eight principles

The Eight Principles consist of four dualities and are used in TCM to help the practitioner form a diagnosis. The four dualities are yin/yang, interior/exterior, deficiency/excess, and cold/heat. These principles guide the practitioner in determining the location, nature, and pathogenic factors of the disease. In addition to the Eight Principles, the four basic diagnostic skills used in TCM are observation, listening and smelling (in Chinese this is one character), inquiring, and palpation.

Expectations and what can occur in a typical TCM treatment

TCM diagnosis is pattern-based, and to make an accurate diagnosis, an acupuncturist gathers the patient's health history and thoroughly questions, listens, observes, and palpates the patient. In TCM, thorough questioning about the subtleties of her symptoms occurs. An example for pregnancy-related nausea and vomiting would be, "What time of day are you vomiting or most nauseous?" "Are you dizzy or light-headed?" "Do you tend to feel cold or hot?" "Do you have heartburn or other accompanying symptoms?" "Does pressure around your stomach make you feel better or worse?" From these questions, in addition to palpation of her pulses and observation of her tongue, a diagnosis will be made. Some common patterns in nausea and vomiting are Phlegm Heat, Liver overacting on the Spleen, or Yang Rising; each of these patterns is treated with a different acupoint prescription. Once the point prescription is determined, needles are inserted into the patient and retained for 20–40 minutes depending upon the therapeutic goal and constitution of the patient. Some common feelings that arise from needle sensation or "de qi" can be numbness, tingling, itching, pulsing, and warmth while the acupuncturist feels a "grasping" of the needle. A common "de qi" sensation elicited by acupressure is a dull

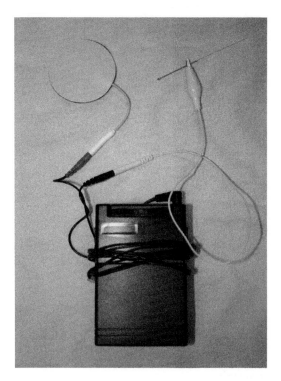

Figure 11.3 TENS equipment.

ache. Most people find acupuncture and acupressure very relaxing and can even fall asleep during the session.

The therapeutic relationship between provider and patient is itself seen as an opportunity for the promotion of healing. Herbs can also be incorporated for medicinal purposes. In pregnancy, a common example is the use of ginger and peppermint. Other physical methods can be incorporated, such as massage (tui na), electro-acupuncture, transcutaneous electrical nerve stimulation (TENS) to acupoints (Figure 11.3), auricular (ear) acupuncture (Figure 11.4), cupping (applying heated glass cups that give slight suction to acupoints (Figure 11.5), and moxibustion (Figure 11.6). Lastly, lifestyle counseling can be included on such topics as diet, exercise, emotions, and the use of mind-body therapies such as qi-gong and tai chi, both of which utilize breathing and meditation practices.

Mechanism of action: Western perspective/theories

The effects of acupuncture and acupressure are complex and the mechanism of action is not entirely clear. Acupuncture or acupressure is a physical stimulus and the human body elicits a response to this stimulus. It is hypothesized that acupoints have a correlation to known neural structures and elicit a variety of effects or responses in the body and the brain in ways not yet completely understood [8].

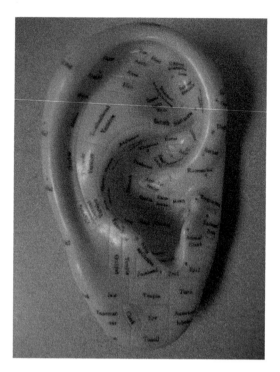

Figure 11.4   Auricular acupuncture.

Within the TCM paradigm, acupuncture impacts qi and the yin/yang relationship to create balance, while in Western terms this balance could be analogous to homeostasis. Homeostasis of the internal human environment depends on three basic components: (1) sensory mechanism, (2) integrating mechanism, and (3) effector mechanism [11]. Once the acupuncture needle is inserted into the body or acupressure is applied, it can begin to evoke physiologic change. These physiologic changes allude to both the mechanisms of action and the therapeutic goals of acupuncture and acupressure, which can include the control of pain, the resolution of inflammation, the support of regeneration, the restoration of physical function, or the normalization of the autonomic nervous activities [11,12].

Acupoints are places on the skin that have lower resistance to the passage of electricity than the surrounding skin. In 1972, Dr. Chan Gunn identified seventy acupoints using an ohm-meter, an instrument that can measure this skin resistance [13]. He classified the acupoints according to their relationship to known neural structures such as superficial nerves to the skin, nerve plexi (main junctions of nerves), points where segmental nerves coming off the spinal cord meet in the midline of the body, at the joining of muscles and tendons, and at motor points. It is suspected that the meridians, the TCM energetic pathways, and actual acupoints correspond mainly to the distribution of the peripheral nervous system by coinciding with nerve endings or points of bifurcation.

(a)

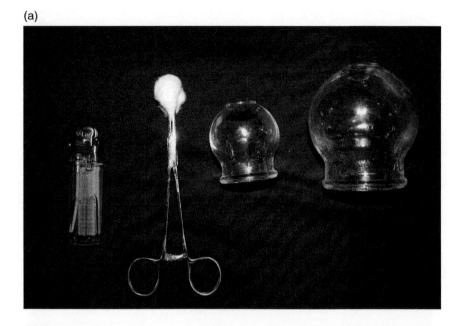

(b)

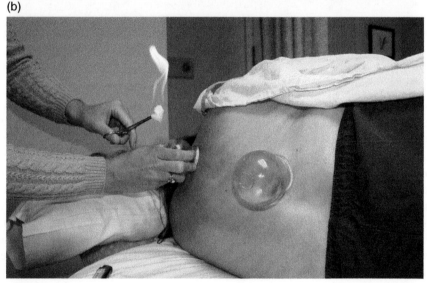

Figure 11.5   (a) Cupping equipment, and (b) cupping with patient.

Western health care providers trained in acupuncture often use an anatomical approach. Rather than using a TCM paradigm, the practitioner combines knowledge of acupuncture with her/his knowledge of anatomy, physiology, and pathophysiology [12,14]. The selection of stimulation sites is based on geographically relevant acupoints, anatomically relevant acupoints (peripheral nerves or spinal or ventral segmental nerves according to dermatomes, myotomes, and sclerotomes), acupoints considered sympathetic or

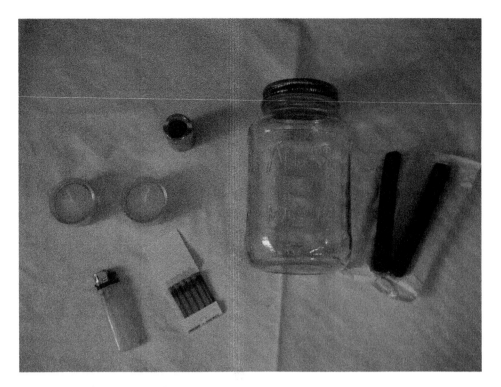

Figure 11.6   Moxibustion equipment.

parasympathetic "switches," relevant cortical sites, motor points, musculotendinous junctions, points related to joints, or relevant projectional sites (microsystems such as the external ear in auricular acupuncture, nose, hand, and foot) [12,14].

Acupuncture stimulation could be seen as an irritant or small microinjury to cells, causing the cells to produce or release a number of chemicals such as bradykinin, substance P, and prostaglandins. The acupuncture needle is seen as a foreign body, and this sensitization would mount a reaction. If there is sufficient activation, an action potential is generated and transmitted to the spinal cord and the brain through nerve axons. A number of steps or synapses would ensue until the stimulus signals arrive at the brain. Activation of the central nervous system (CNS) elicits changes in neurotransmitters, hormones (including cortisol and oxytocin), the immune system, biomechanical effects, and other biochemical substances (endorphins, immune system cells such as cytokines). This is believed to have a normalizing, modulating, or balancing effect.

The interconnections between the higher, intermediate, and lower brain are a large focus for scientists conducting basic science acupuncture research [15]. The limbic system, especially the amygdala together with the hypothalamus, is hypothesized to play the central role in the acupuncture mechanism, including pain control. The hypothalamus is the master controller of the autonomic system. Located in the center of the brain, it has endocrine functions that control hormonal balance and autonomic functions (sympathetic and parasympathetic) together with neurochemical effects. The hypothalamus integrates external and internal stimuli to regulate the internal body environment and homeostatic functions. The amygdala is the major mediator between the sensory and motor hierarchy.

Examination of the mechanism of acupuncture action has also been revolutionized by the use of functional magnetic resonance imaging (fMRI), which has demonstrated that stimulation of specific acupuncture points may have regionally specific, quantifiable effects on relevant structures of the human brain [16–19]. The activation of various brain areas such as the visual and auditory cortices has led to the hypothesis that signals from the brain project through the limbic structures, such as the amygdala, and descend to the hypothalamic center to stimulate endocrine, autonomic, and other functions for the purpose of homeostasis.

It must be remembered that multiple processes occur in a healing encounter. The specific effects of acupuncture are considered to arise from the site of needling and the technique of needling. Some of the influences or nonspecific therapeutic effects (placebo effect) could include the individual's faith and belief or expectations in a treatment modality, focused attention from a provider, or a provider that focuses her/his intention for healing purposes. Nonspecific physiologic effects (nonplacebo effect) could include the relaxation effects, microcirculatory effects, or diffuse noxious inhibitory control mechanism. Nontreatment-related nonspecific effects such as regression to the mean can impact outcomes. Acupuncture is a complex holistic intervention, and research in this area includes the basic science of the mechanism of action as well as the influence of clinical applications.

One controversial aspect within acupuncture research is the choice of an appropriate control condition. Options include "placebo" needles that do not puncture the skin, "sham" acupuncture that does puncture the skin (but at alternate points or nonpoints, near or far from true acupoints), TENS or laser devices with the power "off," placebo ointments, usual care, or alternative treatments. The impact or mechanics involved with any touch or needling of an acupoint has a physiologic effect. The sham needling with acupuncture may not be different in effect from "true" acupuncture, and even the placebo needling is problematic. Despite no skin penetration, the placebo needle tip exerts a mechanical stimulation that may also excite nociceptive primary afferents. With any touch or needling, even to nonacupoint locations, there is a mechanical stimulation that can excite primary afferents and evoke a physiological response. The sensory stimulation still generates impulses that target the brain, regardless of the site of stimulation or the degree of invasiveness. Although the pattern and degree of response to these stimulations may vary, no skin location can be considered "inert" [20].

Safety

Acupuncture is a safe treatment when performed by qualified practitioners. Adverse effects are largely preventable if a patient has recently eaten, is treated while lying down, and practitioners are cognizant of underlying anatomy. Major complications are *extremely* rare but would include perforation of viscus (lung, bowel, bladder), viral infection (hepatitis, HIV), or the masking of serious organic conditions by relieving pain. Minor adverse effects are often unavoidable and include bruising, temporary aggravation or worsening of symptoms, syncope, and nausea. However, there are minor effects such as broken or forgotten needles that are considered avoidable. Hazards with electro-acupuncture include interference with cardiac pacemakers (if improperly placed) and pain if excessive stimulation is applied. It is much safer to avoid the use of electro-acupuncture in people with cardiac pacers. Hazards with TENS would entail skin reactions to tape or electrodes or temporary aggravation of symptoms. Hazards with acupressure could theoretically be bruising.

White [21] conducted a cumulative review from 1994 to 2004 to summarize the range and frequency of significant adverse events associated with acupuncture. Data were extracted from all available types of publications including case reports, reviews of the literature, population surveys, prospective surveys of acupuncture practice, and textbooks that had been cited in case reports or otherwise come to the author's attention. A total of 715 adverse events were reported from either a primary source (the clinician) or a secondary source (another author). Trauma and infection were the most common serious adverse events. There were 90 primary and 137 secondary reports of trauma (most common was pneumothorax, representing over 80% of cases) and 204 primary and 91 secondary reports of infection (most common was hepatitis B representing over 60% of cases). According to the evidence from twelve prospective studies in which more than a million treatments were examined, the risk of a serious adverse event with acupuncture is estimated to be 0.05 per 10,000 treatments and 0.55 per 10,000 individual patients. White concluded the risk of serious events occurring in association with acupuncture is *very low*, below that of many common medical treatments.

MacPherson and colleagues [22] conducted a postal survey of prospectively identified acupuncture patients. Baseline information and consent were obtained from 9,408 patients and 6,348 (67%) completed the 3-month follow-up questionnaires. The 3-month questionnaires provided data on patients' reporting on what they perceived to be adverse events, either caused directly by the acupuncture treatment or indirectly as a result of following the acupuncturist's advice about medication or from delayed conventional diagnosis or treatment. At least one adverse event over the 3 months was reported by 682 patients, a rate of 107 per 1,000 patients (95% CI 100–115). The most common events reported were severe tiredness and exhaustion, pain at the site of needling, and headache.

Incorporating acupuncture and acupressure into pregnancy

Pregnancy is a major life transition for a woman where immense anatomic, physiologic, and psychological changes occur. Women are often motivated to seek knowledge about safe options for care to assist them in achieving optimal health for their babies and themselves. Acupuncture and acupressure are therapeutic modalities for the whole woman: mind, body, and spirit. These therapies can relieve discomforts and help prepare the body for being in optimal balance.

Health care providers can help by understanding basic background and the presumed mechanism of action of a therapy, being cognizant of any safety issues, and being informed about current evidence. Common uses of acupuncture and acupressure during pregnancy and postpartum can be found in Table 11.2.

Table 11.2 Common uses of acupuncture and acupressure in pregnancy and postpartum.

Antepartum	Intrapartum	Postpartum
Digestive discomforts: nausea, vomiting, morning sickness, heartburn, constipation, and hemorrhoids Mental health issues: stress, anxiety, depression, and insomnia Sinus congestion, edema, bladder and urinary issues, and fatigue Pain: sciatica, carpal tunnel syndrome, headaches, migraines, back and pelvic pain Breech presentation Cervical ripening and labor encouragement	Postdate induction of labor Labor augmentation and regulation of uterine contractions Malposition of the fetus Labor discomfort or pain Anxiety	Postpartum discomfort Lactation issues Enhancing energy levels Postpartum anxiety, depression, or stress Urinary concerns

Specific care when treating pregnant women

During pregnancy, it is important to avoid certain contraindicated acupoints or certain combinations of acupoints until term because the acupoints may be involved with cervical ripening or uterine contraction stimulation or are in close proximity to the growing uterus. Therefore, points on the abdomen should generally be avoided. Exceptions include acupoints Xiawan/Ren 10, Jianli/Ren 11, and Zhongwan/Ren 12, which are located *on the abdomen above the umbilicus* and can be used in early pregnancy for nausea and vomiting. Additional abdominal acupoint exceptions, located below the umbilicus, are those used early in pregnancy for threatened miscarriage or spotting and include Zhongji/Ren 3, Guanyuan/Ren 4, and Qihai/Ren 6.

Acupoints and combinations of acupoints that promote cervical ripening or stimulate uterine contractions should be avoided until term gestation; therefore, they are not used prior to 37 weeks gestation. These acupoints include lumbosacral points and points considered "sympathetic switches": Taichong/Liver 3 (LR3) and Hegu/Large Intestine 4 (LI4); Kunlun/Urinary Bladder 60 (UB60), Zhiyin/Urinary Bladder 67 (UB67), Sanyinjiao/Spleen 6 (SP6), and Jianjing/Gallbladder 21 (GB21). Point combinations that are particularly contraindicated unless a woman is at term include SP6 in conjunction with LI4, LR3, or UB60.

Certain conditions, if present during pregnancy, would necessitate caution or avoidance of acupuncture use. Acupuncture can be used with caution as an adjunct to care if the woman has high blood pressure, cancer (symptom management), varicosities (above or below the varicosity is permitted), and fractures (above or below the fracture is permitted). Acupuncture and acupressure are best avoided if there is a blood clotting disorder, thrombosis, herniated vertebral discs, or over skin that has open sores, burns, ulcerations, or a current active skin disease.

Acupuncture and acupressure are very beneficial for pregnancy, labor, and the puerperium as an adjunct to obstetrical and midwifery care. Relief for common pregnancy discomforts and other conditions can be provided with a high success rate. Certain acupressure techniques are easily learned by a provider, may be taught to a woman or her partner, and are safe, easy to administer, and inexpensive. However, care providers must realize their limitations in training and education and refer women to a qualified, reputable practitioner when application beyond basic techniques is warranted.

Selected uses during pregnancy

Several examples of acupuncture and acupressure are provided to demonstrate the potential of this treatment modality, and research evidence is reviewed.

Nausea and vomiting

Most health care providers are aware of the benefits of acupuncture and acupressure use for nausea and vomiting. One of the most commonly used points in a point prescription for nausea and vomiting is Neiguan/Pericardium 6 (PC6). Stimulation of PC6 can be by acupuncture, acupressure [by fingers or using wrist bands; see Figure 11.7(a) and (b)], or a nerve stimulator (Relief Bands). PC6 is located three finger-breadths above the palmar wrist crease between the palmaris longus and flexor carpi radialis tendons. It is important to use the finger-breadth of the woman being treated; acupuncture points are located on a proportional scale specific to the individual. Acupressure can be self-administered, and the acupressure wristbands or nerve stimulators do not require a prescription. The wristbands can be purchased or handmade by taping an uncooked bean (i.e., pinto bean) to the acupoint. These techniques have not been associated with any adverse effects on pregnancy outcomes, hence there should be no hesitation to make this recommendation. See Box 11.1 for specific provider information.

Several systematic reviews have evaluated information regarding the effectiveness and safety of acupuncture, acupressure, and nerve stimulators for nausea and vomiting. Festin [23] concluded that acupressure at P6 is likely beneficial for early nausea and vomiting when compared to sham acupressure and reduces vomiting associated with hyperemesis gravidarum compared to sham acupressure. However, it is unknown if acupressure is more effective then pyridoxine at reducing nausea and vomiting. Results are varied with acupuncture resulting in the conclusion of unknown effectiveness for decreasing nausea and vomiting in early pregnancy or decreasing vomiting with hyperemesis gravidarum. The strong placebo effect with those receiving sham therapy might account for these findings, as there still may be a physiologic response when sham acupuncture is performed. A meta-analysis by Helmreich et al. [24] of acupressure, electro-stimulation bands, and manual acupuncture for nausea and vomiting in pregnancy examined fourteen trials including 1,655 women. Similar conclusions that acupressure and electro-stimulation had greater impact than manual acupuncture in the treatment of nausea and vomiting were reported. Smith et al. [25] found that women receiving *individualized* TCM diagnosis and acupoint selection had the fastest relief of their nausea and dry-retching compared to women that received sham acupuncture, only PC6 needling, or no treatment.

(a)

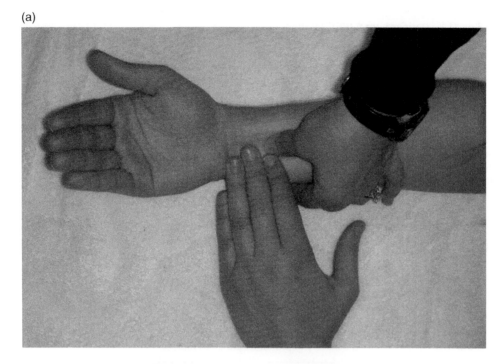

(b)

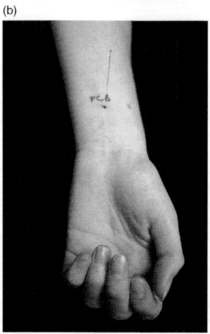

Figure 11.7   (a) P6 acupressure, and (b) acupuncture.

Box 11.1   Pericardium 6 (P6)/Neiguan

Indication: Useful acupoint for nausea and vomiting during pregnancy or labor.
Point location: Locate the transverse wrist crease on the inner aspect of the arm. Then place the woman's ring finger, middle finger, and index finger at the transverse crease of the wrist with the ring finger's outer edge level even with the transverse wrist crease. Two tendons (palmaris longus and flexor carpi radialis) are palpable beneath the three fingers. The point is located between these two tendons on the outer edge of the index finger.
Technique for acupressure: With your thumb or the patient's free thumb, press the point until a sensation is elicited. Women usually report feeling a tingling, heavy, or achy sensation. Apply pressure to this point until the nausea resolves or for approximately 3–5 minutes. Pressure can be applied to the other arm if the nausea persists.
   It can be helpful to use the thumbnail (instead of the pad of the thumb) to accurately get between the two tendons to apply pressure. Apply firm perpendicular pressure to the acupoint, using firm pressure.
   A wristband that is commonly used for seasickness can be purchased and used to provide a low level of pressure to the acupoint. If nausea worsens, push on the bead that is over the P6 acupoint (again for 3–5 minutes) and then apply acupressure to the bead on the other arm. Also, nerve stimulator(s) (looks somewhat like a watch) can be placed bilaterally over P6 acupoint. The stimulation can be increased or decreased as needed with the presence or absence of nausea.
Referral: Practitioners should refer to a qualified licensed acupuncturist when the woman desires strategies beyond acupressure, is not getting results with acupressure, and/or her quality of life is being impacted. Always review warning signs related to nausea/vomiting so the woman knows when to contact her prenatal care provider.

Carpal tunnel syndrome

Carpal tunnel syndrome (CTS) etiology is characterized by compression of the distal median nerve due to elevated interstitial fluid pressure in the carpal tunnel. The median nerve supplies sensation to the 1st, 2nd, 3rd, and a portion of the 4th metacarpals, and impingement of the nerve results in numbness, weakness, or tingling sensations. In pregnancy, the increased production and retention of fluid in the woman's body can cause CTS. This pregnancy discomfort can be very debilitating, impacting physical comfort, sleeping patterns, and functioning. During pregnancy, points are needled locally over the median nerve to relieve the pain and tingling, as well as distally to promote fluid metabolism and address the woman's overall edema. Local acupoints YangChi/SJ4 and Waiguan/SJ5 on the posterior aspect of the forearm and Neiguan/PC6 and Daling/PC7 on the anterior aspect of the arm, utilized for treatment of CTS, are shown in Figure 11.8.

   Acupuncture most likely affects CTS pathology and symptomatology through both peripheral and central mechanisms. Because CTS is due to ischemic neuropathology, the ability of acupuncture to induce increased blood flow both superficially and deep to the surface may improve microcirculation to the impacted median nerve within the carpal tunnel. The vasodilatory effect of acupuncture may result from the release of calcitonin gene-related peptide (CGRP) and other vasodilatory neuropeptides. In future studies, researchers should assess peripheral effects of acupuncture concurrently with central effects. Napadow and colleagues [26] used fMRI imaging to evaluate acupuncture and sham acupuncture stimulation in CTS nonpregnant patients and healthy controls. They

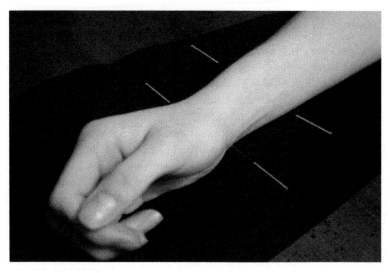

Figure 11.8   CTS treatment.

examined short- and long-term brain response (retesting after 5 weeks of treatment) and found that participants with CTS responded to acupuncture with more pronounced fMRI signal decrease in the amygdala and signal increase in the lateral hypothalamic area. The functional connectivity found between the amygdala and hypothalamus suggests that a coordinated limbic response to acupuncture stimuli may underlie the efficacy of this healing modality.

There are no studies that specifically investigated acupuncture and CTS during pregnancy; however, a recent systematic review and meta-analysis concluded that the evidence for acupuncture as a symptomatic therapy of CTS is encouraging and that further rigorous studies are required [27].

Low back pain, pelvic girdle, and sciatica

Pain in the lower back and pelvic area are common discomforts during the latter months of pregnancy due to weight gain and the shifting center of gravity. The degree of discomfort can range from mild to debilitating. Acupuncture and acupressure can offer pain relief and management of the pain without pharmaceutical use throughout the pregnancy. The specific point prescriptions vary and are dependent upon the location of the pain and the individual.

Authors of two systematic reviews of pelvic and back pain [28,29] reported that acupuncture as an adjunct treatment was superior to standard treatment alone and physiotherapy in relieving pain. Both acupuncture and stabilizing exercises relieved pelvic pain more than standard prenatal care, and acupuncture resulted in more relief of pain occurring in the evening than exercises. Women with both pelvic and back pain found acupuncture more effective than physiotherapy in reducing the intensity of their pain. The acupuncture group reported less intense pain than the usual standard of care group.

Breech presentation

In approximately 3–4% of pregnancies, the fetus will present in the breech position at term. Use of acupuncture-type interventions on acupuncture point Zhiyin/UB 67 has been shown to be beneficial in inducing correction of a breech presentation, reducing the number of cesarean sections, and decreasing cost when compared to expectant management, including external cephalic version (ECV) [30]. Acupuncture-type interventions include the use of moxibustion, combining acupuncture and moxibustion, or acupuncture alone to the acupoint. Zhiyin/UB 67 is located on the lateral side of the 5th metatarsal, just inferior to the bottom outer corner of the toenail.

The frequency of moxibustion that needs to be administered requires that the technique be taught to the woman and administered at home herself or by a partner (Figure 11.9). The acupuncturist provides an initial treatment, teaches the technique, and provides written instructions and moxibustion supplies, and then the woman returns for follow-up care. This technique is noninvasive, effective, safe, and can be encouraged. Optimal circumstances for using moxibustion are approximately 33–34 weeks gestation; smaller fetuses can turn more easily. Typically women would have the treatment daily for 10 days, 20 minutes each day. If the 10-day course is not successful, there is time to repeat the treatment. If moxibustion continues to be unsuccessful, we have anecdotally found that the ECV is much easier with less discomfort having had the moxibustion treatment. Some acupuncturists administer moxibustion with the woman in the "on all fours" position to try to allow for maximal fetal movement. Finally, if the fetus does turn to the cephalic presentation, an abdominal binder can be applied.

Moxibustion is hypothesized to increase corticoadrenal secretion, resulting in increased placental estrogens and changes in the prostaglandin levels. These alterations are thought to impact the myometrial sensitivity and contractility, resulting in an

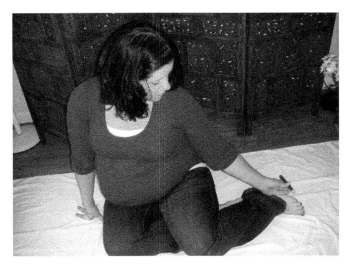

Figure 11.9 Self-administration.

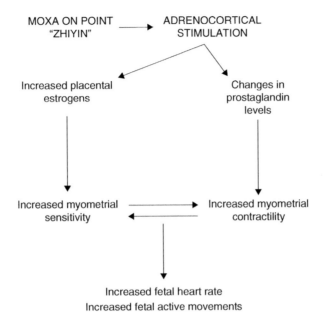

Figure 11.10 Proposed mechanism of action for moxibustion.

increase in fetal activity movements [31]. Increased fetal activity heightens the chance of spontaneous rotation (see Figure 11.10).

A recent Cochrane review by Coyle, Smith, and Peat [32] concluded that moxibustion resulted in fewer noncephalic presentations at birth compared with acupuncture alone. When combined with acupuncture, moxibustion resulted in fewer noncephalic presentations at birth and fewer births by cesarean section compared with no treatment. Moxibustion, when combined with a postural technique, was also found to result in fewer noncephalic presentations at birth compared with the postural technique alone. Postural techniques are often suggested by physicians and midwives to promote spontaneous version of a breech presentation. Postural techniques include knee to chest or lifting the buttocks onto several pillows while lying on the back.

Cervical ripening and labor encouragement

Prebirth treatment is a series of weekly acupuncture or acupressure treatments that begin at 37 weeks gestation. The treatments prepare the mind and body for labor at term. Acupuncture, electro-acupuncture, TENS to acupoints, acupressure, or combinations of the four modalities are administered. The treatment is administered while in the semi-Fowler's or side lying position for approximately 20–30 minutes. Both women and their partners can be briefly trained on locating points and encouraged to apply acupressure, focusing on tender points, several times a day.

If a woman is approaching 41–42 weeks gestation or an indication arises for a medical induction, treatments can commence to assist with cervical ripening and to encourage uterine contractions. If possible, use of these techniques can be helpful when done for several days prior to a scheduled medical induction of labor. Treatment duration would be approximately 30 minutes and can be extended up to several hours. Acupoints commonly stimulated for cervical ripening and labor encouragement include the following: GB21, Ciliao/UB 32, Sanyinjiao/SP6, Yanglingquan/GB 34, Zusanli/ST 36, Shenmai/UB 62, Jiaoxin/Kidney 8, and KI 3. To promote an optimal position (occiput anterior), Kunlun/ UB 60 and Zhiyin/UB 67 can also be administered. Additional acupoints may be added for individualized situations.

The mechanism of action of acupuncture for cervical ripening or initiating uterine contractions is unknown. The selected acupoints may be activating afferent nerve fibers and influencing hormonal changes through the ascending pathways to the hypothalamus, or reflex activation of autonomic efferents to the uterus. Alternatively, it may be a commonality of the spinal cord segment of the parasympathetic outflow and the spinal reference of the acupuncture point selected for treatment [33]. SP6 is an acupoint that is often used in prebirth treatments, labor initiation, and labor augmentation (Figure 11.11). SP6 is located on the medial side of the lower leg, four of the patient's finger-breadths superior to the prominence of the medial malleolus. The Spleen meridian traverses the dermatomes of the areas of L1 to L5 and then upward toward T12 to T5. The sympathetic nerves controlling the uterus through the pelvic plexus receive the preganglionic fibers out of T5 to L4.

Lim et al. [33] conducted a comprehensive search of literature from 1970 to 2008, and although the definitive role of acupuncture in inducing labor is still yet to be established, existing studies suggested that acupuncture may stimulate the onset of labor, with all the preliminary findings demonstrating some positive effects in reduction of labor duration. Smith & Crowther [34] conducted a systematic review of acupuncture for cervical ripening or induction of labor and concluded that acupuncture for induction of labor appeared safe, had no known teratogenic effects, and compared to standard obstetric care resulted in fewer methods of induction. Electro-acupuncture may be especially helpful in cervical ripening and reducing complications. Griebel et al. [35] randomized sixty-seven women into two groups, one using electro-acupuncture and one using the cervical ripening agent misopristol. Although the group using electro-acupuncture experienced a longer duration of labor, they felt more positive about their birth, had a higher frequency of vaginal births, and no obstetric complications.

Acupuncture can be utilized for labor augmentation. Guadernack et al. [36] randomized one hundred healthy pregnant women with spontaneous rupture of membranes into two groups, acupuncture and no acupuncture. The acupuncture group had a significant reduction in the need for oxytocin to augment labor ($p = 0.018$), and their duration of labor was significantly reduced (mean difference of 1.7 hours, $p = 0.03$). In addition, when induction was necessary for participants in either group, the women given acupuncture experienced a shorter duration of active phase labor.

Only one study involving shiatsu (the Japanese equivalent to acupressure) as a pre-birth treatment has been published [37], yet it demonstrated encouraging outcomes with a significantly lower induction of labor rate (17% lower) and a higher spontaneous onset of labor rate (68% vs. 46%, $p = 0.038$). Acupressure can be used for augmenta-tion, and Lee and colleagues [38] randomized seventy-five women to acupressure at

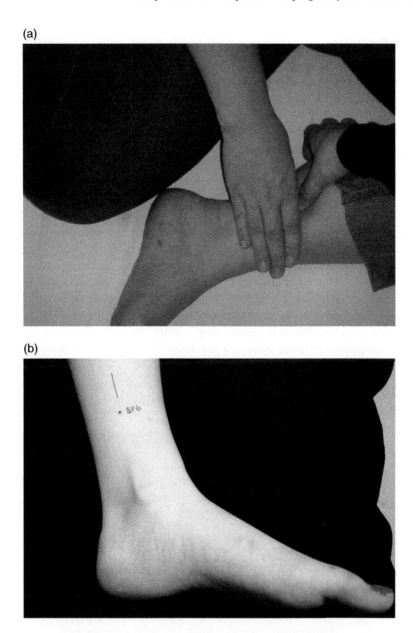

Figure 11.11 (a) Spleen 6 (acupressure) and (b) Spleen 6 (acupuncture).

SP6 versus SP6 touch control group. The authors reported that the acupressure group experienced a significantly decreased level of anxiety pre- to posttreatment; decreased labor pain immediately posttreatment, 30 minutes, and 60 minutes posttreatment; significantly shorter duration of first stage of labor; and shorter overall total length of labor (p = 0.006).

Labor pain

Acupuncture and acupressure can assist women seeking an unmedicated birth or who desire options to help them cope during labor. Tension, anxiety, apprehension, and fear can impact and influence a woman's perception of discomfort or pain, which impacts a woman's labor and birth experience. Pregnant women and their partners, as well as health professionals, can download an instructional acupressure booklet (available in several languages) from the Debra Betts website. The website includes YouTube videos to assist with proper acupoint location and information about an instructional DVD that demonstrates acupressure techniques for labor discomfort [39].

Spleen 6 is an acupoint that has been documented to decrease labor pain with the application of electro-acupuncture [40], acupressure [41], or even ice (Figure 11.12) [42]. Auricular acupuncture may be practical for women that find it difficult to remain still for acupuncture. Stainless beads or intradermal needles with plaster are applied to one ear and a woman stimulates the points by applying enough pressure to elicit the "de qi" sensation. Stimulation of the points can be during a contraction or between contractions or as often as the woman finds helpful. On average, 10–15 minutes time is required for effects to be felt [43]. Effective auricular points include Shenmen, Endocrine, and Uterus (seen in Figure 11.4).

It has been proposed that acupuncture may modify the perception of pain or alter physiologic functions. Dr. Bruce Pomeranz has described the most convincing hypothesis

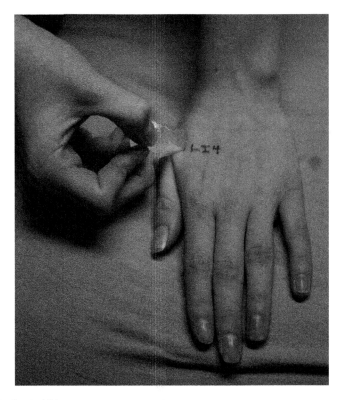

Figure 11.12   Ice to LI4.

of acupuncture analgesia [44]. In the model, it is proposed that the acupuncture needle acti-vates a sensory receptor stimulating small diameter nerves in muscles, which send impulses to the spinal cord and activate three centers (spinal cord, midbrain, and hypothalamus-pituitary) to cause analgesia. The centers are activated to release transmitter chemicals (spinal cord: enkephalin or dynorphin; midbrain: enkephalin and monoamines such as serotonin and norepinephrine; hypothalamus-pituitary: β-endorphins) that block pain messages.

The most recent Cochrane review [45] included thirteen trials with data reporting on 1,986 women. Nine trials examined acupuncture and four trials examined acupressure. Less intense pain was reported from acupuncture compared with no intervention (one trial, 163 women). One trial found increased satisfaction with pain relief compared with placebo control (150 women). Reduced use of pharmacologic analgesia was found in one trial of acupuncture compared with placebo (136 women) and compared with standard care. Following acupuncture treatment, fewer instrumental deliveries were found compared with standard care (three trials, 704 women); however, there was significant heterogeneity of methods and treatments among the trials. Pain intensity was reduced in the acupressure group compared with a placebo control (one trial, 120 women) and a combined control (two trials, 322 women). The authors concluded that acupuncture and acupressure may have a role in reducing pain, increasing satisfaction with pain management, and reducing use of pharmacologic management but call for further high-quality research.

Depression, anxiety, and emotional health

Emotional lability is very common during pregnancy. Many women experience fatigue, lethargy, irritability, or a reduction in libido. Depression during pregnancy and the postpartum period is a difficult clinical problem. It is critical to offer assistance to women, as maternal depression can have adverse effects on the mother-infant bonding as well as child development and behavior [46–51]. Women and their health care providers may be concerned about how pharmacologic treatments may affect the mother and the developing fetus. There is a need to balance the risks and benefits of antidepressant medications with the risk of untreated depression. Acupuncture may be an option that can be offered for care or as an adjunct with other modalities. Within the framework of TCM, acupuncture, diet, and light exercise are all important to nourish the mother's mind and body during this time of great demand and change and for at least a month postpartum.

Two major acupoints used to treat depression and anxiety are DU/GV 20 and Yintang [Figure 11.13(a) and (b)]. The acupoints (and others located on the head and ear) have been shown to increase blood flow in the brain and have sedative effects [52,53]. See Box 11.2 for additional provider information.

The exact mechanism of action of acupuncture treatment for depression or anxiety is unknown. Acupuncture may alleviate symptoms of depression through central effects, such as the release of noradrenaline and serotonin [54], an increased release of pituitary beta-endorphins and adrenocorticotropic hormone [55], other unknown mechanisms, or potentially as a result of patient expectations. Hui and colleagues [56], using fMRI, reported deactivation of the amygdala and hypothalamus during acupuncture. The limbic structures are central to the regulation and control of emotion, cognition, bio-behavior, endocrine, and autonomic nervous functions. The limbic structures are also activated by

(a)

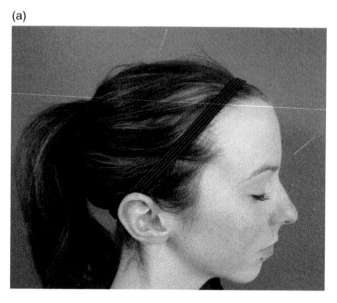

(b)

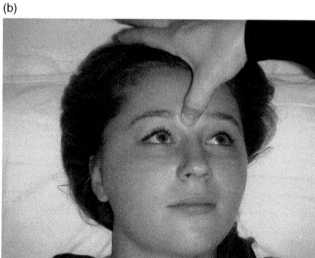

Figure 11.13   (a) Yintang (acupuncture with both points) and (b) Yintang with acupressure.

stress, pain, and negative emotions. Mood disorders, including major depression, are characterized by amygdala hypersensitivity to activation by negative emotional stimuli. This suggests a specific role that acupuncture may play on these major limbic structures.

Clinical studies of the efficacy of acupuncture to treat depression and anxiety can be convincing but remain inconclusive. The limitations of small sample sizes and methodological issues are common; however, enough evidence exists to support a role for this treatment modality.

> **Box 11.2   Yintang/hall of impression (extra point)**
>
> *Indication*: Can be used with mild anxiety or to calm emotions during pregnancy, labor, or during the postpartum period. Stimulation of this acupoint is also often incorporated during prebirth treatments. The acupoint is in close proximity to the pituitary gland.
> *Point location*: At the midpoint between the inside edges (closer to your nose) of the eyebrows, there is a slight dip or divot at the top of the nose.
> *Technique for acupressure*: With your thumb or the patient's free thumb, press the point until a sensation is elicited. Women usually report feeling a tingling, heavy, or achy sensation. Apply pressure to this point for approximately 3–5 minutes.
>   This acupoint would be used in conjunction with advice regarding adequate sleep, diet (avoiding stimulants such as caffeine, sugary snacks; avoiding fatty and fried foods) and exercise, breathing exercises, stretching, creative outlets that may be helpful, and mind-body techniques.
> *Referral*: Practitioners should refer to a qualified licensed acupuncturist when the woman desires strategies beyond acupressure, is not getting results with acupressure, and/or her quality of life is being impacted.

Cost

Women wishing acupuncture or clinicians who recommend the option can locate cost information at the local level. At the current time acupuncture is typically paid out of pocket unless private insurers offer a set number of treatments per annual year for reimbursement.

Training, licensure, and certification: Acupuncture

It is essential that clinicians refer women to individuals that have completed formal education, training, and either licensure or certification to incorporate acupuncture into their clinical practice. Also, it is important that acupuncturists are knowledgeable and experienced in obstetrical acupuncture. Each state varies in its licensure and certification requirements. The midwife or physician should be familiar with local laws and develop a preferred provider list of individuals with proper education, knowledge, training, and experience with obstetrical acupuncture. Clinicians would refer a woman to either a licensed nonphysician clinician (Licensed Acupuncturist) or a health-related professional educated and certified to incorporate acupuncture within her/his scope of practice. National acupuncture organizations may provide names for practitioners in specific areas.

Licensed acupuncturists

At present in the United States, forty-three states regulate the practice of acupuncture and forty-nine states require successfully passing the National Certification Commission for Acupuncture and Oriental Medicine (NCCAOM) exam [57]. Licensed Acupuncturists have the professional designation of L.Ac. In addition, some practitioners may also have a Master's of Oriental Medicine (M.OM), which means they have further education in administering Chinese herbs. The U.S. Department of Education recognizes the Accreditation Commission for Acupuncture and Oriental Medicine (ACAOM) as the accrediting agency for master's-level programs in acupuncture and Oriental medicine [58]. In choosing an acupuncturist, it is important to find an individual that has completed a program recognized by the ACAOM. Currently, sixteen states require continuing education units with an average of 15 hours per year [59]. The NCCAOM website provides information regarding state licensure requirements.

Other regulated health providers

There are programs in North America that educate regulated multidisciplinary health providers in order to integrate acupuncture into their clinical practice. It is important that the health professional has attended a reputable program that meets the World Health Organization (WHO) and the World Federation of Acupuncture and Moxibustion Societies (WFAS) established standards for acupuncture education and training for Western regulated health providers. WHO and WFAS recommend that health professionals who practice acupuncture have completed a minimum of 200 hours of training. The rationale for the difference in hours of education between a Licensed Acupuncturist (1,905 hours or 3 years in length) or M.OM (2,625 hours or 4 years in length) is that regulated health providers have already completed extensive education in human anatomy and physiology, along with basic and clinical sciences.

Health professionals who practice acupuncture should comply with their professional regulatory body, adhere to their profession's scope and standards of practice, adhere to their profession's code of ethics, identify their correct professional designation or the use of protected titles with respect to acupuncture, and maintain continuing competency requirements of this extended practice role [60]. When choosing an acupuncturist it is recommended to determine if they have completed a program approved by the American Board of Medical Acupuncture (ABMA) [61]. It is essential to inquire about education, training, and certification, as some states allow physicians to practice acupuncture without any training. Board certification identifies physicians who have completed a minimum of 200 hours of acupuncture training from an approved educational program, successfully passed the board examination, incorporated medical acupuncture for a minimum of 2 years, performed a minimum of 500 medical acupuncture treatments, and provided three confidential letters of reference from physician colleagues who attest to their character, professionalism, and adequacy of the standards of clinical practice.

Training, licensure, and certification: Acupressure

Individuals can obtain training in Asian Bodywork Therapy, which includes tuina, shiatsu, and many other forms, all of which have their roots in Chinese medicine. The American Organization for Bodywork Therapies of Asia (AOBTA) is a nonprofit organization that recognizes a Certified Practitioner as someone who has completed curriculum requirements of 500 hours and an Associate as someone who has completed a minimum of 150 hours. AOBTA's website has links to accredited schools and additional information [62]. Each state determines its own requirements for massage therapy. Health care providers along with women and their partners can learn some basic massage techniques to incorporate into care.

In conclusion, knowledge of state and local laws and maintaining a referral list of properly licensed or certified acupuncture/acupressure professionals with further education, training, and experience in obstetrical acupuncture or acupressure will help maternity care providers assure the best care to women during pregnancy.

References

1. Yates S & Anderson T. (2003). *Shiatsu for midwives*. London: Elsevier.
2. Gach MR. (1990). *Acupressure's potent points: A guide to self-care for common ailments*. New York: Bantam Doubleday Dell.
3. Bauer C. (1987). *Acupressure for women*. Freedom, CA: Crossing Press.
4. Ma K. (1992). The roots and development of Chinese acupuncture: From prehistory to early 20th century. *Acupuncture in Medicine 10*(Suppl), 92–99.
5. Ni M. (1995). *The yellow emperor's classic of medicine*. Boston: Shambala.
6. Osler W. (1892). *The principles and practices of medicine*. New York: Appleton.
7. Reston J. (1971). Now, about my operation in Peking. *New York Times*, July 26, p. 1.
8. National Institutes of Health. (1997). Acupuncture. *NIH Consensus Statement, 15*, 1–34.
9. Beinfeld H & Korngold E. (1991). *Between heaven and earth: A guide to Chinese medicine*. New York: Random House.
10. Deadman P, Al-Khafaji M, & Baker K. (2001). *A manual of acupuncture*. East Sussex, UK: Journal of Chinese Medicine Publications.
11. Wong J. (2003). *A manual of neuro-anatomical acupuncture*. Vol. III, *East meets West: A review of TCM with western medicine interpretation*. Toronto: Toronto Pain and Stress Clinic.
12. Acupuncture Foundation of Canada Institute. (2005). *Level CAFCI 1, Part 1 Manual*. Toronto: Acupuncture Foundation of Canada Institute.
13. Gunn CC. (1976). Acupuncture loci: A proposal for their classification according to their relationship to known neural structures. *American Journal of Chinese Medicine, 4*(2), 183–195.
14. Wong J & Rapson L. (1999). Acupuncture in the management of pain. *Complementary Therapies in Physical Medicine and Rehabilitation, 10*(3), 531–545.
15. Cho ZH, Wong EK, & Fallon JH. (2001). *Neuro-acupuncture*. Vol. 1, *Neuroscience basics*. Anaheim, CA: Q-puncture.
16. Cho ZH, Chung SC, Jones JP, Park JP, Park HJ, Lee HI, et al. (1998). New findings of the correlation between acupoints and corresponding brain cortices using functional MRI. *Proceedings of the National Academy of Sciences, 95*, 2670–2673.
17. Cho ZH, Lee SH, Hong IK, et al. (1999). Further evidence for the correlation between acupuncture stimulation and cortical activation. Proceedings, New Directions in the Scientific Exploration of Acupuncture, University of California, Irvine.
18. Hui KKS, Liu J, Marina O, et al. (2005). The integrated response of the human cerebro-cerebellar and limbic systems to acupuncture stimulation at ST 36 as evidenced by fMRI. *Neuroimage, 27*, 479–496.
19. Lewith GT, White PJ, & Pariente J. (2005). Investigating acupuncture using brain imaging techniques: The current state of play. *Evidence-Based Complementary and Alternative Medicine, 2*, 315–319.
20. Lund I & Lundeberg T. (2006). Are minimal, superficial or sham acupuncture procedures acceptable as inert placebo controls? *Acupuncture in Medicine, 24*(1), 13–15.
21. White A. (2004). A cumulative review of the range and incidence of significant adverse events associated with acupuncture. *Acupuncture in Medicine, 22*(3), 122–133.

22. MacPherson H, Scullion A, Thomas KJ, & Walters S. (2004). Patient reports of adverse events associated with acupuncture treatment: A prospective national survey. *Quality & Safety in Health Care, 13*, 349–355.
23. Festin M. (2009). Nausea and vomiting in early pregnancy. *Clinical Evidence* (online), June 3, 1405.
24. Helmreich RJ, Shiao S, Dune LS. (2006). Meta-analysis of acustimulation effects on nausea and vomiting in early pregnancy. *Explore, 2*, 412–421.
25. Smith C, Crowther C, & Beilby J. (2002). Acupuncture to treat nausea and vomiting in early pregnancy: A randomized controlled trial. *Birth, 29*(1), 1–9.
26. Napadow V, Kettner N, Liu J, Li M, Kwong KK, Vangel M, Makris N, Audette J, & Hui KK. (2007). Hypothalamus and amygdala response to acupuncture stimuli in carpal tunnel syndrome. *Pain, 130*(3), 254–266.
27. Sim H, Shin BC, Lee MS, Jung A, Lee H, & Ernst E. (2011). Acupuncture for carpal tunnel syndrome: A systematic review of randomized controlled trials. *Journal of Pain, 12*(3), 307–314.
28. Pennick V & Young G. (2007). Interventions for preventing and treating pelvic and back pain in pregnancy. *Cochrane Database of Systematic Reviews*, issue 2. Art. No.: CD001139. DOI: 10.1002/14651858.CD001139.pub2.
29. Ee CC, Manheimer E, Pirotta MV, White AR. (2008). Acupuncture for pelvic and back pain in pregnancy: A systematic review. *American Journal of Obstetrics and Gynecology, 198*, 254–259.
30. van den Berg I, Kaandorp GC, Bosch JL, Duvekot JJ, Arends LR, & Hunink MG. (2010). Cost-effectiveness of breech version by acupuncture-type interventions on BL 67, including moxibustion, for women with a breech foetus at 33 weeks gestation: A modelling approach. *Complementary Therapies in Medicine, 18*(2), 67–77.
31. Co-operative Research Group on Moxibustion Version. (1984). Clinical observation on the effects of version by moxibustion. Abstracts from the Second National Symposium on Acupuncture and Moxibustion and Acupuncture Anaesthesia, All-China Society of Acupuncture and Moxibustion, Beijing, p. 150.
32. Coyle ME, Smith CA, & Peat B. (2012). Cephalic version by moxibustion for breech presentation. *Cochrane Database of Systematic Reviews*, issue 5. Art. No.: CD003928. DOI: 10.1002/14651858. CD003928.pub3.
33. Lim C, Wilkinson J, Wong W, & Cheng, N. (2009). Effect of acupuncture on induction of labor. *Journal of Alternative and Complementary Medicine, 15*(11), 1209–1214. DOOI:10.1089/acm.2009.0100.
34. Smith CA & Crowther CA. (2004). Acupuncture for induction of labour. *Cochrane Database of Systematic Reviews*, issue 1. Art. No.: CD002962. DOI: 10.1002/14651858.CD002962.pub2.
35. Gribel GP, Coca-Velarde LG, Moreira de Sá RA. (2011). Electroacupuncture for cervical ripening prior to labor induction: A randomized clinical trial. *Archives of Gynecology and Obstetrics, 283*(6), 1233–1238.
36. Gaudernack LC, Forbord S, & Hole E. (2006). Acupuncture administered after spontaneous rupture of membranes at term significantly reduces the length of birth and use of oxytocin. *A randomized controlled trial. Acta Obstetricia et Gynecologica Scandinavica, 85*(11), 1348–1353.
37. Ingram J, Domagala C, & Yates S. (2005). The effects of shiatsu on post-term pregnancy. *Complementary Therapies in Medicine, 13*(1), 11–15.
38. Lee MK, Chang SB, & Kang DH. (2004). Effects of SP6 acupressure on labor pain and length of delivery time in women during labor. *Journal of Alternative and Complementary Medicine, 10*(6), 959–965.

39. Debra Betts website: http://acupuncture.rhizome.net.nz/acupressure/download.aspx.
40. Ma W, Bai W, Lin C, Zhou P, Xia L, Zhao C, Hao Y, Ma H, Liu X, Wang J, Yuan H, Xie Y, & Lu A. (2011). Effects of Sanyinjiao (SP6) with electroacupuncture on labour pain in women during labour. *Complementary Therapies in Medicine, 19*(Suppl 1):S13–18.
41. Hjelmstedt A, Shenoy ST, Stener-Victorin E, Lekander M, Bhat M, Balakumaran L, & Waldenström U. (2010). Acupressure to reduce labor pain: A randomized controlled trial. *Acta Obstetricia et Gynecologica Scandinavica, 89*(11), 1453–1459.
42. Waters BL & Raisler J. (2003). Ice massage for the reduction of labor pain. *Journal of Midwifery & Women's Health, 48*(5), 317–321.
43. Budd S, Yelland S, & Maciocia G. (1998). Acupuncture and herbal treatment in midwifery. *Obstetrics and Gynecology in Chinese Medicine*, 559–564.
44. Stux G, Berman B, & Pomeranz B. (2003). *Basics of acupuncture*, 5th ed. New York: Springer.
45. Jones L, Othman M, Dowswell T, Alfirevic Z, Gates S, Newburn M, et al. (2012). Pain management for women in labour: An overview of systematic reviews. *Cochrane Database of Systematic Reviews, 3*. DOI: 10.1002/14651858.
46. Grace SL, Evindar A, & Stewart DE. (2003). The effect of postpartum depression on child cognitive development and behavior: A review and critical analysis of the literature. *Archives of Women's Mental Health, 6*(4), 263–274.
47. Moehler E, Brunner R, Wiebel A, Reck C, & Resch F. (2006). Maternal depressive symptoms in the postnatal period are associated with long-term impairment of mother-child bonding. *Archives of Women's Mental Health, 9*(5), 273–278.
48. Forman DR, O'Hara MW, Stuart S, Gorman LL, Larsen KE, & Coy KC. (2007). Effective treatment for postpartum depression is not sufficient to improve the developing mother-child relationship. *Development and Psychopathology, 19*(2), 585–602.
49. Hollins K. (2007). Consequences of antenatal mental health problems for child health and development. *Current Opinion in Obstetricss and Gynecology, 19*(6), 568–572.
50. Deave T, Heron J, Evans J, & Emond A. (2008). The impact of maternal depression in pregnancy on early child development. *BJOG, 115*(8), 1043–1051.
51. McGrath JM, Records K, & Rice M. (2008). Maternal depression and infant temperament characteristics. *Infant Behavior and Development, 31*(1), 71–80.
52. Byeon HS, Moon SK, Park SU, Jung WS, Park JM, Ko CN, Cho KH, Kim YS, & Bae HS. (2011). Effects of GV20 acupuncture on cerebral blood flow velocity of middle cerebral artery and anterior cerebral artery territories, and CO_2 reactivity during hypocapnia in normal subjects. *Journal of Alternative and Complementary Medicine, 17*(3), 219–224.
53. Litscher G. (2005). Shenting And Yintang: Quantification of cerebral effects of acupressure, manual acupuncture, and laserneedle acupuncture using high-tech neuromonitoring methods. *Medical Acupuncture, 16*(3), 24–29.
54. Han JS. (1986). Electroacupuncture: An alternative to antidepressants for treating affective diseases? *International Journal of Neuroscience, 29*(1–2), 79–92.
55. Malizia E, Andreucci G, Paolucci D, Crescenzi F, Fabbri A, & Fraioli F. (1979). Electroacupuncture and peripheral beta-endorphin and ACTH levels. *Lancet, 2*(8141), 535–536.
56. Hui KK, Marina O, Liu J, Rosen BR, & Kwong KK. (2010). Acupuncture, the limbic system, and the anticorrelated networks of the brain. *Autonomic Neuroscience, 157*(1–2), 81–90.
57. National Certification Commission for Acupuncture and Oriental Medicine. (2012). Retrieved from: www.nccaom.org.
58. Accreditation Commission for Acupuncture and Oriental Medicine. (2012). Retrieved from: www.acaom.org.

59. National Center for Complementary and Alternative Medicine. (2012). Retrieved from: www. nccam.nih.gov.

60. Acupuncture Foundation of Canada Institute (AFCI). (2012). Retrieved from: http://www. afcinstitute.com/AboutAFCI/CodeofProfessionalPractice/tabid/68/Default.aspx.

61. American Board of Medical Acupuncture (ABMA). (2012). Retrieved from: http://www. aobta.org/.

62. American Organization for Bodywork Therapies of Asia (AOBTA). (2012). Retrieved from: http://www.aobta.org/.

Section 3

Organizational approaches to supporting physiologic pregnancy and birth

Chapter 12

Rethinking care on the hospital labor unit

Emily Higdon, Rachel Woodard, Kristin Rood and Heidi Jean Bernard

---

Key points

- Change on hospital labor units is needed to affect maternity care and outcomes in the United States.
- Implement a low-intervention strategy using the six Lamaze practices.
- Adapt the labor unit environment to a welcoming and home-like environment.
- Identify a formal change process and involve all staff in planning for change.
- Identify key leaders and possible barriers to change.
- Nurses are key to leading change in labor unit practices and environment.
- Provide education for staff regarding physiologic labor support practices.
- Evaluate change and document care practices including national perinatal quality measures.

The key to change . . . is to let go of fear.

Rosanne Cash

Introduction

Fundamental change in maternity care in the United States must begin on hospital labor and birth units across the country, where 99% of births occur. Current trends in birth care and U.S. outcomes would probably surprise the average recipient of maternity care. The United States ranks forty-sixth in maternal mortality in the world [1] and in 2008 ranked forty-ninth in infant mortality in the world [2]. Infant mortality, a commonly used measure of the general health of a nation, improved to 6.05 per 1,000 live births in the United States in 2011, a decline of nearly 10% from 6.71 in 2009 [3]. The epidural rate was reported to be at least 61% in 2008, a number that does not include women who had a cesarean section, either scheduled or unscheduled [4]. The cesarean rate was 32.8% in 2010 [5]; therefore, adding a proportion of the 32.8% of cesarean births to the

Supporting a Physiologic Approach to Pregnancy and Birth: A Practical Guide, First Edition.
Edited by Melissa D. Avery.
© 2013 John Wiley & Sons, Inc. Published 2013 by John Wiley & Sons, Inc.

61% epidural rate would result in an epidural rate even higher. The U.S. rate of labor induction was 23% of all live births in 2007 [6]. As evidenced by these statistics, many maternity health care providers tend to forget that giving birth is a normal human physiologic experience, viewed as the norm long before the use of so many interventions in maternity care was common. Supporting women through labor and birth is an art that has been practiced since long before the emergence of modern-day obstetrical care [7].

At the same time as intervention rates are high in hospitals, home births (specifically among Caucasian women) increased by 23% from 1990 to 2006 [8], a message that some women are looking for a different kind of experience. Home birth rates have been trending upward as women seek a childbirth experience that is less interventional, less controlled by health care providers, and that takes place in an environment that is more home-like and less institutional. Birth centers (free-standing alternatives to hospital labor units) have been increasing as a choice in response to the desire by pregnant women and their families to have a birth experience that is more personalized with fewer medical interventions [9]. Health care providers have a responsibility to try and accommodate the preferences of the women they serve whenever possible. One common reason for mothers planning a home birth to transfer to the hospital is the desire for epidural anesthesia. Hospitals can provide an environment with fewer routine medical interventions and more labor support interventions in a home-like environment that is desirable to women who prefer a hospital birth, who require higher levels of care, and those who desire epidural or spinal anesthesia, including women who transfer from an out-of-hospital birth environment.

Empowering women by providing a woman-centered environment that allows women to take charge of their care should be the gold standard on labor and birth units. For a woman with a healthy and uncomplicated pregnancy, labor and birth is a natural process that requires minimal intervention in most cases. Certain circumstances during pregnancy or labor may require that birth occur in a more controlled environment. However, it is important for maternity care providers to remember that when caring for women with uncomplicated pregnancies and labors that studies have demonstrated similar safety comparing home and hospital births [10]. Women want something else. While most women desire the safety they associate with hospital births, they also want hospital staff to work with them to create a birth experience as close to their preferences as possible. The hospital labor and birth unit staff must focus its attention on providing quality, safe labor and birth experiences for each woman that enters their doors.

This chapter will focus on approaches to care on the labor and birth unit—reviewing recent evidence and trends in birth care; the change process—discussing methods to implement change; and finally a vision of the new labor and delivery unit—descriptions of what the experience of labor and birth can look like on the new labor unit. To illuminate the possibilities by implementing evidence-based changes on the hospital labor unit, a case study in three parts will be presented throughout the chapter. Kristi is a primigravida with a healthy, uncomplicated pregnancy at 39 weeks 6 days gestation and has begun spontaneous labor. She received care at a community hospital after the changes discussed in this chapter were implemented. The Lamaze care practices have been adopted as a framework for care by all clinicians practicing on the unit; women are cared for in a physiologic manner unless there is a reason for higher levels of care. Data are collected to document and report care provided. This case study highlights the opportunities for improvement in care to women and the potential to increase their satisfaction through the birth experience. Evidence supports that the care strategies proposed here to decrease interventions for women with uncomplicated pregnancies are safe and may result in improved maternal and infant outcomes, including decreased induction and cesarean section rates.

Approaches to care

First, let's acknowledge that large-scale changes in maternal and infant care related to labor and birth will require that hospital units across the country adopt significant culture change. This includes labor and birth units in large, teaching, tertiary care hospitals as well as smaller, private community hospitals. The place to start is to minimize unnecessary medical interventions such as elective induction of labor and increase supportive interventions such as one-to-one nursing care. Implementation of continuous labor support and other supportive interventions represents change that can be implemented through strong hospital nursing leadership. A call to action for quality care in labor and birth was issued jointly in 2011 by the American Academy of Family Physicians, the American Academy of Pediatrics, the American College of Nurse-Midwives, the American College of Obstetricians and Gynecologists, the American College of Osteopathic Obstetricians & Gynecologists, the Association of Women's Health, Obstetric, and Neonatal Nurses, and the Society for Maternal-Fetal Medicine. The document acknowledges pregnancy, labor, and birth as normal physiologic processes requiring minimal intervention in most cases. The organizations called for "effective communication, shared decision-making, teamwork, and data-driven quality improvement initiatives" [11, p. 1]. This document would be useful on hospital labor units across the country and could really jump start a collaborative change project.

Physical support

It is possible to support women experiencing uncomplicated, healthy pregnancies through a woman-centered, low-intervention, home-like birth experience that promotes physiologic birth. What is physiologic birth? Physiologic birth can be defined by the practices used to promote it. The World Health Organization identified four care practices that promote, protect, and support physiologic birth, and Lamaze International has recommended two additional practices. Together these six care practices can be employed as a framework to promote the normal physiologic process of birth [12]:

• Allowing labor to start on its own.
• Freedom of movement during labor.
• Continuous labor support.
• Spontaneous pushing in nonsupine positions.
• No separation of mother and baby.
• No routine interventions.

The sixth care practice, no routine interventions, helps to promote labor without disruption of the normal physiologic process. Hospital labor units can provide optimal services by making safe, evidence-based changes that can both increase women's satisfaction and improve outcomes. Adopting these practices in caring for the laboring woman is a change that does not require much, if any, financial investment. What is required is that the new approach be accepted as the standard of care by all maternity care providers. Adopting the Lamaze six birth care practices is a key first step in changing the approach to care for the low-risk laboring woman in the hospital labor and birth unit.

In 2008, Childbirth Connection published a report that examined multiple systematic reviews and other sources of evidence to inform the need for change on labor units across the United States. The report identified key areas of improvement in maternity care that would better position the country to be at or near the top in world rankings [13]. Aiming to provide maternity care resulting in "least-harm" can decrease overused maternity care practices. Increasing the use of underused maternity care practices not only improves birth outcomes but also decreases the cost of birth care dramatically in the United States. Overused maternity practices include labor induction, epidural analgesia, and cesarean section. The authors concluded that mothers, newborns, and payers of health care would benefit from utilizing effective, safer care paths and using riskier interventions only when clearly indicated. Underused maternity practices include continuous labor support, nonpharmacologic techniques that decrease pain and facilitate the progress of labor, non-supine pushing positions, and early mother-baby skin-to-skin contact. These and other techniques will be discussed further in the chapter.

Another resource that hospital staff can utilize is the Coalition for Improving Maternity Services (CIMS) Mother-Friendly Childbirth Initiative [14]. In 1996, a number of organizations and individuals endorsed an effort to promote mother-friendly services. Included are a philosophy of pregnancy and birth as normal, women's empowerment and autonomy, doing no harm, and responsible care provision. Birth locations can carry out the identified ten steps to mother-friendly care, which include the WHO/UNICEF steps to promote breastfeeding [14].

Environmental support

Environmental support can enable staff to provide care that promotes physiologic birth. Physical attributes of the hospital labor and birth room can affect women's health outcomes during and after labor and birth as well as their satisfaction with their birth experience. Hospital labor rooms associated with improved patient outcomes are those that offer privacy, promote social support, allow freedom and control, are calming, and include scenes of nature and other visual and auditory stimuli that elicit positive emotional responses [15]. In the typical labor and birth room, the bed is positioned as the focal point in the room surrounded by medical equipment including IV poles, oxygen tanks, fetal monitors, and more. Locating the bed centrally in the room sends the message that the bed is the appropriate place for a woman to labor. As many as 70–80% of laboring women remain in bed for all or most of their labor [15].

Hodnett et al. [15] devised an approach to creating a more home-like hospital room using the acronym PLACE (Pregnant and Laboring in an Ambient Clinical Environment).

The PLACE labor room is a hybrid space based on a reconceptualization of an optimal environment for labor and birth in the hospital. First, the authors suggested moving the bed into the corner of the room. Hospital beds can be replaced with standard double beds on wheels with comfortable mattresses. The bed can then be moved to the middle of the room as needed based on the condition of the woman. Hospital beds with bed rails that can be concealed, equipped with comfortable hospital bed mattresses, and/or covered with brightly colored sheets and multiple pillows can also help to make the room feel more like home and less like the hospital. Comfortable rocking chairs, birthing balls, and large pillows to kneel on, as well as a private area to walk around in, can facilitate movement during labor and birth. Medical equipment should be concealed as much as possible. The availability of telemetry monitors and handheld Dopplers for fetal monitoring will support nurses in providing care that encourages freedom of movement. Dimming the lights creates a calming environment that can promote relaxation. Music has also been shown to reduce pain and decrease anxiety among laboring women [16, p. 367]. Providing CD players or MP3 player docks in labor rooms and encouraging women to bring their own music is a simple change to help promote a relaxing environment and distraction for laboring women. DVDs with relaxing nature sounds can help create an ambient atmosphere in the labor room. Hanging a framed poster of upright labor positions can also be helpful to women in labor. Architectural designs that include private showers and tubs provide nonpharmacological alternatives for pain relief during labor and birth. While some of these changes would require financial investment, many would require minimal to no financial investment at all. Finally, alternative hospital-based settings that focus on a physiologic approach to labor and birth for low-risk women have been associated with fewer medical interventions, more vaginal births, and improved maternal satisfaction [17].

The "Nuts and Bolts" of change on the labor unit

Change strategies must be thoughtfully implemented to affect clinician attitudes toward birth care as well as change the physical environment of the labor unit. An intentional approach to change will help promote acceptance of change by those providing birth care support. Bingham [18] outlined strategies and tactics for implementing change on maternity units, including communication (discourse), education (formal and informal), and data (audit). Communication or discourse strategies include multidisciplinary staff meetings and group discussions, one-to-one discussions between a change leader and another individual on the unit, reviews of academic research either one on one or in groups, reminders such as checklists, order sets, newsletters, or formal written updates distributed to staff periodically, posters and bulletin boards, group and individual e-mails, rewards for individuals or the group, and feedback and disciplinary discussions. Education strategies include the use of grand rounds or educational sessions often held once a week, conferences on the topic of interest, competency fairs, tests and demonstrations, and online learning tools. Data strategies include audits and feedback (both group and individual), and public release of care pattern and outcome data [18]. This approach to the change process can be modified and adapted as needed to support individual labor unit staff. Data should also be collected in order to report important perinatal outcomes and document the results of changes implemented. The National Quality Forum has endorsed twelve perinatal measures [19], five of which are included in the Joint Commission set of perinatal care measures [20]. Hospitals could choose to report the Joint Commission set of five perinatal measures; Elective Delivery, Cesarean Section, and Exclusive Breast Milk Feeding would be of greatest interest to a project promoting a physiologic approach to labor and birth.

The change process

Identifying leaders

Considerable effort is required to change one aspect of labor and birth care and effective leadership is crucial. Leadership representatives from physicians, midwives, nurses, and other health care practitioners from the labor and birth hospital unit should meet together to brainstorm the steps to create and implement a process to change current unit practice to an approach that better supports a physiologic, more home-like birth experience. Graham, Logan, Davies, & Nimrod [21] found that nurses perceived that their nurse managers championed for change on the obstetrical unit, while similar leadership failed to emerge from obstetricians. It is of utmost importance that all disciplines partner and commit to change their practice to support physiologic labor and birth. Without support from all disciplines change is difficult to implement and sustain. Individuals selected to provide leadership can help facilitate change by demonstrating, assisting, answering questions, and helping to maintain positive attitudes on the hospital labor unit [22]. Regardless of the specific frameworks and tools that are used in implementing change, it is important that all of the individual practitioners working on the hospital labor unit recognize that change can be difficult and time consuming. Resistance will be encountered and problems will arise. However, with persistence, committed leadership, and motivation, barriers that could prevent hospital labor units from adopting physiologic support practices in a more home-like birth environment can be overcome. Labor units can change over time to better meet the needs of laboring women and their families.

Selecting the change process/initial data collection

Selecting a theoretical framework for change provides a tool to develop and evaluate the project. One example of a change process is the FOCUS tool. FOCUS is an acronym for Find a process, Organize a team that knows the process, Clarify current knowledge of the process, Understand sources of process variation, and Select the process improvement [23, p. 108]. Another tool available to help facilitate change and identify barriers is the Plan, Do, Check, and Act (PDCA) cycle developed by Edward Deming in the 1950s [24]. This cycle is conceptualized as a circle with each step connecting to the next until it comes full circle. First, an improvement is planned and data collection is undertaken. Next, the improvements are implemented and further data are collected. The next step is reviewing the data to discover if the project led to expected improvements, uncovering what worked well and what did not. Finally, the last step is to standardize the parts of the project that worked and send the parts that didn't work as expected back into the PDCA cycle [23]. (See Box 12.1.)

Box 12.1   Strategies for change

FOCUS
F – Find a process
O – Organize a team
C – Clarify current knowledge of the process
U – Understand sources of process variation
S – Select the process for improvement

PDCA
P – Plan
D – Do
C – Check
A – Act

Box 12.2   Key change concepts

1. Key leaders identified.
2. Select change process.
3. Collect necessary data.
4. Determine barriers.
5. Determine resources/education needed.
6. Determine changes to unit/equipment needed.
7. Implement change.
8. Evaluate success of change.

When using the PDCA cycle on a labor unit to facilitate change, each area or care process that a unit wishes to change must be approached individually. For example, if the labor unit staff wants to address the overuse of continuous electronic fetal monitoring and increase utilization of intermittent auscultation, the first step includes the recognition that a problem exists and creation of a team charged with assisting the staff to make the change. This is coupled with an examination of the medical records to understand the rates of electronic fetal monitoring utilization on the labor unit and surveying individual maternal care providers about their attitudes toward the use of intermittent auscultation. Following analysis of the initial data, results are presented to the unit employees and other staff. Education, including current research, is presented to those practicing on the unit. Posters and bulletin boards are prepared and displayed in areas commonly used by physicians, nurses, and midwives. Checklists and pocket cards that assist care providers to remember the details related to intermittent auscultation are provided. The electronic health record can be updated to provide more detailed information regarding the characteristics of the auscultated fetal heart rate and pattern. Finally, after a period of 30–60 days, the health record is examined again for documentation of the use of intermittent auscultation and maternal and fetal outcomes during the period of change, and maternal care providers are surveyed regarding their attitudes toward intermittent auscultation. Once the data analysis is complete the unit employees are updated about the results. Those aspects of fetal monitoring that aren't working well (e.g., poorly working handheld Dopplers, or poor nurse understanding of the use of a Pinnard stethoscope/fetoscope) are reevaluated and addressed in another PDCA cycle. (See Box 12.2.)

Determining barriers to change

Multiple barriers may inhibit change to increase the use of care practices that promote, protect, and support the physiologic processes of labor and birth in the hospital. Identifying, understanding, and potentially removing barriers are necessary steps in the process of implementing change. Potential barriers can include lack of knowledge of physiologic birth among pregnant women and health care providers (often perpetuated by the media), difficulty translating evidence into practice, and environmental factors such as insufficient nursing staff to provide the necessary care to facilitate physiologic birth and lack of necessary equipment or funding to make environmental changes.

In order to supplement information received from their physicians and midwives, women seek information about pregnancy and childbirth from a variety of sources. As many as 97% of women use the Internet to search for pregnancy-related information and 83% use this information to make decisions regarding their pregnancy and birth [25]. Using the Internet as a source for health-related information may be a barrier to providing an appropriate physiologic birth experience, especially if this information is not from a credible website. Although women are aware that quality standards exist for websites, few are able to name those standards [25]. As consumers of information, pregnant women and their families looking for information regarding pregnancy and birth need to know who is sponsoring the website, how often the information provided is updated, and the credibility of the source. Health care providers can suggest high-quality websites for the women in their care. If women search for and find information about pregnancy and birth from trust-worthy sites they will be better able to make informed decisions. Discussing the information they find with their provider is a positive step that indicates women are motivated to learn about their pregnancy and want to play an active role in their decision making and should not be seen as a threat to the provider's credibility.

Another source of media information is childbirth literature. Reading books about pregnancy and childbirth can encourage women to value their own needs and to learn as much as possible about the birthing process and options, enabling women to make informed decisions. However, this information is often comprised of lists of prenatal diagnostic tests, pregnancy disorders, and discussions of worst-case scenarios, making it difficult for women to discern how birth can be achieved without a great deal of medical intervention [26, p. 210]. Texts that promote physiologic birth that are honest about the risks involved in pregnancy and birth while still reinforcing the fact that birth is a natural, physiologic process are available to women. *Our Bodies, Ourselves: Pregnancy and Birth* [27] is an excellent example. The nonjudgmental tone, with quotes from other women, can inspire confidence and reassure women that childbirth is a normal, healthy process. Maternity care providers can be aware of similar books and recommend positive texts to the women in their care.

Another source of pregnancy and birth information is found in childbirth education classes. Difficulty scheduling classes into families' busy lives is certainly a barrier to these important classes. Childbirth education classes vary in length spanning a weekend to multiple sessions over several weeks. The valuable information provided can guide a woman and her family's expectations for birth as well as assist her in developing a birth plan appropriate for the individual pregnant woman. For example, Simpson, Newman &

Chirino [28] found that when perinatal education classes included the topic of the risk of elective inductions, the rate of elective induction decreased for women who attended the classes, indicating that the classes were influential in their decisions.

Just as lack of knowledge about physiologic birth is a barrier to pregnant women, it is also a barrier to health care providers. Lack of knowledge about physiologic birth and the research related to promoting physiologic birth can make implementing evidence into practice difficult. The six practices supported by Lamaze International [12] are based on research evidence. Allowing labor to start on its own, freedom of movement during labor, continuous labor support, and spontaneous pushing in nonsupine positions improve birth outcomes. Applying these practices requires behavior and environmental changes that are possible only with the support and cooperation of all groups of health care providers. With high-level support from all provider groups and hospital administration, the resources needed to provide appropriate nurse staffing and funding to improve the labor unit environment can be implemented in a way that labor is first viewed as a normal process and supported as such unless clear information indicates that other actions are required.

There is a culture of fear on labor and birth units across the United States. Obstetricians are sued more frequently than physicians in most other specialties, and liability insurance premiums are highest for obstetricians [29, p. 2]. Fear of litigation can affect health care providers' decision making and result in overuse of medical interventions in the labor and birth setting. When these medical interventions are used prematurely, the needs of the provider are placed above those of the laboring woman and her family. Providers and staff can create guidelines for women with low-risk labor that support physiologic birth and are evidence-based such as the six Lamaze healthy birth care practices. These guidelines can help facilitate the decision-making process, minimize risk to mother and baby, and help to support the health care provider in the event of an adverse outcome.

Determining educational needs of labor unit staff

Before strategies and tactics to effect change can be implemented, it is important to assess the perceived capabilities of the nursing staff to provide the care measures that support physiologic birth. Social cognitive theory [30] is one framework that can be utilized to assess and change behaviors. This theory addresses self-efficacy and the relationships between individuals, their environment, and their behavior. Self-efficacy is defined as "people's judgments of their capabilities to organize and execute a course of action required to attain designated types of performances" [30, p. 605]. Davies and Hodnett [31] created a fourteen-item self-efficacy scale that rates labor and delivery nurses' confidence and skills in providing labor support (emotional support, physical comfort advice, and information). This type of survey can help identify areas where education and improvements in care are needed related to the use of practices that promote physiologic birth. Implementing change through data collection can include surveys asking how often skills that promote physiologic birth were used by nurses and other health care providers. Examples include how often clinicians encouraged women to be upright and mobile during labor, support techniques used during first stage labor, the positions used during second stage labor, and whether staff encouraged women to delay pushing until having an urge to push. The survey can be followed up with an audit of data documenting those labor support activities including specific comfort measures used (hydrotherapy, massage, birthing balls). This information will provide feedback to staff about the implementation of evidenced-based practices. Information obtained through audits can be discussed during monthly educational meetings with nursing, midwifery and medical staff and communicated in unit-based newsletters, e-mails, or posters.

Strategies used to update nurses, midwives, and physicians about physiologic birth practices could include formal presentations and case discussions at grand rounds, introducing evidence related to specific care practices at staff meetings, online learning, and informal poster presentations. Empowering labor and delivery nurses is a key step in implementing change on the labor unit. Nurses need opportunities to learn and practice labor support techniques and understand that their role in the support of physiologic birth is valued by their colleagues and the unit manager. After all, research has documented that one-to-one nursing support for the laboring woman has improved health outcomes for both mothers and newborns, including lower rates of epidural, spinal, and other pharmacologic analgesia and anesthesia, a lower cesarean rate, shorter labors, increased 1- and 5-minute Apgar scores, and increased maternal satisfaction with the birth experience [32].

Labor and delivery nurses can increase confidence in their ability to provide labor support by attending a doula course or similar education program focused on nonpharmacologic interventions that can be utilized in providing labor support. These support techniques could become part of required nursing competencies, similar to fetal monitoring and newborn resuscitation, including regular updates and documentation. In addition, adapting the electronic health record to allow for easy documentation of labor support methods could naturally increase the number and diversity of support techniques offered to women. Possible support methods to include in the medical record are counterpressure, massage, position changes, encouragement and reassurance, heat, whirlpool or bath tub, walking, squatting, birthing ball, ice packs or cool washcloths, music, humming or moaning, and many others. The documentation itself would serve as a reminder to use multiple labor support methods and provide an opportunity to document change on the unit.

Implementation and evaluation

Each labor unit must adapt its approach to implementing change to fit the needs of the individual unit. An assessment of possible champions, personalities, and willingness to change on the unit as well as the barriers to change must be completed before the change can be implemented. Engaging each staff member in planning and executing the change and assembling a strong committed leadership team will be helpful in the effort to implement positive and sustainable changes.

When the preparation work is complete, implementation dates will be set and the project will be ready to "go live." Be sure all staff are aware of implementation dates and that equipment, materials, and supplies needed are ready and in place. Champions should be available to assist the implementation process on all shifts for the first several days to weeks depending on the degree of change implemented. Data collection as planned by the leadership team should be in place with dates determined in advance to report on evaluation of progress, maintain enthusiasm of the staff, and adjust the process as needed depending on the specific change process selected. (See Box 12.3.)

Box 12.3   The "Nuts and Bolts" of change

Communication or discourse strategies:

- Multidisciplinary staff meetings/group discussions.
- One-to-one discussions between a change leader and another individual on the unit.
- Reviews of academic research either one on one or in groups.
- Reminders such as checklists.
- Order sets.
- Newsletters or formal written update that is distributed periodically.
- Posters and bulletin boards.
- E-mails (either one to one or group).
- Rewards for individuals or the group.
- Feedback and disciplinary discussions.

Education strategies:

- Use of grand rounds or educational sessions often held once a week.
- Conferences on the topic of interest.
- Competency fairs.
- Tests and demonstrations.
- Online learning tools.

Data strategies:

- Audits and feedback (both group and individual).
- Public release of care pattern and outcome data.

Picturing a transformed labor unit

To understand what this transformed labor unit might look like, simple care changes implemented for each stage of labor will be presented. But first let's consider what a woman might experience when she enters the labor unit. On arrival to the unit she would find a clean, quiet, and inviting atmosphere. Ideally, the health care providers on the labor unit would be anticipating her arrival after consulting with the woman by phone during early labor. She would be greeted by name by her nurse, who has already reviewed her prenatal record and birth plan and spoken with her physician or midwife. Required paperwork and consents for care on the labor unit have been completed during a prenatal visit to decrease the number of people entering her room and requiring her attention during a time when she needs to focus on labor. The labor room has been prepared for her arrival with the lights dimly lit; the bed is decorated with bright, pleasing covers and is located on the side of the room, and a cool glass of ice water is on a table next to the bed. A comfortable rocking chair is near the table, other comfortable chairs are available, and labor support devices such as a birthing ball can be found in the room. Quiet music is playing in the background.

First stage of labor

As the longest stage of labor, first stage offers multiple opportunities to adjust common hospital procedures to accommodate women and their families to expect a normal labor

Case Study 12.1

First stage labor

Kristi calls the labor unit reporting spontaneous labor contractions every 5–7 minutes lasting 40–70 seconds for the last hour and a half. She reports good fetal movement, no leaking of amniotic fluid or vaginal bleeding. The nurse advises her to drink plenty of fluids including water, apple or orange juice, or an electrolyte drink such as Gatorade, to lie down and/or take a warm shower or bath, and to continue to monitor her contractions and fetal movement. She asks Kristi to call back when her contractions are less than 5 minutes apart for 2 consecutive hours, or if she has other questions.

Kristi calls the labor unit 5 hours later stating her contractions are every 2–3 minutes and last 50–70 seconds, and she tells the nurse that she thinks it is time to come in. She is audibly in pain during her contractions over the phone; listening, the nurse agrees with Kristi's perception. Kristi arrives at the unit to find a quiet, clean entry to the labor unit, is greeted by her nurse at the registration desk, and is accompanied to a labor room where the lights are dimmed, quiet relaxing music is playing, and a cool glass of water sits on the table. Kristi sits in a comfortable chair while her nurse gently palpates several contractions, listening to the fetal heart between contractions. After Kristi and her partner have a chance to adjust to the hospital environment and the nurse observes her labor pattern, a quick cervical exam reveals Kristi's cervix is 4 cm dilated, completely effaced, with the fetal head at a 0 station. She is given a menu and orders some toast and a yogurt. After Kristi changes into her own comfortable nightgown, her nurse encourages her to sit on the birthing ball in the center of the room. She moves around the room, changing positions as needed with the assistance of her partner and nurse. She utilizes the recliner, hands-and-knees position on a yoga mat, the birthing ball, and the whirlpool bathtub. Her membranes spontaneously rupture 4 hours after her admission with clear amniotic fluid. The nurse intermittently auscultates the fetal heart rate and palpates uterine contractions every 15–30 minutes. She encourages Kristi with relaxation techniques including counterpressure for her lower back and massage. Shortly after the rupture of her membranes, Kristi's pain becomes nearly unbearable. The nurse sits with Kristi, breathing with her, massaging her back, providing counterpressure and encouragement and assistance with position changes. Her nurse then assists Kristi into a warm bath and continues to intermittently auscultate fetal heart tones and monitors the water temperature to ensure the water does not get too cool but is not so warm as to raise her body temperature. Two hours later Kristi begins to feel intermittent rectal pressure and is assisted out of the bath. Upon cervical exam she is completely dilated, with the vertex at a +1 station. Her midwife is notified and her nurse encourages and assists Kristi to change positions as needed for comfort until rectal pressure is constant.

in a more home-like environment. Multiple changes that are easily implementable during the first stage of labor are presented. (See Case Study 12.1.)

Nutrition, fluids, and IV access

Many hospital protocols call for the laboring woman to be NPO (nothing by mouth) or on a clear liquid diet to reduce the risk of aspiration of the stomach contents in the event of the use of general anesthesia. The risk of death from aspiration from 1979 to 1990 during childbirth was 0.667 per million or approximately 7 in 10 million births [33, p. 508]. Fasting during labor depletes the carbohydrates available to do the work of labor, causing the body to metabolize fat for energy. Laboring women can be viewed as healthy and in a temporary state of extreme exertion, similar to an athlete during strenuous exercise

[33, p. 510]. Athletes are encouraged to eat high-carbohydrate/low-fat meals with frequent breaks to replace depleted fluids. Not allowing a laboring woman to eat or drink can also be frustrating for the woman and her family. Given the small risk of aspiration, women may be encouraged to eat and drink small amounts of carbohydrates and protein as they wish. Authors of a Cochrane review of current evidence concluded that there was no justification for the restriction of food and fluids to low-risk laboring women [34, p. 2].

If a woman is able to drink fluids during first stage labor, is GBS negative, and is not requesting an epidural, placing an IV catheter is unnecessary. The insertion and placement of an IV catheter is usually painful, and the IV catheter is irritating. Running continuous IV fluids results in attaching the woman to an IV pole, and the IV tubing can often be frustrating to a woman trying to change positions and move freely while in labor. Many physicians may prefer to have IV access to be prepared in case of an emergency. However, life-threatening emergencies are rare in low-risk pregnancies [35, p. 24]. Given this low risk, Enkin et al. [36] concluded that the routine use of IVs is unlikely to be beneficial. Each labor unit can provide either a private or shared space with beverages and snacks such as water, orange and/or apple juice, milk, and soda like Sprite or Diet Sprite, crackers, popsicles, Jell-O, soups (like chicken noodle), light salads or vegetable trays, and sandwiches or wraps.

Intermittent fetal monitoring

Electronic fetal monitoring was implemented in the 1970s, used in 45% of all U.S. births in 1980, and by 1998 continuous fetal monitoring was used in 84% of all births in the United States [34, p. 3]. Continuous fetal monitors are confining for women who desire to be mobile while in first stage labor. Intermittent auscultation is preferable for women with a low-risk labor to encourage freedom of movement and allows the woman to utilize multiple labor positions. No differences have been identified in Apgar scores, admission to the NICU, stillbirths, or early neonatal deaths when comparing intermittent and continuous fetal monitoring. However, the risk of a cesarean was increased by 40% with continuous fetal monitoring, and the risk of operative vaginal birth increased by 20% [38, p. 367]. Despite the evidence, many labor units continue to use continuous fetal monitoring for low-risk women. Current standards for intermittent auscultation involve using a handheld Doppler or Pinnard stethoscope/fetoscope to auscultate fetal heart tones every 30 minutes in early labor, every 15 minutes in active labor, and every 5 minutes during second stage. Contractions can be palpated by hand or traced with a tocodynameter. Fetal heart tones should be evaluated before, during, and after a contraction [39]. If a woman requires continuous fetal monitoring, telemetry (or wireless) monitors can be placed. These wireless monitors allow the woman to move unrestricted and to easily change positions as needed throughout her labor.

One-to-one nursing care

Perhaps the most important component of a safe, minimal-intervention childbirth is the provision of one-to-one nursing care for the woman in active labor. If labor units are to decrease medical interventions and increase support, nurses must become more involved in the labor process. To make a properly informed assessment of a laboring woman the labor nurse must be present with the woman and be able to lay hands on for assessments.

Intermittent fetal monitoring requires a nurse to be present in the room at least every 15 minutes during active labor. Continuous support in labor is supported by a Cochrane review that found that women receiving continuous support were more likely to have a vaginal delivery, less likely to use pharmacologic pain control, were more satisfied with their birth experience, had shorter labors, fewer instrumental births, and were less likely to have a baby with a low 5-minute Apgar score [40].

By being present in a more supportive environment, the nurse can assist the laboring woman with relaxation techniques including encouragement and reassurance, counterpressure, counting and breathing exercises, suggestions on position changes, and motions to decrease the pain sensation. These techniques can reduce or delay the need for pharmacologic pain relief and can shorten the duration of labor by helping the woman maintain an upright position. The confidence that a nurse can provide to a laboring woman is key to maximizing the laboring woman's satisfaction with her experience [41, p. 72]. Nursing support with an epidural, when needed, can also decrease the length of labor and increase patient satisfaction.

Women can be encouraged to experience early labor at home as much as possible, reducing the average length of stay on the labor unit, thus decreasing the opportunities for unnecessary intervention. Reduction in time spent on the labor unit could better enable nurses to provide one-to-one care in active labor. Current AWHONN guidelines call for one-to-one nursing care for women choosing a "low-tech" birth or receiving oxytocin for induction or augmentation of labor [42].

Epidural support

It is possible for women who choose an epidural to have virtually a pain-free labor or to have relief from a protracted tiring labor. Some labor and birth units report epidural rates as high as 80–90% in the United States [43, p. 153]. Despite women with epidurals being confined to bed, many labor and birth positions can be utilized to promote a more normal experience. Women can be assisted into positions such as the throne position, upright side-lying position, kneeling, and hands-and-knees positions, and depending on the strength of the epidural women can be assisted on the side of the bed to dangle, allowing gravity to assist in fetal descent and cervical dilatation. AWHONN recommends the assessment of motor ability after the epidural is placed [44, p. 41]. According to the individual woman's motor capabilities, positions should be utilized that maximize the diameter of the pelvis, decrease the duration of labor, minimize pain intensity, decrease perineal trauma, and increase maternal satisfaction with the birth experience [43, p. 157].

Second stage of labor

Second stage labor is a critical time to continue one-to-one nursing care and provide ongoing support to the laboring woman and her family or support persons. The duration of second stage is typically between 20 minutes and 2 hours [45, p. 24]. Current efforts are to eliminate the time limits often used to define second stage labor. Rotation and descent of the fetus through the birth canal can be slow, and as long as mother and baby are tolerating second stage labor, evidence does support allowing labor to progress without medical intervention [46]. (See Case Study 12.2.)

Case Study 12.2

Second stage labor

Kristi's nurse witnesses her involuntarily pushing and verifies that she is having constant rectal pressure. Kristi's nurse asks her what position feels best for pushing and assists her to a comfortable squatting position. Her partner is shown how to squat behind Kristi, so that he can help provide support, also offering her sips from a popsicle as she pushes. Kristi's nurse stays close to her and encourages pushing as she wishes with contractions. Her midwife monitors the descent of the fetal head with pushes. Ten minutes later Kristi states that her knees feel unstable. She is assisted into a hands-and-knees position on the bed with her nurse and husband near the head of the bed supporting her while the midwife supports the perineum for birth of the fetal head. Kristi is encouraged to do what comes naturally, bearing down as she is comfortable. Quiet music continues in the background. The nurse auscultates heart tones intermittently between pushing efforts. Five minutes later the baby is born. Her nurse and partner assist her to turn into a high Fowler's position, careful to avoid the umbilical cord. Kristi is encouraged to reach down and receive the baby from the midwife. She pulls the baby to her chest as the nurse helps her lay back. The baby is cleaned with warm, dry blankets on Kristi's chest, while her partner cuts the umbilical cord after it stops pulsating. The baby is then placed skin to skin with the mother while the midwife awaits the birth of the placenta. The nurse immediately assists Kristi in getting the baby to the breast and the baby begins nursing.

Pushing positions

Commonly, once a cervical exam confirms complete dilatation women are asked to start pushing regardless of their having a definite urge to push. However, it is beneficial to encourage women to begin pushing only when they have an urge even if that means resting during the early passive phase of second stage labor [46]. Women may expect that they will push in low Fowler's or lithotomy positions, positions that can seem unnatural and uncomfortable. In reality, women experiencing the second stage of labor will typically change positions frequently on their own. Upright positions such as squatting, kneeling, or hands and knees utilize gravity and can help the fetus rotate if in an occiput posterior position [47, pp. 188–193].

Dorsal lithotomy (low Fowler's) puts the birth canal in an "uphill" orientation. Lateral lying positions place the birth canal in a gravity-eliminated orientation. Semi-prone, side-lying, and side-lying lunge are examples of alternative second stage labor positions [47, p. 187]. Additionally, blood flow is optimized in a left side-lying position by avoiding uterine compression of the inferior vena cava. The need for perineal sutures was decreased when the lateral lying position was assumed during birth with epidural anesthesia [48].

Second stage with epidural analgesia

The term "laboring down" is commonly used to refer to allowing for fetal descent without active maternal pushing. The term is usually used for women with epidural anesthesia where the urge to push is blunted. This practice is associated with research at Queen Charlotte's and Chelsea Hospital, where women with epidurals labored down for an hour during the passive phase of second stage, allowing fetal descent without active maternal pushing. Some women were assisted to maintain a recumbent position and others an upright position. Once descent occurred, pushing was initiated during the active phase of second stage labor. A reduction in second stage labor of approximately 20 minutes was observed in women who were encouraged to be upright [49, p. 20]. Authors of a randomized controlled trial three decades ago [50] examined delayed pushing in women with epidural analgesia and concluded that delayed pushing was associated with an increase in vaginal births and a decrease in instrumental deliveries. Delayed pushing was not associated with an increase in fetal heart rate decelerations or decreases in Apgar scores [51, p. 32].

Low Fowler's position with knees pulled back has been shown to be the most common position used during the second stage for women with epidural analgesia [44]. Women are commonly encouraged to push in this position because epidurals restrict their movement; they may become frustrated, especially if they do not have an urge to push. Changing positions every 20–30 minutes can help promote fetal descent [47, p. 186]. Upright positions are usually achievable with an epidural and proper support, thus using gravity to help with descent of the baby. Examples of upright positions include semi-sitting, kneeling, and supine with leg supports [47, p. 187]. Women birthing in the half-sitting position delivered babies with higher Apgar scores and experienced an increased number of early fetal heart rate decelerations, fewer late fetal heart rate decelerations, fewer instrumental deliveries, and increased maternal satisfaction. Authors of this study found no difference in pushing duration [51]. Some women with epidurals can be assisted into the squatting position with the use of a squat bar. The squatting position widens the pelvic outlet, requiring less bearing down effort. Pushing in the squatting position decreased the length of the second stage of labor, including decreasing the need for oxytocin to enhance contractions and fewer and less severe perineal lacerations than when in the semi-recumbent position [48]. The use of upright positions by women with epidurals should be carefully considered on an individual basis, assessing the individual's risk for falling, and only used when deemed safe.

Third stage of labor

Changes that can be implemented in the third stage of labor and immediate postpartum period can maximize patient satisfaction, bonding between parents and infant, and facilitate early breastfeeding. These changes are relatively easy to implement on the hospital labor unit. (See Case Study 12.3.)

Active versus expectant/physiologic management of third stage

Usually within minutes of the birth of the infant, the placenta is delivered. Postpartum hemorrhage is the most common and most fatal complication of the third stage of labor [52], occurring in up to 18% of women [53]. Authors of the most recent Cochrane review on active versus expectant management of third stage labor, while acknowledging a lack of high-quality evidence for primary outcomes, concluded that active management (prophylactic uterotonic, early cord clamping, controlled cord traction) reduced the incidence of primary

Case Study 12.3

Third stage labor

Kristi delivered a healthy baby boy weighing 3,726 grams, who was immediately placed in skin-to-skin contact with her and breastfeeding was initiated during the third stage of labor. She had no risk factors for postpartum hemorrhage and preferred a physiologic third stage, so the placenta is allowed to deliver spontaneously while Kristi continues to breastfeed her infant in an upright position with the guidance of her nurse. The midwife inspects the perineum and no lacerations are noted. The placenta delivers spontaneously with no excess bleeding and an immediately firm fundus. Fundal checks are completed every 15 minutes while Kristi continues to breastfeed and/or bond with her baby. Her nurse makes sure that Kristi has plenty of oral fluids in the immediate postpartum period to ensure hydration and blood pressure stabilization. Infant vital signs are taken, and medications are administered (per protocol) while the baby remains skin to skin with Kristi with her partner at her side. Approximately 60 minutes after giving birth, Kristi is assisted to the bathroom to void, cleanse the perineal area, and change her gown. During the second hour after the birth, the family holds the baby and Kristi breastfeeds for 15 more minutes. After transfer to the postpartum unit the infant has a head-to-toe assessment by the pediatric team. Upon discharge from the labor unit Kristi has held her baby for 90 minutes and has breastfed for 35 minutes. Following family transitions, the care providers document the final information about the birth into the electronic health record anticipating hospital reporting of the Joint Commission perinatal measures set.

postpartum hemorrhage of 1,000 ml, mean maternal blood loss at birth, and hemoglobin less than 9 in the first 72 hours postpartum in a mixed-risk population. Similar results were noted for women at low risk of postpartum hemorrhage, although there were no significant differences in severe hemorrhage or hemoglobin less than 9 at 72 hours postbirth. Adverse effects of active management such as hypertension, vomiting, and increased postpartum pain and analgesic use were also identified [54]. Women should be provided with their risk status for postpartum hemorrhage and an explanation of the care management choices and be allowed to make an informed choice about third stage care [54,55]. It has been argued that expectant management is not necessarily the same as physiologic management of third stage labor, and further research is needed to compare active and physiologic management of third stage [56].

Maximizing maternal/newborn bonding

For women and their families, the first hour after giving birth is an emotional and amazing experience, the beginning of their new family. To the maternity and neonatal health care staff attending the birth and postpartum care, the first hour after delivery is about assessing both mother and newborn to assure healthy transition following birth. Creating a home-like environment that maximizes bonding and breastfeeding should be a priority for the hospital labor unit, especially in that critical first hour of life when the infant is most alert. Head-to-toe infant assessments can wait until after the first hour of life in a healthy infant. Uterine fundal assessments, neonatal vital sign measurement, and neonatal injections and heel sticks can all be performed while the mother holds her infant. Multiple studies have found that women breastfeed for a longer duration when breastfeeding is initiated within the first hour of life. DiGirolamo, Grummer-Strawn, and Fein [57] found a statistically significant protective effect against early termination of breastfeeding when initiated within the first hour of life. Early initiation of breastfeeding also protects against neonatal hypoglycemia, assists with thermoregulation of the infant, and facilitates bonding between mother and infant [57]. Placing an infant skin to skin with the mother for the first hour of life can maximize positive outcomes for both mother and infant. Early skin-to-skin contact between mother and newborn has also been shown to improve breastfeeding with no harmful effects [58].

Conclusion

Evidence supports a minimally interventive environment for labor and birth for low-risk women. Low-intervention births can occur in a hospital setting while providing a safe, quality birthing experience for women with a healthy, uncomplicated pregnancy. By identifying the evidence-based changes supported by the Lamaze six birth care practices and the potential barriers to making these changes, labor units can overcome barriers and create a birth experience that is as home-like as possible. Modern labor and birth units can accommodate these changes to provide a twenty-first-century birthing environment that is both safe and provides the mother and family with the high-quality, high-value experience they desire. By assisting low-risk women to have a low-intervention birth in a home-like environment, a shorter and more satisfying labor, birth, and postpartum experience is possible for the mother, the infant, and the family. A similar approach to care can also be useful and appropriate for women with a more complex pregnancy or labor while also providing the required level of care.

Change is not easy. Strong leadership, time, patience, and the participation of everyone involved in the labor unit are required. A specific change process should be followed and adapted to the individual needs of the labor unit to increase the chances of success. The hospital labor unit is where substantial change is necessary to positively affect the care for laboring women and their families and improve outcomes in the United States.

References

1. World Health Organization. (2012). *Maternal mortality ratio*. Retrieved from: http://apps.who. int/ghodata/?vid=250.
2. Central Intelligence Agency. (2012) Country comparison: Infant mortality rate. Retrieved from: https://cia.gov/library/publications/the-world-factbook/rankorder/2091rank.html.
3. Hoyert DL & Xu J. (2012). Deaths: Preliminary data for 2011. *National Vital Statistics Reports*, *61*(6). http://www.cdc.gov/nchs/data/nvsr/nvsr61/nvsr61_06.pdf. Accessed November 17, 2012.
4. Osterman MJ & Martin JA. (2011). Epidural and spinal anesthesia use during labor: 27-state reporting area, 2008. *National Vital Statistics Report*, *59*(5), 1–16.
5. Hamilton BE, Martin JA, & Ventura SJ. (2011). Births: Preliminary data for 2010. *The National Vital Statistics Reports*, *60*(2), 1–26.
6. Martin JA, Hamilton BE, Sutton PD, Ventura SJ, Mathews TJ, Kirmeyer S, & Osterman MJ. (2010). Births: Final data for 2007. *National Vital Statistics Reports*, *58*(24), 1–86.

7. Dye NS. (1980). History of childbirth in America. *Signs*, *6*(1), 97–108.
8. MacDorman MF, Declercq E, & Menacker F. (2011). Trends and characteristics of home births in the United States by race and ethnicity, 1990–2006. *Birth: Issues in Perinatal Care*, *38*(1), 17–23.
9. MacDorman MF, Menacker F, & Declercq E. (2010). Trends and characteristics of home and other out-of-hospital births in the United States, 1990–2006. *National Vital Statistics Reports*, *58*(11).
10. Boucher D, Bennett C, McFarlin B, & Freeze R. (2009). Staying home to give birth: Why women in the United States choose home birth. *Journal of Midwifery & Women's Health*, *54*(2), 119–126.
11. American Academy of Family Physicians; American Academy of Pediatrics; American College of Nurse-Midwives; American College of Obstetricians and Gynecologists; American College of Osteopathic Obstetricians & Gynecologists; Association of Women's Health, Obstetric and Neonatal Nurses; & the Society for Maternal-Fetal Medicine. (2011). Quality patient care in labor and delivery: A call to action. Retrieved from: http://www.acog.org/~/media/Departments/Patient%20Safety%20and%20Quality%20Improvement/Call%20to%20Action%20Paper.pdf?dmc=1&ts=20130223T1729565571.
12. Lamaze International. (2009). Lamaze healthy birth practices. Retrieved from: http://www.lamaze.org/Default.aspx?tabid=90.
13. Sakala C, & Corry M. (2008). *Evidence-based maternity care: What it is and what it can achieve*. New York: Childbirth Connection.
14. Coalition for Improving Maternity Services. (1996). Mother-friendly childbirth initiative. Retrieved from: http://www.motherfriendly.org/MFCI. Accessed November 6, 2012.
15. Hodnett ED, Stremler R, Weston JA, & McKeever P. (2009). Rec-conceptualizing the hospital labor room: The PLACE (pregnant and laboring in an ambient clinical environment) pilot trial. *Birth*, *36*(2), 159–166.
16. Zwelling E, Johnson K, & Allen J. (2006). How to implement complementary therapies for laboring women. *Maternal Child Nursing*, *31*(6), 364–370.
17. Hodnett ED, Downe S, Walsh D, & Weston J. (2010). Alternative versus conventional institutional settings for birth. *Cochrane Database of Systematic Reviews*, issue 9. Art. No.: CD000012. DOI: 10.1002/14651858.CD000012.pub3.
18. Bingham D & Main EK. (2010). Effective implementation strategies and tactics for leading change on maternity units. *Journal of Perinatal & Neonatal Nursing*, *24*(1), 32–42.
19. National Quality Forum. 2012. Endorsement summary: Perinatal and reproductive health measures. Retrieved from: http://www.qualityforum.org/Projects/n-r/Perinatal_Care_Endorsement_Maintenance_2011/Perinatal_and_Reproductive_Healthcare_Endorsement_Maintenance_2011.aspx.
20. Joint Commission. (2010). Perinatal care measures. http://manual.jointcommission.org/releases/TJC2011A/PerinatalCare.html. Accessed November 6, 2012.
21. Graham ID, Logan J, Davies B, & Nimrod C. (2004). Changing the use of electronic fetal monitoring and labor support: A case study of barriers and facilitators. *Birth*, *31*(4), 293–301.
22. Scott T, Mannion R, Davies HT, & Marshall MN. (2003). Implementing culture change in health care: Theory and practice. *International Journal for Quality in Health Care*, *15*(2), 111–118.
23. Roberts L, Culliver B, Fisher J, & Cloyes KG. (2010). The coping with labor algorithm: An alternate pain assessment tool for the laboring woman. *Journal of Midwifery & Women's Health*, *55*(2), 107–115.
24. Shaw PL, Elliott C, Isaacson P, & Murphy EE. (2009). *Quality and performance improvement in healthcare*. Chicago: American Health Information Management Association.

25. Lagan BM, Sinclair M, & Kernohan WG. (2010). Internet use in pregnancy forms women's decision making: A web-based survey. *Birth, 37*(2), 106–115.

26. Pincus J. (2001). Childbirth advice literature as it relates to two childbearing ideologies. *Birth, 27*(3), 209–213.

27. Boston Women's Health Book Collective. (2008). *Our bodies, ourselves: Pregnancy and birth.* New York: Touchstone.

28. Simpson KR, Newman G, & Chirino OR. (2010). Patient education to reduce elective inductions. *MCN: American Journal of Maternal and Child Nursing, 354*, 188–196.

29. Yang YT, Mello MM, Subramanian SV, & Studdert DM. (2009). Relationship between malpractice litigation pressure and rates of cesarean section and vaginal birth after cesarean section. *Med Care, 47*, 234–242.

30. Bandura A. (1997). *Self-efficacy: The exercise of control.* New York: Freeman.

31. Davies BL, & Hodnett E. (2002). Labor support: Nurses' self-efficacy and views about factors influencing implementation. *JOGNN, 31*(1), 48–55.

32. Sauls DJ. (2002). Effects of labor support on mothers, babies, and birth outcomes. *JOGNN, 31*(6), 733–741.

33. Sleutel M & Sherrod Golden S. (1999). Fasting in labor: Relic or requirement. *JOGNN, 28*(5), 507–512.

34. Singata M, Tranmer J, & Gyte GM. (2010). Restricting oral fluid and food intake during labor. *Cochrane Collaboration, issue* 1, 1–93.

35. Lothian JA, Amis D, & Crenshaw J. (2004). Care practices that promote a normal birth #4: No routine interventions. *Journal of Perinatal Education, 13*(2), 23–29.

36. Enkin M, Kierse MJC, Neilson J, Crowther C, Duley L, Hodnett E, et al. (2000). *A guide to effective care in pregnancy and childbirth.* New York: Oxford University Press.

37. Alfirevic Z, Devane D, & Gyte GML. (2008). Continuous cardiotocography as a form of electronic fetal monitoring for fetal assessment during labour. *Cochrane Collaboration, issue* 4, 1–97.

38. Albers LL. (2001). Monitoring the fetus in labor: Evidence to support the methods. *Journal of Midwifery & Women's Health, 46*(6), 366–373.

39. American College of Nurse-Midwives. (2010). Intermittent auscultation for intrapartum fetal heart rate surveillance. *Journal of Midwifery & Women's Health, 55*(4), 397–403.

40. Hodnett ED, Gates S, Hofmeyr GJ, Sakala C, & Weston J. (2011). Continuous support for women during childbirth. *Cochrane Collaboration*, issue 2, 1–104.

41. Gagnon AJ, Waghorn L, & Covell C. (1997). A randomized trial of one-to-one nurse support of women in labor. *Birth, 24*(2), 71–77.

42. Association of Women's Health, Obstetric and Neonatal Nurses. (2011). Guidelines for professional registered nurse staffing for perinatal units executive summary. *JOGNN, 40*(1), 131–134.

43. Mayberry LJ, Strange LB, Suplee PD, & Gennaro S. (2003). Use of upright positioning with epidural analgesia: Findings from an observational study. *MCN: American Journal of Maternal Child Nursing, 28*(3), 152–159.

44. Gilder K, Mayberry LJ, Gennaro S, & Clemmens D. (2002). Maternal positioning in labor with epidural analgesia. *AWHONN, 6*(1), 40–45.

45. Perry J. (2011). *Understanding birth.* Longmont, CO: In Joy Publishers.

46. Roberts J & Hanson L. (2007). Best practices in second stage labor: Maternal bearing down and positioning. *Journal of Midwifery & Women's Health, 52*(3), 238–245.

47. Simkin P & Ancheta, R. (2011). *The labor progress handbook: Early interventions to prevent and treat dystocia*, 3rd ed. West Sussex, UK: Wiley-Blackwell.

48. Blaz A. (2011). Pushing during 2ⁿᵈ stage of labor: Dorsal lithotomy vs. squatting. Retrieved from: http://www.scienceandsensibility.org/?author=92.

49. Golara M, Plaat F, & Shennan AH. (2002). Upright versus recumbent position in the second stage of labour in women with combined spinal-epidural analgesia. *International Journal of Obstetric Analgesia*, 11, 19–22.

50. Maresh M, Choong KH, & Beard RW. (1983). Delayed pushing with lumbar epidural analgesia in labour. *British Journal of Obstetrics and Gynaecology*, 90(7), 623–627.

51. Hansen SL, Clark SL, & Foster JC. (2002). Active pushing versus passive fetal descent in second stage of labor: A randomized controlled trial. *Obstetrics & Gynecology*, 99(1), 29–34.

52. Afolabi EO, Kuti O, Orji EO, & Ogunniyi SO. (2010). Oral misoprostol versus intramuscular oxytocin in the active management of the third stage of labor. *Singapore Medical Journal*, 51(3), 207–211.

53. Anderson JM & Etches D. (2007). Prevention and management of postpartum hemorrhage. *American Family Physician*, 75(6), 875–882.

54. Begley CM, Gyte GML, Devane D, McGuire W, & Weeks A. (2011). Active versus expectant management for women in the third stage of labour. *Cochrane Database of Systematic Reviews*, issue 11. Art. No.: CD007412. DOI: 10.1002/14651858.CD007412.pub3.

55. International Confederation of Midwives. (2011). Role of the midwife in physiological third stage labor (position statement). Retrieved from: http://www.nurse.or.jp/nursing/international/icm/definition/pdf/shoshin/f-31.pdf.

56. Fahy KM. (2009). Third stage of labour care for women at low risk of postpartum haemorrhage. *Journal of Midwifery and Women's Health*, 54, 380–386.

57. DiGirolamo AM, Grummer-Strawn AM, & Fein SB. (2008). Effect of maternity-care practices on breastfeeding. *Pediatrics*, 122(Supplement), S43–S49.

58. Moore ER, Anderson GC, Bergman N, & Dowswell T. (2012). Early skin-to-skin contact for mothers and their healthy newborn infants. *Cochrane Database of Systematic Reviews*, issue 5. Art. No.: CD003519. DOI: 10.1002/14651858.CD003519.pub3.

Chapter 13

Out-of-hospital birth

Marsha E. Jackson and Alice Bailes

Key points

- Consumer interest in out-of-hospital birth (home and free-standing birth center settings) is on the rise.
- A home birth consensus summit in 2011 resulted in nine statements agreed to by individuals from consumer organizations, multiple health professions, health care administrators, health policy experts, and public health researchers and educators.
- Giving birth in the home or birth center setting limits technologic interventions and increases the authority, centrality, and privacy of the client, enhancing the opportunity for her to birth normally.
- Out-of-hospital practice includes enhancing women's confidence to give birth and the expectation that nonpharmacological strategies are effective in supporting labor and birth.
- A consulting network and seamless access to a care continuum are essential for out-of-hospital birth practice.
- Collegial communication between hospital staff and home birth and birth center providers when hospital transfer is necessary promotes more effective care and may contribute to better outcomes.

[T]he art of doing 'nothing' well.

Holly Powell Kennedy

Introduction

The Consensus Statement Supporting Healthy and Normal Physiologic Childbirth jointly authored by the American College of Nurse-Midwives, the National Association of Certified Professional Midwives, and the Midwives Alliance of North America describes a normal birth as "one that is powered by the innate human capacity of the woman and fetus" and that "supporting the normal physiologic processes of labor and birth . . . has the potential to enhance best outcomes for the mother and infant" [1].

Supporting a Physiologic Approach to Pregnancy and Birth: A Practical Guide, First Edition.
Edited by Melissa D. Avery.
© 2013 John Wiley & Sons, Inc. Published 2013 by John Wiley & Sons, Inc.

In both the home and birth center environments, the laboring mother and practitioner deliberately put increased technology at a distance, supporting a physiologic approach. The mother has greater control, and the providers around her bolster her sense of empowerment. She labors in an environment that is private, familiar, and small, where encountering unexpected interruptions and unknown personnel are very unlikely. Home birth and birth center providers, usually serving one laboring client at a time, are able to give more hands-on support and can take the time to support the woman's birth preferences while monitoring her condition to assure safety [2].

In this chapter we provide a brief overview of the history of home birth and birth center birth in the United States, including the consensus statements from the 2011 summit "The Future of Home Birth in the United States: Addressing Shared Responsibility." Research supporting home birth for low-risk women as well as a philosophic framework are discussed. We provide basics of safe out-of-hospital birth including the use of consultation networks, safe transfer and receiving of clients, quality improvement, and two case studies illustrating these principles. Finally system barriers to successful out-of-hospital birth are presented.

Background

History

The roots of American midwifery and birth are firmly planted in the home. During early colonial times, before the creation of a medical system, midwives functioned without regulation in homes. Childbirth was known as women's work and a mother's efforts to give birth were supported by other women in her community. Women who assisted others during childbirth called themselves midwives. In colonial times, midwives were held in high esteem in their communities [3].

The American population growth in the eighteenth and nineteenth centuries was concentrated in urban centers, providing opportunities for sharing ideas, including major advances in the science of obstetrics and the education of physicians. Hospitals were created to care for wounded soldiers, the chronically ill, and the poor. Although middle-class and rural women continued to stay at home to have their babies, indigent and unwed pregnant women found maternity assistance in hospitals, thus providing physicians easy access to groups of women. These women often became the subjects of experiments as physicians and medical students developed, refined, and learned obstetrical techniques. Although these experiments sometimes resulted in harm or even death to the mother or baby, advances were made in the use of forceps, cesarean birth, and analgesia and anesthesia. These interventions in combination with the use of antibiotics to combat puerperal fever and ergot to control hemorrhage changed the face of obstetrical care for the better. However, the price paid in life and health of mothers and babies was high [4,5].

As new advances in obstetrics evolved, information was not shared with the midwives and they were excluded from the education process. They were also excluded from working in hospitals where these new interventions were put into practice. The low status of women in society, lack of financial resources, racism, sexism, language barriers, transportation difficulties, and restrictive laws kept midwives isolated. Thus, midwives were unable to advocate for themselves. They were unable to share information, set up education programs, or form midwifery associations that may have increased their influence [6,7].

The shift from midwife-attended home birth to physician-attended hospital birth began in the twentieth century. Physicians initiated a successful campaign to enhance their practice and to discredit the midwives. Women were led to believe that childbirth was now a pathologic process and that they were better served by medical and surgical interventions in the hospital.

Eventually, middle-class women began to opt for what seemed to be beneficial interventions and gave birth in hospitals. They left the comforting presence of the midwife in the familiar environment of their own homes in exchange for drugs used to create a painless childbirth and take advantage of what was believed to be a modern and scientific medical approach in hospitals. A Harvard professor of obstetrics, Frederick Irving, MD, expressed concern regarding the overuse of unnecessary interventions in the hospitals. In 1937 in the *New England Journal of Medicine* he stated, "We have prophylactic forceps, prophylactic version, and even prophylactic rupture of membranes. It is not evident against what the prophylaxis is directed, unless it be against normal childbirth" [8].

The migration of birth into the hospital occurred fairly rapidly. Midwife-attended births dropped from about 40% in 1915 to less than 11% by 1935 [9]. However, the practice of midwifery in the rural south remained intact with "granny" midwives. Because most hospitals by law barred blacks from admission, black women who experienced complications and needed hospital services were often distant from the few hospitals that would allow them admission. The granny midwives served their communities, attending approximately 54% of births in 1935, primarily for black women. Despite limited resources, the granny midwives had good outcomes and were indispensable in their communities [6,7,9,10].

In the 1950s and 1960s, the concept of "natural childbirth" was introduced to the United States through British physician Grantly Dick-Read's *Childbirth without Fear*. Dr. Dick-Read believed that pain in childbirth was due to the fear-tension-pain cycle and that interference with the birth process was one of the greatest dangers with which mother and child had to contend. In the mid-1960s, Elizabeth Bing and Marjorie Karmel brought the Lamaze method of childbirth to the United States from France. The American Society for Psychoprophylaxis in Obstetrics (now Lamaze International), an organization including childbirth instructors, physicians, and parents, advocated for the father's presence in the delivery room and for a reduction in intervention. By the 1970s a movement to demedicalize birth in order for women and families to maintain their authority in the birth process escalated. Women also started self-help groups to demystify their health care experience. Consumer groups maintained that childbirth was not a disease process and women did not need hospitalization if the mother was healthy and the pregnancy was normal. Families sought alternatives for childbirth, including more control over their care, and some sought home and birth center settings [11].

Home birth practices began serving families in the early 1970s. The midwives collective in Santa Cruz, California, the Maternity Center Associates midwives in Maryland, the Farm Midwives Center in Tennessee, and Greggory White and Robert Mendelsohn— physicians in Chicago—provided home birth services. Consumer-oriented books on home birth were published, including one of the most well-known childbirth books of this era, *Spiritual Midwifery*, by Ina May Gaskin [7].

Ruth Lubic, EdD, CNM, led the effort at Maternity Center Association in New York City to open a model birth center as an alternative to hospital and home births. The birth center offered safe, sensitive, cost-effective care with minimal intervention in a home-like environment. The birth center movement grew and was successful in providing a satisfying birthplace for healthy pregnant women. In 1983, Kitty Ernst, CNM, was a driving force in the creation of the American Association of Birth Centers (AABC), formerly the National Association of Childbearing Centers (NACC). Ruth Lubic, Edie Wonnell, and Sr. Angela Murdaugh supported Ernst's efforts in promoting the birth center concept. AABC established standards and gave workshops that guided practitioners and consumers to start and maintain high-quality centers. Ernst remains active promoting the birth center mission [12].

The American College of Nurse-Midwives adopted a policy statement in 1991 called "The Appropriate Use of Technology in Childbirth," advocating nonintervention in normal processes. The college published the *ACNM Home Birth Practice Handbook* providing guidance to midwives who wished to include home birth in their practice. Together these documents provided an endorsement of low-intervention home births [13,14]. The Midwives Alliance of North America (MANA), incorporated in 1982, provided an organization for midwives who emphasized low-tech home and birth center practice. MANA also stressed unity among midwives and acted as the springboard for promoting a new credential, the Certified Professional Midwife (CPM), who functions primarily in home and birth center environments [15,16].

Recent films such as *The Business of Being Born* (2008) have increased public awareness about the safety and satisfaction of birth outside the hospital setting. Internet resources such as the Transforming Maternity Care project of Childbirth Connection,and the blog "Science and Sensibility" have brought more information about normal birth to the attention of childbirth consumers and care providers [17,18]. According to the National Center for Health Statistics data, there has been a 29% increase in home birth from 2004 to 2009 [19].

A home birth consensus summit was convened in 2011 titled "The Future of Home Birth in the United States: Addressing Shared Responsibility." The participating stakeholders represented consumers, representatives of consumer organizations, home birth midwives, maternal-child health collaborating providers, obstetricians, pediatricians and family practice physicians, health care administrators, health policy experts, and public health researchers and educators. The purpose of the summit was to reach consensus in order to improve the safety of maternal and newborn care for families choosing home birth. Progress was made toward cooperation among participants, who reached mutual agreement as individuals adopting the following nine landmark statements on which the participants in the summit could agree.

STATEMENT 1

We uphold the autonomy of all childbearing women. All childbearing women, in all maternity care settings, should receive respectful, woman-centered care. This care should include opportunities for a shared decision-making process to help each woman make the choices that are right for her. Shared decision making includes mutual sharing of information about benefits and harms of the range of care options, respect for the woman's autonomy to make decisions in accordance with her values and preferences, and freedom from coercion or punishment for her choices.

STATEMENT 2

We believe that collaboration within an integrated maternity care system is essential for optimal mother-baby outcomes. All women and families planning a home or birth center birth have a right to respectful, safe, and seamless consultation, referral, transport and transfer of care when necessary. When ongoing inter-professional dialogue and cooperation occur, everyone benefits.

STATEMENT 3

We are committed to an equitable maternity care system without disparities in access, delivery of care, or outcomes. This system provides culturally appropriate and affordable care in all settings, in a manner that is acceptable to all communities.
We are committed to an equitable educational system without disparities in access to affordable, culturally appropriate, and acceptable maternity care provider education for all communities.

STATEMENT 4

It is our goal that all health professionals who provide maternity care in home and birth center settings have a license that is based on national certification that includes defined competencies and standards for education and practice. We believe that guidelines should:

- allow for independent practice,
- facilitate communication between providers and across care settings,
- encourage professional responsibility and accountability, and include mechanisms for risk assessment.

STATEMENT 5

We believe that increased participation by consumers in multi-stakeholder initiatives is essential to improving maternity care, including the development of high quality home birth services within an integrated maternity care system.

STATEMENT 6

Effective communication and collaboration across all disciplines caring for mothers and babies are essential for optimal outcomes across all settings. To achieve this, we believe that all health professional students and practitioners who are involved in maternity and newborn care must learn about each other's disciplines, and about maternity and health care in all settings.

STATEMENT 7

We are committed to improving the current medical liability system, which fails to justly serve society, families, and health care providers and contributes to:

- inadequate resources to support birth injured children and mothers;
- unsustainable healthcare and litigation costs paid by all;
- a hostile healthcare work environment;

- inadequate access to home birth and birth center birth within an integrated health care system;
- restricted choices in pregnancy and birth.

STATEMENT 8

We envision a compulsory process for the collection of patient (individual) level data on key process and outcome measures in all birth settings. These data would be linked to other data systems, used to inform quality improvement, and would thus enhance the evidence basis for care.

STATEMENT 9

We recognize and affirm the value of physiologic birth for women, babies, families and society and the value of appropriate interventions based on the best available evidence to achieve optimal outcomes for mothers and babies [20].

Midwives and physicians in the United States and worldwide are disseminating information and issuing policy statements about the benefits of low-tech births in the home, birth center, and even in the hospital [1,21–24]. It appears that birth has come full circle. Birth began in the home, moved to the hospital, and now more women and families with healthy pregnancies are planning births at home and in free-standing birth centers. Increasingly these environments outside the hospital are recognized as places where low-intervention birth is fostered. Policy efforts at the national level to improve the quality and value of maternity care include removing barriers to out-of-hospital birth for healthy women and improving care options in the hospital setting [25].

Review of evidence for out-of-hospital birth

In the United States, published reliable data regarding home birth first emerged in the early 1900s through data focusing on maternal and neonatal mortality collected by health departments and the federal government [26]. Maternity Center Association in New York, staffed by midwives doing home births, reported a 0.9/1,000 maternal mortality rate in a geographic area where maternal mortality was reported as 10.4/1,000 [6]. Metropolitan Life Insurance Company reported on births at Frontier Nursing Service, where 60% of births occurred at home in rural Kentucky. The neonatal death rate was 17.3/1,000 compared to an overall U.S. neonatal death rate of 19.6/1,000 [27,28]. In the 1930s, two government studies compared midwifery outcomes favorably to physician outcomes, attributing the good outcomes to the midwives' maternal focused management style. The report stated physician care was associated with harm to mothers and newborns caused by procedures calculated to hasten delivery and illustrated that a practice style of too much intervention in normal physiologic birth interfered with healthy outcomes [3,5,8,9].

Following these early studies, there was a long pause before U.S. researchers collected, examined, and published home birth data. In the early 1970s, Lewis Mehl and Nancy Mills reviewed outcome statistics during the early days of the home birth renaissance. Their descriptive, retrospective research documented a low incidence of intrapartum and neonatal problems associated with home birth, although a hospital comparison group was not included in the research design [29].

Literature in the 1980s and early 1990s focused on safety of birth at home. Research documenting home births that were planned demonstrated that they were much safer than home births that were unplanned or took place accidentally at home. During that time, researchers were concerned with outcome comparisons of home versus hospital birth, but not necessarily with care processes. Essential principles for safe home birth began to become evident. Safe home birth is promoted when the:

- Birthing mother is healthy.
- Plan to birth at home is made before the onset of labor.
- Birth is attended by a skilled provider.
- Pregnancy is continuously evaluated to assure normalcy throughout pregnancy and labor.
- Arrangements are in place for hospital transfer should a complication arise requiring hospital-based personnel and equipment [11,30–37].

More research was conducted examining home birth and birth center birth. Homes and birth centers were recognized as settings where fewer interventions took place and where low-intervention care supported normal physiologic birth [38–40].

Studies of birth out of the hospital in the mid-1990s began to include rates of obstetric interventions. These interventions included narcotic and epidural analgesia, augmentation or induction of labor, and assisted vaginal or cesarean birth [41–47]. The focus on safety continued to be an ongoing concern. Two significant home birth studies were published in 2009. DeJonge et al. analyzed Dutch national perinatal and neonatal registration data from 2000 to 2006. The study was significant due to the very large number of subjects: 529,688 low-risk planned home and hospital births. The authors concluded that rates of intrapartum death, neonatal death, and NICU admissions were not higher in the low-risk planned home birth group compared to the low-risk planned hospital group [48]. Janssen et al. compared outcomes of low-risk women who would be eligible for home birth. The authors prospectively studied three cohorts of women: 2,802 who planned to give birth at home with a midwife, 5,984 who planned hospital birth with a midwife, and 5,985 who planned hospital birth with a physician. Similar perinatal death rates were observed in all three groups. Women who planned to give birth at home, including those who required intrapartal hospital transfer, encountered fewer complications and interventions such as analgesia, augmentation or induction of labor, assisted vaginal or cesarean birth, postpartum hemorrhage, fever, and third- or fourth-degree lacerations. Their newborns were less likely to have Apgar scores less than 5 at 1 minute or need medications for resuscitation [41].

In November 2011, the *British Medical Journal* published the findings of Great Britain's National Perinatal Epidemiology Unit (NPEU), the National Health Service (NHS), and the National Institute for Health and Clinical Excellence (NICE) study utilizing a data set of over sixty-four thousand prospectively identified mothers who labored between April 2008 and April 2010. The results showed that "the odds of receiving individual interventions (augmentation, epidural or spinal analgesia, general anaesthesia, ventouse or forceps delivery, intrapartum Caesarean section, episiotomy, active management of the third stage)" were lower in midwifery managed cases, "with the greatest reductions seen for planned home and freestanding midwifery unit births . . . The proportion of women with a 'normal birth' (birth without induction of labour, epidural or spinal analgesia, general anaesthesia, forceps or ventouse delivery, Caesarean section, or episiotomy) varied from 58% for planned obstetric unit births to 76% in alongside midwifery units, 83% in freestanding midwifery units, and 88% for planned home births" [49].

Women are more satisfied with their birth experiences when their sense of control is enhanced. To obtain this sense of control while giving birth, more consumers are choosing to remain at home or receive care at a free-standing birth center [50]. Many women believe that communication with their providers will be enhanced, their wishes will be respected, and fewer unnecessary technologic interventions will be implemented in these environments. They also believe that with reduced interventions they will be safer; the literature supports their beliefs [51,52].

Factors motivating clients to seek out-of-hospital birth—authority, centrality, and privacy

Michel Odent is a physician who founded a birthing clinic in the South of France. He learned from the midwives who worked for him that the most experienced midwives simply brought their inconspicuous quiet presence and did very little at births. The woman would find her own way to work with her labor, undisturbed. Odent became a vocal proponent of undisturbed birth. When speaking at conferences and other events, he would say repeatedly in his thick French accent, "The most important thing is not to disturb, do not disturb" [53].

Many maternity care providers have adopted this important tenet. Sara Buckley, an Australian family physician, further expands this concept: "Undisturbed birth is exceedingly rare in our culture, even in birth centers and home births. Two factors that disturb birth in all mammals are firstly being in an unfamiliar place and secondly the presence of an observer. Feelings of safety and privacy thus seem to be fundamental. Yet the entire system of Western obstetrics is devoted to observing pregnant and birthing women, by both people and machines, and when birth isn't going smoothly, obstetricians [and other care providers] respond with yet more intense observation. It is indeed amazing that any woman can give birth under such conditions" [54]. When the birth environment respects the mother's innate abilities to birth, there are fewer disturbances to disrupt the hormonal levels that dictate labor's ebbs and flows. It is this protection from disturbance of the woman in labor that aids in maintaining a productive hormonal balance for labor.

Midwives who work in the home and in birth centers believe that the mother's hormonal balance creates the labor pattern. Any interaction with a woman during labor constitutes an intervention that can enhance or interfere with that hormonal balance, altering labor's course. An intervention can be as simple as offering a drink of water or as complex and technologic as placing epidural anesthesia. In the environment of the client's home or in a birth center, technologic interventions that have the potential to cause complications are deliberately limited or avoided. Providers develop highly perfected skills to support the mother's efforts to birth without these technologies.

Professional health care organizations (ACNM/MANA/NACPM Joint Statement, WHO, ICM, Joint Statement of Canada, Joint Statement of Great Britain) have issued statements describing factors or interventions supportive of normal, physiologic birth. These include a gentle nonthreatening environment, labor free of time limits, pain relief through nonpharmacologic means, encouragement of eating and drinking, spontaneous rupture of membranes, freedom of movement, intermittent auscultation of the fetal heart, vaginal exams limited in frequency, and episiotomy performed judiciously [1,21–24]. Although these factors can be easily implemented in the home or birth center setting, with increased awareness and effort, hospital staff and administration can incorporate these factors into the plan of care in the hospital setting as well.

Giving birth in the home or birth center setting not only purposefully limits technologic interventions but also increases the *authority, centrality, and privacy* of the client, enhancing the opportunity for her to birth normally. The shift away from a hospital immediately changes the balance of power, with the locus of control shifting toward the client. A woman and her family can more easily feel a sense of familiarity and control in the small and intimate birth center environment. In the home setting, familiarity and control are enhanced even further. The care provider is the guest, and the client is the host. Distractions that occur in an environment unfamiliar to the client are decreased, improving her ability to focus her energy on the work of labor. The woman and her family significantly increase their authority, centrality, and privacy in a smaller setting. "Smallness appears to be attuned to labor physiology, which inherently manifests biological rhythms based on hormonal pulses of activity rather than regular clock time rhythms" [55, p. 181].

Authority has been defined as "the power to control, command or determine" [56]. Women have described their feelings regarding control, or lack of it, over the events of labor, and are outsiders to the complex, bureaucratic structure of a hospital. There, valuable energy is wasted as each woman tries to figure out who to ask for a washcloth, and "Where is the bathroom?" When authority is thus diminished, even her ability to recognize her own needs is diminished. In the smaller, simpler birth center or home setting, she is relieved of the task of figuring out what is going on in an unfamiliar environment and more easily directs her attention to choosing effective comfort measures, understanding options, and taking an active role in clinical decisions.

In the hospital setting, the needs of many (staff as well as patients) must be served, so the *centrality* of the laboring woman is necessarily diminished. In the home environment, there are no other clients to be served, and birth centers do not often serve more than one laboring client at a time. Thus, the laboring woman is the central focus of all who interact with her during labor.

Privacy in the hospital setting may be difficult for the client to attain. There is the ritual of staff knocking on the labor room door, pausing, and saying, "May I come in?" but the client refusing entry to staff is rarely an option. The client really does not have ownership of the labor room space. Taking hold of the hospital space outside of the labor room is certainly not possible. In the out-of-hospital environment, privacy allows the woman to fully relax and respond to the demands of labor with fewer inhibitions. She may feel less self-conscious expressing herself as she works with her labor in her own way.

Hospital rules and procedures may not be congruent with the mother's needs. The woman may be separated from her partner, who may be directed to registration to complete admission paperwork. Labor companions who are important to the mother may be barred from the labor and birth unit if hospital policy limits the number of visitors or when

Case Study 13.1

Multipara—planned home birth

AH is a 31-year-old G4 P2012, married female of mixed race at 38 weeks gestation and planning a home birth. She has had one previous home birth and one previous birth center birth. Her husband, KH, and their extended families are supportive of their decision to stay home to birth. She started her prenatal care at 12 weeks gestation and her prenatal course has been uncomplicated. AH has a history of short labors and wants to include her other children in the birth.

04:00—AH is awakened with contractions and calls to alert her CNM that labor is starting. AH is concerned about impending rush hour and CNM getting to her on time. AH is able to go back to sleep.

09:00—AH discouraged. No change in contractions (q7–10 min X30–40 sec—mild). Previous labors were 4–5 hours total. CNM checks to be sure AH has eaten breakfast, continues to hydrate well, and has notified her birth assistant that labor may be starting. Her husband stayed home from work today.

12:00—AH experiences no change in contractions but notices some pinkish, mucousy discharge. She notifies CNM who encourages normal activities of the day and to try to take a nap.

17:00—A&K pick up children from school/daycare, have dinner, and notice an increase in contractions (q5–7 min X50 sec—mild/mod intensity). AH is very excited that contractions are changing. AH notifies CNM and birth assistant of change and AH requests that her birth team assemble at her home.

19:00—CNM and birth assistant arrive at client's home. Initial vital signs and FHTs are recorded. CNM and birth assistant review written birth plan, organize supplies, and set up for the home birth. AH beginning to work with contractions. A&K had wanted their children to be involved in the birth but decide to put them to bed at their regular time. Their friend Jan is on her way to their home to be with the children.

20:00—CNM observes that the household is still very busy and the children are excited.

20:15—Jan arrives to care for the children.

20:30—Children in bed.

21:00—Now that household is quiet, AH focuses more easily on labor. Contractions q4–5 min X60–75 sec. BOW intact, having some backache, needing to breathe with contractions.

22:00—AH expresses frustration with this labor. Needing KH to put a lot of pressure on back. Thought the baby would have been born by now. CNM listens and expresses that each labor is different. Offered SVE. AH wants exam.

22:10—SVE 100%/5/-2 LOP+bloody show. Labor progressing slowly. AH glad she has dilated but somewhat disappointed.

01:00—all vital signs remain WNL.

02:00—AH labor dancing with KH. AH beginning to feel pressure in her pelvis.

02:30—AH begins to spontaneously bear down. FHT 130s after every other contraction.

03:00—CNM does not see any evidence of making progress with pushing. Suggests SVE.

03:10—SVE C/rim/-1, unable to reduce cervix, LOP persists. AH encouraged not to push. AH to tub to aid relaxation. Plan to auscultate FHT q15 min if client not actively pushing.

03:30—More comfortable in tub (listening to music, dim lights, drinking fluids) and experiencing less urge to push.

04:15—AH wants out of tub, feeling stronger urge to push. Contractions now q5–6 min X75 sec—strong.

04:20—AH spontaneously bearing down and BOW visible slightly with contractions. KH supporting her standing. FHTs 130s.

04:30—Making slow progress with pushing. Baby still posterior.

04:35—AH to hands and knees. Pushing.

04:40—AH states back pain is gone.

04:55—Progressing. SROM, clear fluid. FHTs 140s. Starting to crown. Baby spontaneously rotating.

05:12—SVD of living female born OA. While AH remains on hands and knees, CNM passes baby through AH's legs enabling her to receive her baby. Apgars 9/10. AH, with her baby in her arms, is assisted to comfortable semireclining position on the bed. Baby nuzzling at the breast. Baby's vitals done while she remains in AH's arms. AH crampy but no signs of placental separation.

05:30—KH cuts the cord after it stops pulsating.

05:37—AH squats for birth of placenta while KH holds his newborn.

05:45—AH settling down with baby who has good latch and nurses well. Vital signs stable for both.

07:00—Postpartum all going well. AH ate, showered. No repair was needed. Kids awaken and welcome new baby.

Comments

AH's labor was different from previous labors, needed lots of encouragement and support to accept this unexpectedly long labor. Contractions never got very close, but the space between contractions and AH's changing positions and labor dancing gave the baby time to turn. The CNM was able to observe labor progress by the intensity of the contractions and AH's response.

CNM considered potential rapid birth with rush hour traffic as factor; contractions remained mild, so CNM felt comfortable waiting.

A&K were flexible with their birth plan. They wanted to include the children in the birth but decided to put them to bed at their regular time to enable AH to concentrate on working with labor. Their friend Jan slept at their home in case a transfer was needed.

To help control the premature urge to push, CNM suggested AH get into the tub and suggested/implemented other relaxation techniques.

Membranes remained intact and the fluid helped assist rotation of the baby. When AH got up on her hands and knees, the baby spontaneously rotated and her back pain was relieved.

hospital staff performs certain procedures. If membranes rupture, policy may restrict the mother to bed, limiting her freedom of movement and ability to find positions of comfort. (See Case Study 13.1.)

Enhancing empowerment of the birthing woman and family

In home and birth center settings, there is an expectation and dependence on nonpharmacologic labor management. Providers are familiar with and promote other methods to support and manage labor. Medications to relieve pain and stimulate labor have side effects and can decrease the effectiveness of uterine contractions and inhibit the newborn initiation of respiration. Medications to stimulate labor can cause tetanic contractions leading to uterine rupture, premature separation of the placenta, or fetal hypoxia and can make labor more difficult for the mother to manage. These pharmaceuticals are not used in the out-of-hospital birth setting.

Out-of-hospital practitioners convey an attitude of confidence, with the expectation that nonpharmacologic methods work to support labor. Providers encourage clients to prepare themselves for birth through childbirth education and make sure they have information upon which to base clinical management decisions. These providers offer liberal doses of presence and patience, avoiding artificial timetables as the process of labor unfolds at its own speed. They balance this presence with providing privacy for the mother and her partner for intimacy or private conversation. Sensitive to the mother's efficient use of labor energy, the providers observe carefully for the mother's needs to replenish her energy with rest and food, and assist the mother to move around to promote labor progression. They are well versed at assisting the mother with position changes that favor maternal comfort and fetal descent. Out-of-hospital clinicians are accustomed to utilizing practical strategies such as water immersion, massage, visualization, and the use of bright or subdued lighting or changing activities to match the circadian rhythms of the day. Sometimes the provider can help by suggesting a move to another room or suggesting moving to the outdoors. The living room is more social, the kitchen conveys the energy of work, the bedroom more rest and privacy. All of these "interventions" are commonly part of home birth or birth center providers' repertoire.

The confidence that a client gains by partnering with trusted providers brings with it yet another level of laboring undisturbed. She knows that her providers will avoid offering the more complex technologies, since they are expert at and supportive of nontechnologic labor support and management. She can avoid feeling defensive and does not have to be on guard, ready to decline offers of interventions not consistent with her preferences. She knows that her providers are not only accustomed to respecting and assuring implementation of the family's birth plans but that they will add coping tools as needed and promote the ability to birth normally and physiologically. Finally, she has the confidence that all useful natural techniques and appropriate technology would be attempted before a cesarean birth would be performed.

The client has control over the number and choice of people present at her birth. This includes family and friends as well as professional support, and she can anticipate that only those with whom she is already acquainted will be present. Usually the providers emphasize continuity of care to limit shift changes and reduce the efforts the mother must make to adjust to a new provider's style. No unfamiliar lab technician disturbs the environment to collect a specimen; no housekeeping staff interrupts to do chores. In most cases, certainly not in her own home, she does not have to adapt to the needs of other laboring families. The bacterial environment in home and birth center settings is less pathogenic than the hospital. In the home, the mother has antibodies to her own family's familiar bacteria. She protects the baby with these antibodies to prevent infection, promoting good health by reducing stress on the immune systems of the pair.

In the home birth setting, family life is less disturbed during labor. In most home and birth center settings, the family invites a special childcare provider to enable the children to go about their usual activities while the client and her birth partner are busy working with labor. Many times, the mother enjoys having the busy-ness and distraction of the usual activities of home life until labor requires her full attention. Then she will depend on help from her birth partner, usually her baby's father, and often a grandparent or trusted familiar babysitter takes care of sibling needs. The mother sets the boundaries on the children's participation, and the children may participate as much or as little as they wish within those boundaries. Even toddlers can offer help to their laboring mother with a cool washcloth or sips of water from a sports bottle. When oriented to the sights and sounds of labor, children can do quite well when allowed to choose according to their own comfort level. All participants must understand that they are welcome only as long as the mother wants their presence. They must respect that she may need privacy and/or have a special need to focus during labor. Occasionally providers may notice that the mother's labor is distracted by too much socializing and may suggest decreasing traffic within the birthing space. Perceptiveness and sensitivity on the part of the providers in these cases is very important; the balance between client choice and provider experience is delicate.

In home and birth center settings, separation from the baby does not usually occur unless there is a medical problem or it is a part of the family's birth plan. In most cases, there is no interruption from the baby's exit from the vagina into the mother's arms. Breastfeeding begins as soon as the mother and baby are ready and continues as long as they both desire. Newborn procedures are delayed and usually done with the baby in the mother's arms. Most providers view the parents and siblings as the appropriate caretakers of their baby, and the baby remains skin to skin with the mother or in the arms of another family member.

Key considerations for safe out-of-hospital birth

Develop a consultation network

Although most planned home or planned birth center births proceed as intended with excellent outcomes [41,48,57], there are times when consultation about a problem during pregnancy or transfer to the hospital during labor is necessary. The number one priority of midwifery practice, regardless of birth site, is the safety of the mother and her baby. Safety criteria for home or birth center births include establishing a supportive consultation network should hospital-based services become necessary. These services can be accessed through private physicians, through midwives with hospital privileges, directly through the hospital via a hospitalist or an on-call hospital provider, or through privileges maintained by the home or birth center provider herself.

A pathway for communication that flows easily is essential to create seamless consultation or transfer without fragmentation or disruption of services. Specific recommendations for establishing a consultation network should include a number of parameters that are highlighted in Box 13.1.

Box 13.1   Consultation network parameters

- A relationship among providers of mutual trust and respect.
- An arrangement for consultation made well in advance of need.
- An understanding of a well-defined scope of practice for every participant.
- Open communication of clinical management among providers on a regular basis so that management of care is agreed upon and the midwifery model of care is supported.
- Groundwork laid for a midwife/physician pathway of communication if physician services are needed for surgical or medical problems.
- Regular review of cases including positive and negative concerns.
- Knowledge of state laws and regulations enabling practice for each type of provider.
- Mutual understanding of differences and similarities of practice within each system.

The receiving hospital staff and providers can gain insight into the structure of a home or birth center practice through documents such as the *ACNM Handbook on Home Birth* or AABC's *Standards for Birth Centers* [12,14].

If transfer to hospital-based care is necessary, nursing staff plays an important role. Nurses coordinate availability of nursing personnel, obstetrical and anesthesia staff, and labor or operating room availability. If the on-call service for labor and delivery and/or hospitalists is the identified consultant service, the out-of-hospital providers should know consultant preferences regarding notification of impending transfers. It is important to note that the majority of transfers are nonurgent and women are usually transported via the family car.

Making time to create a positive working relationship is very worthwhile. Consultants have experienced harassment for working with out-of-hospital providers. Occasionally, consultants have been the focus of lengthy investigations regarding hospital privileges, attempts to impose a surcharge on professional liability premiums, or loss of professional liability insurance altogether [58]. One way to nurture consultant relationships is to provide relief by developing a pool of available consultants. Not only does this help to prevent overburdening a primary individual consultant, but it can reduce the vulnerability of that consultant in an environment that may not be welcoming to home and birth center birth. In some states, legislation limits midwifery practice, and midwives are unable to provide services without a consultation agreement. If the midwife loses the consultant arrangement, she may lose her right to practice.

Care continuum when transfer is necessary

What can be done to help the client who has planned an out-of-hospital birth and finds she needs to transfer to a hospital birth? How can out-of hospital and hospital-based professionals offer a more seamless transfer of care when a laboring woman needs hospital-based technologic intervention? Prenatal preparation for transfer to the hospital for services if needed is important and should include discussion with the out-of-hospital provider and a written hospital birth plan prepared by the client.

A simple start for women planning an out-of-hospital birth may be to visit the hospital birthing unit where she would be transferred if needed. A staff nurse could provide a unit tour, ending the tour in a birthing room and providing a labor rehearsal. The labor rehearsal could provide expectant parents with an opportunity to try out the squat bar, to find comfortable places in the birthing room to labor out of the bed, to practice contractions sitting on a birth ball or on the bath bench in the shower stall, to learn where the patient nutrition center is, and to become oriented to policy for NICU care if there is a neonatal problem. Thus, valuable labor energy is saved should the client need to return for her birth by being familiar with the labor unit and its policies.

Collegial transfer communication between hospital staff and home birth and birth center providers promotes more effective care and probably contributes to better outcomes. When a home birth or birth center client is in labor, the provider may notify the receiving hospital. The client's name can then be placed on the birthing unit's board so the staff is aware that a client is in labor. When the client gives birth, the hospital is notified, and the client's name is taken off of the board. Because only 11% of clients require an in-labor transfer, the hospital staff thus becomes aware of the other 89% of clients who do not need hospital services and give birth as planned in their home or a birth center [39,40]. The call when a mother is in labor, also gives staff a "heads up" that there is another client in labor that potentially may need the hospital's services.

If a transfer becomes necessary, arrangements have ideally already been made for providers to contact the hospital staff by telephone. The receiving provider may be a hospital-based midwife, a physician, or a member of the nursing staff. The transferring provider brings the client's chart including prenatal record, a birth plan, a description of labor's course, and identification of the problem that needs attention. Transferring providers usually accompany the client, acting as a bridge, providing technical information to the hospital staff and emotional and labor support to the family, thereby easing the transition on both ends. Transferring providers often remain with the client through the baby's birth, giving additional assistance with initiating breastfeeding. Hospital staff can offer support to transferring providers as well. Many times a transfer is made after a long labor that has deprived transferring providers as well as the client of sleep. If an epidural is placed to give the client enough comfort so she can sleep, staff can quiet the room environment and can help assure that the transferring providers also have an opportunity to rest.

When the hospital staff receives a client with respect, she feels reassured that she may maintain some *authority*, and that she and her baby are safe under the care of that staff. The client's safety is augmented when there is a respectful previously agreed-upon method of communication between hospital staff and her home or birth center providers. Transfer usually occurs due to a problem, so the client may be worried about her health and/or her baby's health in addition to her feelings of disappointment over the loss of her planned home or birth center birth. The receiving staff has a dual role: to show empathy for the client's disappointment and to assess for and implement the care needed to resolve the presenting problem. Usually there is time for this process to occur because most transfer cases are initiated for slow labor progress or maternal exhaustion.

Hospital staff reassurance can help the client to reenergize and to increase her ability to cope with labor and the change in planned birth site. Reviewing her birth plan and preferences for care following transfer can also reassure the client that the staff respects her authority. A method for the client's access to her hospital chart could be devised, and she could be encouraged to review notes entered during her hospital stay if desired.

One-to-one nursing care offers the client a feeling of *centrality*. Ideally, the staff assigned to the client will be familiar with techniques supportive of normal physiologic birth. The staff can explain their philosophy of care, and the client can be reassured that the staff's philosophy is congruent with the client's ideas about her labor and birth care. The client's centrality is augmented if shift changes can be kept to a minimum, and the primary nurse can take care of registration tasks in the labor room, draw blood and start IVs if indicated, and monitor the baby using intermittent auscultation. When the fetus is monitored with Doppler instead of electronic fetal monitor, the personal interaction through touch, eye contact, and conversation between client and staff enhances the relationship and reinforces the client's feeling of centrality.

The importance of basic *privacy* cannot be overemphasized. The processes of labor and birth are centered in the sexual anatomy of the woman. Her native oxytocin is enhanced by privacy, while corticosteroids are increased with anxiety. A client may want privacy that includes only her partner, she may be reassured by the presence of a consistent staff member, or she may feel comfort in continuity of care with her transferring providers. An awareness of the client's response to labor as it progresses allows the staff to provide the appropriate balance of privacy and presence.

The mother's preferences for clothing during labor depend on the way she perceives the privacy offered. She may choose to be clad in her own soft oversized tee shirt that opens in the front for breastfeeding easy access, she may prefer a hospital gown that she doesn't have to take home to launder, or she may wish to labor naked. When the woman develops confidence that the staff person who manages her care and the traffic in and out of her birthing room can be trusted, she may be able to reach a deeper level of relaxation. Speaking at a conference, Ina May Gaskin once told of a couple that posted a sign stating "Caution, kissing in progress." All of the staff on the birthing unit were very conscientious about guarding the couple's privacy [59]!

Quality control/improvement

Keeping careful records of the process of care and outcome statistics can help a practice foster safe physiologic birth. Most home birth and birth center practices implement some form of quality management review, and many integrate the review finding when establishing a practice. The plan takes into account safety, efficacy of service, and client satisfaction. The American Association of Birth Centers' Uniform Data Set (UDS) and the MANA Stats [60,61] serve as two data sets that can be used to collect data prospectively, track process and outcome data, and monitor the effectiveness of the care provided.

Home birth and birth center practices also use evaluation forms to collect client satisfaction data. These forms help practitioners examine their practices through their clients' eyes, identifying ways to improve care. Providing clients with an evaluation form postpartum also gives clients a mechanism to convey thoughts that they may feel uneasy communicating face to face.

Most hospitals have an existing mechanism for evaluation, but the system is often not utilized effectively. Including questions specific to clients who transferred into the hospital during labor would be beneficial in evaluating the process of hospital-based care. Follow-up telephone calls to these clients from the hospital's quality management team may also prove helpful. (See Case Study 13.2.)

Case Study 13.2

Primigravida—planned birth center birth—transfer to hospital

RT is a primigravida G1P0 30-year-old, married, white female. Both RT and her husband, BB, had been planning to conceive for the past 3 months. They were ecstatic to find out they were pregnant. R&B had attended a free information meeting at BirthCare about 6 months before conceiving. They had seen the movie *The Business of Being Born* and were sure that they wanted to explore having their baby either at their home or in a free-standing birthing center not connected to a hospital. R&B were very concerned about the high cesarean birth rate and wanted to do all they could to avoid a cesarean. They had found information about BirthCare online and also had a friend that had a home birth 2 years previous with BirthCare. R&B called to initiate care and they had their 1 hour new prenatal visit at 10 weeks gestation.

Prenatal course

R&B experienced a normal pregnancy and BB accompanied RT for almost all the prenatal appointments. They attended Bradley childbirth classes together and an added benefit was that their childbirth instructor was also a qualified birth assistant. They wasted no time in hiring her to assist the CNM at their birth. At 36 weeks gestation, their birth assistant met with R&B for a home visit to discuss plans for their birth and to check that needed supplies and car seat were ready to be taken to the birth center when labor began.

April 22—40w+2d

02:00—RT awakens during the night with mild, irregular contractions. She is so excited that she awakens BB and they are up for 2 hours. They call to check in with the on-call CNM, who encourages them to go back to sleep.

10:00—R&B slept in late since they were up during the night. RT is not having many contractions and BB decides to go into work (RT had stopped work I week ago). RT checks in with her midwife, who encourages her to have breakfast, take a walk, drink plenty of fluids, and check back with the midwife at 12:00.

12:00—CNM telephones RT but gets no answer.

15:00—RT calls CNM to check-in. RT kept busy most of the day running errands and forgot to drink. She is having irregular crampy contractions.

17:00—RT calls CNM and states she feels better after hydrating and taking a nap.

April 23—40w3d

03:00—RT is awakened again with irregular contractions. She tries not to wake BB but after 45 minutes of contractions, she notices a pinkish vaginal discharge and awakes BB to tell him. They are able to doze off and on with the contractions.

07:00—Contractions are coming in a regular pattern q10–15 min X30 sec. They call the on-call midwife to alert her that labor may be starting. The contractions are noticeable, but RT is able to walk and talk with them. The pinkish show continues. The plan was to eat breakfast, go for a walk, and relax and let labor happen. She was scheduled for a prenatal appointment at 10:00 and plans to keep the appointment if things are the same.

10:30—R&B are in for their prenatal appointment. Reassured all WNL and is informed she is having some prodromal labor. SVE cervix 50% effaced /2 cm/-2 station. R&B are happy that she is starting to dilate but thought she would be further along by now. Questions answered and return home to await labor progress.

21:00—Contractions stronger, unable to talk and needing to focus with contractions q5 min X50 sec for the past hour. R&B want to come into the birth center, but the on-call midwife lives in their neighborhood and decides to check them at home. SVE 100%/2/-2. CNM offers client a prescription for Ambien to help with sleep, but RT declines. CNM reassures them that they are making some progress. Given comfort suggestions and to call back as needed.

April 24—40w4d

02:00—R&B unable to sleep. Contractions now q4–5 min X60 sec and much stronger. Having red mucousy bloody show. Contacts on-call CNM and will meet at the birth center.

03:30—Evaluated at the birth center. Appears to be in an active labor pattern. Membranes intact. R&B working well together with contractions. Vital signs and FHT checked. Observed at birth center for 2 hours. SVE 100%/3/-2, bag of waters not well applied to cervix. Client home to await progress.

07:00—R&B rested some. To grocery store to walk and shop for nutritious snacks. Spoke on phone with parents. Grandparents getting worried that labor taking a long time.

9:30—RT in shower to aid relaxation, but contractions q3–4 min X60 sec and stronger. Ready to go back to the birth center.

10:30—Admitted to birth center. Birth assistant, midwife, and maternal grandparents present. RT sitting on birth ball, breathing and relaxing well with contractions. Checked vital signs and FHTs checked q30 min.

14:00—SVE 100% effaced/5–6 cm/-1 station, vertex is asynclitic. Outside to walk and up and down steps.

16:00—In Jacuzzi—more comfortable with contractions.

21:00—Good labor progress based on maternal signs. Did well eating, walking, and resting, but says she is very discouraged and wants to transfer to the hospital. SVE 100% effaced/9 cm/0 station. RT very encouraged by cervical change. Feels she can continue working at the birth center. RT's mother in to provide emotional support and massage. BB took a nap and is now more energized.

23:00—Used multiple techniques to encourage baby's descent into pelvis (examples: knee chest position, asymmetrical squats, labor dancing, belly dancing on the birth ball). SVE complete dilatation/0 station. RT appearing very tired. Contractions have spaced out to q5–6 min. Encouraged to rest between contractions. No spontaneous bearing down sensations yet. IV-LR started and infusing to hydrate and increase energy. 500 cc bolus given and encouraged to eat honey since RT had no desire to eat.

23:45—Up to bathroom. Beginning to feel pressure in pelvis. Pushing spontaneously with contractions.

April 25—40w5d

00:30—Pushing well. Little progress.

01:00—To Jacuzzi to push and help relax.

02:00—RT feeling discouraged. Contractions not as strong and not all pushy. IV-LR bag #1 infused and bag #2 hung.

03:00—R&B requesting again to go to the hospital. SVE in tub reveals no descent and minimal molding.

03:00—Tx to hospital initiated. CNM places call to hospital-based CNM consultant to advise re: need and reason for transfer to the hospital.

03:15—BB gathers suitcase that had been packed prenatally in case of transfer and some snacks to take to hospital. Midwife and birth assistant put chart, birth bowl containing clamps and scissors in a sterile pack, bulb syringe, cord clamp and deLee, oxygen tank, and blankets in the CNM's car. Saline lock placed on IV catheter. R&B and grandparents to family car. CNM leads caravan to the hospital.

03:30—Arrival at hospital. R&B go directly to L&D as they previously preregistered. Greeted on L&D by pleasant, energetic nurse and CNM. Birth plan reviewed. Their welcoming demeanor, expressions of empathy re: RT's need to transfer established trust. R&B less anxious and more confident that they would be well supported in the hospital and still hoping for a vaginal birth.

04:30—Epidural in place and pitocin infusing slowly. Slept and labored down (fully dilated, no encouragement to push without urge to push). Contractions now q2–4 min X60–75 sec. RT resting and laboring down.

05:30—RT feeling increase in pelvic pressure. Hospital CNM in to evaluate. SVE completely dilated/+1 station. Encouraged to push. Epidural infusion decreased.

05:45—Making good progress and pushing effectively. Grandparents invited into the birth room.

06:13—SVD of living male infant. Apgars 8/9, small first-degree vaginal laceration, not repaired. Baby latched without difficulty. Family happy.

Comments

Primigravidas labor a long time and care is very time intensive. The clients were well prepared through their childbirth classes and accepting of early labor's ebbs and flows. R&B attended prenatal visits together and knew their care providers well. This helped to establish trust with their care providers. RT declined medication during labor to aid relaxation. Many clients desiring home or birth center birth may be adverse to medications when a long prodromal phase is encountered. The CNM should present options and encourage the client to make decisions, thus maintaining authority. Due to the long prodromal phase, RT interacted with several midwives. The midwives maintained communication among themselves by texting each other on their mobile devices. This helps to free the client of the need to repeat the same story for each CNM and helps to maintain continuity of care.

The birth center midwives oriented them to the possibility of transfer during labor. Their prenatal visit to the hospital reduced the stress of the transfer. They were familiar with the facility. Except for the first day of prodromal labor, R&B were both attentive to preserving a good balance of activity, rest, and nutrition. This enabled RT to get to full dilation. Having IV fluids on board before transfer to the hospital helped to expedite placement of the epidural. The baby was low enough in the pelvis so that the receiving providers were willing to proceed with a plan for a vaginal birth. It was clear that her exhaustion was the cause for the needed interventions.

System barriers to out-of-hospital birth

Social constructs and attitudes

The barrier to out-of-hospital birth that is the most difficult to overcome is the most widely disseminated and diffuse: attitude. The early twentieth-century message that promoted birth as dangerous continues to be alive and well today. The belief that birth is inherently dangerous has been repeatedly reinforced and internalized as a societal norm. Medical opinion rather than current evidence, media, a litigious environment, and misinformation have increased fear of out-of-hospital birth, particularly home birth, among expectant parents, their families, and health care professionals. Despite evidence to the contrary, there is a lingering unfounded belief that birth in any place but a hospital is unsafe. Contributing to maintaining this attitude is the 2011 American Congress of Obstetricians and Gynecologists (ACOG) "Statement on Home Birth," which supports birth only in hospitals and birth centers [62].

This negative attitude is enhanced by hospital-based providers' lack of exposure to normal birth. Many have never seen or assisted with a normal physiologic birth. Regrettably, too many hospital-based providers have seen birth only within the cascade of interventions model where labor is often induced and the cesarean section rate is high. These clinicians do not believe that they can practice safely without technology close at hand.

Hospital-based providers do not usually have contact with the 89% of women who choose a home or birth center birth and complete their births without hospital-based assistance. If there is any contact at all, it is usually in the context of receiving a transfer and providing care for women among the 11% who have encountered a problem [39–40]. Tensions can be high. The birthing family is worried about the health of mother and/or baby. They have concerns about negative effects of technology they were trying to avoid in an unfamiliar environment and may not trust the hospital providers.

The receiving providers are being asked to solve a problem whose development they did not observe. They do not know the woman and may perceive her and her family as potentially uncooperative. In addition, the hospital providers may not know the home birth or birth center provider and may be unfamiliar with that provider's qualifications. The staff may also fear litigation. In these situations, it is difficult to accomplish a cooperative seamless transfer [63]. Unfortunately, litigation is a realistic concern that often impacts the decision-making process of the receiving hospital practitioner.

Access to home or birth center services

Another significant barrier to access to home and birth center care is a shortage of providers. There has been a marked increase in home and birth center birth demand from 2006 through 2009 [19,64–65]. An informal survey of home and birth center providers in the Washington, D.C., area revealed that every practice has experienced an increase in client requests for services, with practices creating waitlists for care.

Access to consultant services

Not only has a shortage of home and birth center providers occurred but access is limited to hospital-based providers' willingness to arrange consultation, collaboration, and referral services. This is not a new problem but one that has persisted over many years. Hospital-based providers may find that hospital administrators discourage these relationships. Some hospital-based home birth consultants are discovering that their colleagues are unwilling to cover or share call time for home birth or birth center clients. Hospital legal departments fear malpractice suits and may endorse withdrawing privileges from hospital providers who work with home and birth center providers. Professional liability carriers may attempt to apply surcharges to consultants or set high premium prices that are not actuarially based for out-of-hospital birth.

Lack of hospital response to patient preferences

The Listening to Mothers II 2006 survey revealed another barrier, the failure of hospital-based services to review patient experience surveys. "Many women did not have the childbirth choices or knowledge they wanted. Support for women's intrinsic capacity for physiologic childbirth appeared to be extremely limited. A large proportion of women experienced numerous labor and birth interventions of benefit to mothers with specific risk conditions, but inappropriate as routine measures. These interventions left healthy women immobilized, vulnerable to high levels of surgery and burdened with health concerns while caring for their newborns." Support for breastfeeding was also lacking [50].

Insurance

Inadequate insurance reimbursement is another barrier to low-intervention care provided by home and birth center practices. The 2011 ACOG "Statement on Home Birth" has had repercussions [62]. Health insurance companies cite the lack of ACOG support for home birth in refusing to reimburse home birth providers. Lack of direct reimbursement places a financial burden on families who must then self-pay for their maternity care.

Both professional liability insurance and reimbursement from health insurance companies negatively impact the financial viability of home and birth center practices. The cost of professional liability premiums has increased, and the reimbursement for services rendered has gone down. These changes have limited the financial resources to support the day-to-day operations of a home or birth center practice. As home and birth center providers feel the squeeze of increasing professional liability premiums and decreasing health insurance reimbursement, some practices have been forced to close. In addition, reimbursement for patient education counseling and doula services is limited. Providing support for normal physiologic birth is often time consuming and labor intensive. Yet there is no mechanism for billing for the additional time required for this level of care and not enough statistical data available supporting the cost-effectiveness of this model of care to effect policy change.

Barriers to students for access to education

Students have often requested more home and birth center clinical experiences during their address at the ACNM annual meeting. Unfortunately, home and birth center services are small and few in number, limiting student access to this special kind of clinical experience. Many home and birth center practices are unable to satisfy the professional liability insurance limits of liability required by the educational programs. Although lawsuits are rare in the out-of-hospital setting, some programs will not allow students to even observe due to the programs' fear of litigation. Home and birth center practices are usually small and therefore may not provide a sufficient number of experiences to meet the students' learning needs. In some cases, the time commitment required to provide labor support while attending births, to manage the practice, and to keep up with political challenges may cause potential preceptors to feel they do not have enough time to provide students with appropriate clinical education and supervision in the out-of-hospital setting.

Conclusion

Consumer awareness and desire to give birth in the home and birth center settings are on the rise. Out-of-hospital birth, either in the home or a free-standing birth center, is a safe option when low-risk, well-informed women work with skilled clinicians within a larger network of collaborators and facilities that can extend to hospital-based services if needed. When a birthing woman or her baby needs to be transferred into the hospital setting, clinicians can work respectfully together to share full information and partner to provide a safe and satisfying experience for the woman and her family.

Events such as the home birth summit and efforts by Childbirth Connection to transform maternity care can help practitioners, administrators, and policy-makers in all birth settings "listen to women." The landmark 2013 study of 15,574 women planning a birth center birth "further demonstrates the safety of the midwifery-led birth center model of collaborative care" [66]. More and more research demonstrates the value of normal physiologic birth and shows that a reduction in unnecessary technologic interventions improves both outcomes and satisfaction for healthy women experiencing normal pregnancy. This research gives hospitals an opportunity to develop new evidence-based programs and services that inform and support families during their maternity experience. Although hospitals cannot replicate the experience of families in the home or birth center, the concerns and desires of families planning hospital birth can be addressed. Small changes in the childbirth services offered by hospitals can have a significant impact on families now and in the future. Each positive change will continue the movement to support normal physiologic birth, providing safe and satisfying experiences for all families, while retaining the woman and her support network at the center of the equation.

References

1. Supporting Healthy and Normal Physiologic Childbirth (2012). A consensus statement by the American College of Nurse-Midwives, the Midwives Alliance of North America, and the National Association of Certified Professional Midwives. May 14. Retrieved from: http://www.midwife. org/ACNM/files/ACNMLibraryData/UPLOADFILENAME/000000000272/Physiological%20 Birth%20Consensus%20Statement-%20FINAL%20May%2018%202012%20FINAL.pdf.
2. Bailes A & Jackson ME. (2000). Shared responsibility in home birth practice: Collaborating with clients. *Journal of Midwifery & Women's Health*, *45*, 537–543.
3. Litoff JB. (1978). *American midwives 1860 to the Present*. Westport, CT: Greenwood Press.
4. Wertz RW & Wertz DC. (1989). *Lying-in: A history of childbirth in America*. New Haven, CT: Yale University Press.
5. Litoff JB. (1982). The midwife throughout history. *Journal of Nurse-Midwifery*, *27*, 3–11.
6. Varney H, et al. (2004). *Nurse-midwifery*, 4th ed. Boston: Jones and Bartlett.
7. Rooks JP. (1997). *Midwifery and childbirth in America*. Philadelphia: Temple University Press.
8. Irving FC. (1937). Maternal mortality at the Boston Lying-In Hospital in 1933, 1934, and 1935. *New England Journal of Medicine*, *217*, 693–695.
9. Devitt N. (1977). The transition from home to hospital birth in the United States, 1930–1960. *Birth and the Family Journal*, *4*, 47–48.
10. Robinson S. (1984). A historical development of midwifery in the black community: 1600–1940. *Journal of Nurse-Midwifery*, *29*, 247–250.
11. Jackson ME & Bailes A. (1995). Home birth with certified nurse-midwife attendants in the United States: An overview. *Journal of Nurse-Midwifery*, *40*, 493–507.
12. American Association of Birth Centers. (2012). Retrieved from: http://www.birthcenters.org/. Accessed August 19, 2012.
13. American College of Nurse-Midwives. (1991). Position statement: Appropriate use of technology in childbirth. Updated 2001.
14. Jackson ME & Bailes A, eds. (1997). *ACNM handbook on home birth practice*. Washington, DC: American College of Nurse-Midwives. Updated 2004.
15. Midwives Alliance of North America. (2012). Retrieved from: http://mana.org/index.html. Accessed August 19, 2012.
16. National Association of Certified Professional Midwives. (2012). Retrieved from: http:// nacpm.org/. Accessed August 19, 2012.
17. Childbirth Connection. (2012). Transforming maternity care. Retrieved from: http://transform. childbirthconnection.org/. Accessed August 19, 2012.
18. Lamaze International. Science and sensibility. Retrieved from: http://www.scienceandsensibility. org/. Accessed August 19, 2012.
19. MacDorman MF, et al. (2012). Home births in the United States, 1990–2009. *NCHS Data Brief*, no. 84. Hyattsville, MD: National Center for Health Statistics.
20. Home Birth Consensus Summit. Retrieved from: http://www.homebirthsummit.org/summit-outcomes.html. Accessed August 19, 2012.
21. International Confederation of Midwives. (2008). Position statement: Keeping birth normal. Retrieved from: http://www.nurse.or.jp/nursing/international/icm/definition/pdf/shoshin/f-17. pdf. Accessed August 19, 2012.

22. World Health Organization. (1997). Care in normal birth: A practical guide. Report of a Technical Working Group (online ed).

23. Royal College of Midwives, Royal College of Obstetricians and Gynaecologists, & National Childbirth Trust. (2007). Making normal birth a reality. Consensus statement from the Maternity Care Working Party, November.

24. Society of Obstetricians and Gynaecologists of Canada; the Association of Women's Health, Obstetric and Neonatal Nurses of Canada; the Canadian Association of Midwives; the College of Family Physicians of Canada; & the Society of Rural Physicians of Canada. (2008). Joint policy statement on normal childbirth. *Journal of Obstetrics and Gynaecology of Canada, 221*, 1163–1165.

25. Home Birth Consensus Summit. (2012). Retrieved from: http://www.homebirthsummit.org/. Accessed August 19, 2012.

26. Tom SA. (1982). The evolution of nurse-midwifery: 1900–1960. *Journal of Nurse-Midwifery, 27*, 4–13.

27. Metropolitan Life Insurance Company. (1958). Summary of the tenth thousand confinement records of the Frontier Nursing Service. *Quarterly Bulletin of Frontier Nursing Service*, 45–55.

28. Browne H & Isaacs G. (1976). The Frontier Nursing Service: The primary care nurse in the community hospital. *American Journal of Obstetrics and Gynecology, 124*, 14–17.

29. Mehl L. (1992). Statistical outcomes of home births in the United States: Current status. In D Stewart & L Stewart, eds., *Safe alternatives in childbirth*, 4th ed. Marble Hill, MO: NAPSAC.

30. Northern Region Perinatal Mortality Survey Coordinating Group. (1996). Collaborative survey of perinatal loss in planned and unplanned home births. *British Medical Journal, 313*, 1306–1309.

31. Schramm WF, et al. (1987). Neonatal mortality in Missouri home births, 1978–84. *American Journal of Public Health, 77*, 930–935.

32. Burnett CA, et al. (1980). Home delivery and neonatal mortality in North Carolina. *Journal of the American Medical Association, 244*, 2741–2745.

33. Hinds MW, et al. (1985). Neonatal outcome in planned vs. unplanned out-of-hospital births in Kentucky. *Journal of the American Medical Association, 253*, 1578–1582.

34. Shy KK, et al. (1980). Out-of-hospital delivery in Washington state 1975–1977. *American Journal of Obstetrics and Gynecology, 137*, 547–553.

35. Janssen PA, et al. (1994). Licensed midwife-attended, out-of-hospital births in Washington state: Are they safe? *Birth, 21*, 141–148.

36. Campbell R & MacFarlane A. (1986). Place of delivery: A review. *British Journal of Obstetrics and Gynaecology, 93*, 675–683.

37. Sullivan DA & Beeman R. (1983). Four years' experience with home birth by licensed midwives in Arizona. *American Journal of Public Health, 73*, 641–645.

38. Leslie MS & Romano A. (2007). Birth can safely take place at home and in birthing centers. *Journal of Perinatal Education, 16*(Suppl), 81S–88S.

39. Murphy PA & Fullerton J. (1998). Outcomes of intended home births in nurse-midwifery practice: A prospective descriptive study. *Obstetrics and Gynecology, 92*, 461–470.

40. Rooks JP, et al. (1989). Outcomes of care in birth centers—the National Birth Center Study. *New England Journal of Medicine, 321*, 1804–1811.

41. Janssen PA, et al. (2009). Outcomes of planned home birth with registered midwife versus planned hospital birth with midwife or physician. *Canadian Medical Association Journal, 181*, 377–383.

42. Hutton E, et al. (2009). Outcomes associated with planned home and planned hospital births in low-risk women attended by midwives in Ontario, Canada, 2003–2006: A retrospective cohort study. *Birth, 36*, 180–189.

43. Janssen PA, et al. (2002). Outcomes of planned home births versus planned hospital births after regulation of midwifery in British Columbia. *Canadian Medical Association Journal, 166*, 315–323.

44. Chamberlain G, et al. (1997). *Home births: Report of the 1994 confidential enquiry of the National Birthday Trust Fund.* Cranforth, UK: Parthenon.

45. Ackermann-Liebrich U, et al. (1996). Home versus hospital deliveries: Follow up study of matched pairs for procedures and outcome by the Zurich study team. *British Medical Journal, 313,* 1313–18.

46. Wiegers TA, et al. (1996). Outcome of planned home and planned hospital births in low risk pregnancies: Prospective study in midwifery practices in the Netherlands. *British Medical Journal, 313,* 1309–13.

47. Treffers PE, et al. (1990). Letter from Amsterdam: Home births and minimal medical interventions. *Journal of the American Medical Association, 264,* 2203–2208.

48. deJonge A, et al. (2009). Perinatal mortality and morbidity in a nationwide cohort of 529,688 low-risk planned home and hospital births. *British Journal of Obstetrics and Gynaecology,* DOI: 10.111/j.1471-0528.2009.02175.x.

49. Birthplace in England Collaborative Group. (2011). Perinatal and maternal outcomes by planned place of birth for healthy women with low risk pregnancies: The Birthplace in England National Prospective Cohort Study. *British Medical Journal, 343,* d7400.

50. Declercq ER, Sakala C, Corry MP, & Applebaum S. (2006). *Listening to Mothers II: Report of the Second National US Survey of Women's Childbearing Experiences.* New York: Childbirth Connection.

51. Boucher D, et al. (2009). Staying home to give birth: Why women in the United States choose home birth. *Journal of Midwifery & Women's Health, 54,* 119–126.

52. MacDorman MF, et al. (2011). United States home births increase 20 percent from 2004 to 2008. *Birth, 38,* 185–190.

53. Odent M. (1987). The fetus ejection reflex. *Birth, 14,* 104–105.

54. Buckley S. (2009). *Gentle birth, gentle mothering: A doctor's guide to natural childbirth and early parenting choices.* Berkeley, CA: Celestial Arts.

55. Walsh D. (2008). Promoting normal birth: Weighing the evidence. In S Downe, ed., *Normal childbirth evidence and debate,* 2nd rev. ed. London: Churchill Livingstone.

56. *Random House Dictionary of the English Language,* 2nd edition (unabridged), s.v. "Authority."

57. Fullerton JT, et al. (2007). Outcomes of planned home birth: An integrative review. *Journal of Midwifery & Women's Health, 52,* 323–333.

58. United States Court of Appeals, Sixth Circuit. (2012). Nashville, TN: 918 F.2d 605, 1991. [Online]. Retrieved from: http://bulk.resource.org/courts.gov/c/F2/918/918.F2d.605.88-5842.89-5491.html. Accessed August 22, 2012.

59. Gaskin I. (1994). The spirit and science of home birth. American College of Nurse-Midwives Annual Meeting, Nashville, TN, April.

60. AABC Uniform Data Set. (2012). Retrieved from: http://www.birthcenters.org/data-collection. Accessed August 23, 2012.

61. MANA Stats Project. (2012). Retrieved from: https://www.manastats.org/help_public_about. Accessed August 23, 2012.

62. American Congress of Obstetricians and Gynecologists. (2011). Planned home birth. Committee Opinion, no. 476.

63. Cheyney M. (2009). Narratives of risk speaking across the hospital/homebirth divide. *Anthropology News,* March, 7–8.

64. MacDorman M, Menacker F, & Declercq E. (2010). Trends and characteristics of home and other out-of-hospital births in the United States, 1990–2006. *National Vital Statistics Reports, 58*(11).

65. Martin JA, Hamilton BE, Ventura SJ, Osterman MJK, Wilson EC, & Mathews TJ. (2012). Births: Final data for 2010. *National Vital Statistics Reports, 61*(1).

66. Stapleton S, Osborne C, Illuzi J. (2013). Outcomes of care in birth centers: Demonstration of a durable model. *Journal of Midwifery and Women's Health, 58,* 3–14.

Chapter 14

Educating health professionals for collaborative practice in support of normal birth

Melissa D. Avery, John C. Jennings and Michelle L. O'Brien

Key points

- Federal and private organizations have advocated for interprofessional education (IPE) for health professionals for 40 years; IPE competencies have now been developed by representatives of multiple health professions organizations.
- Acceptance of a team care model, hierarchical conflicts, resource limitations, scope-of-practice issues, and legal and ethical constraints can be barriers to effective IPE.
- Interprofessional education is an essential ingredient in developing a high-quality, high-value maternity care system in the United States.
- A common core curriculum in maternity care could be developed to meet the needs of each profession's programmatic, accreditation, and scope-of-practice requirements.
- Learners in medicine, nursing, midwifery, family medicine, obstetrics and gynecology, and other disciplines can learn together in classroom and online environments, including simulated and real-world clinical experiences, in order to provide high-quality, collaborative, woman-centered maternity care.
- Interprofessional continuing education for all health professionals involved in maternity care should be developed immediately.

All health professionals should be educated to deliver patient centered care as members of an interdisciplinary care team, emphasizing evidence-based practice, quality improvement approaches, and informatics.

IOM 2001

Introduction

In the current era of health care reform debate, the United States is struggling with unsustainable increases in the cost of health care including millions of Americans uninsured or underinsured. The call is loud for a team-based and collaborative interprofessional

Supporting a Physiologic Approach to Pregnancy and Birth: A Practical Guide, First Edition.
Edited by Melissa D. Avery.
© 2013 John Wiley & Sons, Inc. Published 2013 by John Wiley & Sons, Inc.

approach to care, including interprofessional education, as a way to improve the quality of care and care outcomes and to lower the cost of care. Maternity care providers have a tremendous opportunity to examine the possibilities and fundamentally change the basic way care is provided. Meaningful change in the provision of care must be accompanied by a change in health professions education. Learning together is a key ingredient in the recipe for partnering to provide the best care for each woman. For this chapter we examined national calls for interprofessional education and barriers to providing that education, and we collaborated in thinking about where we have come from as health professionals in maternity care as well as what is being asked of us as educators in a reformed health care system. Current examples of health professionals being educated together are provided to help consider possibilities for future education of maternity care providers. We have considered basic education and specific experiences that may be integrated in support of a physiologic approach to pregnancy and birth, anticipating that additional examples and proposals will emerge as this important discussion unfolds.

Background

Maternity care in the United States began as an import of practices from England, carried on by settlers in the "New World." The philosophy of care at that time was one of "social childbirth," and women were supported by a team of women: family, neighbors, and midwives in their homes. This model continued for about 150 years until the Revolutionary War era when the idea of physicians attending births began to gain popularity. Physicians attending births were primarily general practitioners, the predecessors for the present-day family medicine specialty. These general practitioners had very little experience with childbirth compared to the midwives. In order to expand their knowledge and experience, physicians travelled abroad for their education and returned with new knowledge and skills that were dubbed the "new midwifery," This new model of U.S. maternity care was similar to the European model, where birth was viewed as a natural process and allowed to progress without interference. It was believed that interventions should be limited and midwives and physicians worked together. Most providers involved in maternity care believed that "normal" births could and should be managed by midwives and that physicians should be called only for "difficult" deliveries.

With the advent of medical education in the United States, physicians attempted to create a more respected profession. Birth moved from home to hospitals, physicians required that only trained attendants assist with deliveries, and the specialty of obstetrics and gynecology was initiated. In the early 1900s, Dr. Williams, the "father" of obstetrics, suggested that only obstetric specialists were competent to attend hospital deliveries, that general practitioners were able to participate in uncomplicated home births, and that midwives should be abolished. Thus began our health care system's journey into a segregated and siloed approach to maternity care [1].

Maternity care in the United States today is provided by nurses, midwives, and physicians in family medicine and obstetrics. Each health profession has standards, competencies, and requirements for accreditation and certification unique to their respective disciplines. Rarely are the professions formally educated together, and while students of various professions may be in a clinical facility at the same time, requirements for cross-profession interaction are uncommon. National calls for interdisciplinary or interprofessional education that began more than 40 years ago [2] are increasing in intensity. We have reviewed our own professions' standard-setting documents, within the context of broader calls for collaborative education and practice, to look for evidence of requirements for interprofessional education to prepare our learners for the health care system of the future.

National calls for interprofessional education

Recommendations for interprofessional education were published as early as 1972, when the Institute of Medicine (IOM) called for educating health professionals together and recommended that faculty become skilled in this model of teaching [2]. The Pew Health Professions Commission issued five recommendations for all health professions in 1998; recommendation three was to require interdisciplinary competence. The recommendations were accompanied by twenty-one competencies for the twenty-first century, including working in interdisciplinary teams [3]. This recommendation was strengthened in the 2001 landmark IOM report *Crossing the Quality Chasm*. Six aims proposed for improving health care were that care should be safe, effective, patient centered, timely, efficient, and equitable. Inherent in that framework was that clinicians would improve communication and collaboration, including changes in the education of health care clinicians [4]. Following that recommendation, *Health Professions Education: A Bridge to Quality* was published in 2003. Five competencies were recommended for all health professions students: provide patient-centered care, quality improvement, evidence-based practice, informatics, and work in interdisciplinary teams [5].

The Interprofessional Education Collaborative (IPEC), made up of six national education associations including the American Association of Colleges of Nursing (AACN), the American Association of Osteopathic Colleges of Medicine (AACOM), the American Association of Colleges of Pharmacy (AACP), the American Dental Education Association (ADEA), the American Association of Medical Colleges (AAMC) and the Association of Schools of Public Health (ASPH), took the next steps on recommendations from the *Bridge to Quality*. The intent of their partnership was to promote and encourage efforts to advance substantive interprofessional learning experiences to prepare clinicians for team-based patient care. The panel reviewed all relevant statements on interprofessional competency in the United States, Canada, and internationally in order to identify a set of competencies to cross all health professions.

The landmark report *Core Competencies for Interprofessional Collaborative Practice* builds on the specific *Bridge to Quality* competency—working in interdisciplinary teams. The expert panel views working in interdisciplinary teams as central in relationship to the other four identified *Bridge to Quality* competencies [6]. (See Figure 14.1.) The core competencies utilize the WHO definition of interprofessional education (IPE): "When students from two or more professions learn about, from and with each other to enable effective collaboration and improve health outcomes" [6]. The IPEC report examines the foundational core competencies and their relevance to the various professions and

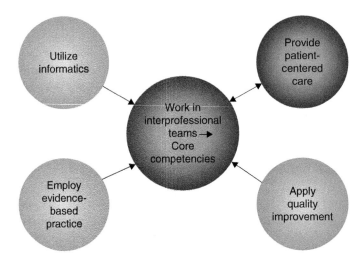

Figure 14.1   Interprofessional teamwork and IOM core competencies. Interprofessional Education Collaborative Expert Panel. (2011). *Core competencies for interprofessional collaborative practice: Report of an expert panel.* Washington, DC: Interprofessional Education Collaborative.

proposes an implementation plan for interprofessional education and practice. These four competency domains with corresponding competencies are as follows:

1   Values and ethics for interprofessional practice: Working with individuals and maintaining a climate of mutual respect and shared values; putting the interest of patients at the center of team function by developing trust relationships based upon respect for dignity, privacy, and culture; team members develop and maintain high standards of ethical conduct, quality of patient care, and competence in their profession.
2   Roles and responsibilities: Having appropriate knowledge and recognition of roles of each profession within the team; patients and families are to be informed of the roles of team members; team collaboration to maximize utilization of knowledge and skills of team members to the benefit of patients.
3   Interprofessional communication: Communication among patients, families, communities, and other health entities conducted in a responsible manner supporting a team approach to care; using communication tools to convey information to patients, exchange knowledge and opinions among team members, and provide performance feedback; effective team communications promote mutual respect, conflict resolution, and positive interprofessional working relationships.
4   Teams and teamwork: Team-based care applies relationship-building values and principles to the dynamics of the team to provide patient-centered care in a safe, timely, efficient, effective, and equitable manner; team leadership supports collaboration, shared accountability, and a team environment of continued process improvement.

The core competencies, as advocated by IPEC, are meant to complement the competencies of individual professions involved in the collaborative team effort with a resultant positive synergism in the delivery of patient-centered care. Strong academic leadership and preparation for faculty to teach interprofessional competencies to students from multiple disciplines is needed. A focus on IPE and interprofessional practice must be integrated by accreditation, certification, and licensing bodies and promoted in health professions continuing education. Accrediting bodies are being asked to place a greater emphasis on outcomes of health professions education programs. The critical task now is to capitalize on these efforts, increasing momentum in the preparation of health practitioners for the future utilizing team-based care to meet the triple aim of better care, better outcomes, and lower cost in the United States [7].

Health professions educational competencies

All health professions education includes external processes to assure quality, consistency, and ultimately public safety. Accreditation and licensure are the regulatory processes on either side of formal education. These bodies and any applicable standard documents for each health profession are displayed in Table 14.1.

Nursing education

Basic nursing education in the United States, in preparation for licensure as a registered nurse, occurs in programs resulting in the awarding of a diploma, the associate degree, or the baccalaureate degree. The associate degree, initiated during a nursing shortage post–World War II, is the educational route for approximately 60% of new RNs. The baccalaureate is the entry point for nearly 40%, with only a few hospital-based nursing diploma programs remaining [8]. In addition, some nursing schools have programs for individuals with an existing baccalaureate degree to enter nursing education and earn a second bachelor's or a graduate degree. The IOM report on the future of nursing recently called for higher levels of education, including more nurses entering the workforce with a baccalaureate degree or completing that degree early in their careers, and specifically that 80% of RNs have a baccalaureate degree by 2020 [8].

AACN "Essentials of Baccalaureate Education for Professional Nursing Practice" [9] Essential VI, Interprofessional Communication and Collaboration, acknowledges the recent national calls related to providing patient-centered care in interprofessional teams. Six outcomes highlight important educational goals for understanding one's own and other health professions roles, communication, and collaborative team-based care. "NLNAC Standards and Criteria—Baccalaureate" requires students to be prepared for "safe practice in contemporary health care environments," and curricula should incorporate professional standards and competencies and reflect interdisciplinary collaboration [10]. These documents reflect the more recent IOM *Future of Nursing* report recommendation that "nurses should be educated with physicians and other health professionals as students and throughout their careers" [8, p. 7].

Table 14.1 Standards and credentialing for nursing, medicine, midwifery, and family medicine and ob/gyn residencies.

Profession	Standard setting body(-ies) and documents	Examining bodies	Accreditation organization
Nursing CCNE	American Association of Colleges of Nursing (AACN) Essentials of Baccalaureate Education for Professional Nursing	National Council of State Boards of Nursing (NCSBN) National Council Licensure Examination for Registered Nurses (NCLEX-RN)	Commission on Collegiate Nursing Education (CCNE)
Nursing NLNAC		NCSBN NCLEX-RN	National League for Nursing Accrediting Commission (NLNAC)
Allopathic medicine (MD)	Functions and Structure of a Medical School	Federation of State Medical Boards (FSMB) National Board of Medical Examiners (NBME) United States Medical Licensing Examination (USMLE)	Liaison Committee on Medical Education (LCME)
Osteopathic medicine (DO)	Osteopathic Core Competencies for Medical Students	National Board of Osteopathic Medical Examiners (NBOME) Comprehensive Osteopathic Medical Licensure Exam (COMLEX-USA)	American Osteopathic Association Commission on Osteopathic College Accreditation (COCA)
Family medicine residency allopathic	ACGME Program Requirements for Graduate Medical Education in Family Medicine	American Board of Family Medicine (ABFM)	Accreditation Council for Graduate Medical Education (ACGME) Family Medicine Residency Review Committee (RRC)
Family medicine residency osteopathic	Basic Standards for Residency Training in Osteopathic Family Practice and Manipulative Treatment	American Osteopathic Board of Family Physicians (AOBFP)	American Osteopathic Association and American College of Osteopathic Family Physicians

Ob/gyn residency allopathic	ACGME Program Requirements for Graduate Medical Education in Obstetrics and Gynecology	American Board of Obstetrics and Gynecology (ABOG)	Accreditation Council for Graduate Medical Education (ACGME) OB/Gyn Residency Review Committee (RRC)
Ob/gyn residency osteopathic	Basic Standards for Residency Training in Obstetrics and Gynecology	American Osteopathic Board of Obstetrics and Gynecology (AOBOG)	American Osteopathic Association and American College of Osteopathic Obstetricians and Gynecologists
Midwifery CNM/CM	American College of Nurse-Midwives Core Competencies for Basic Midwifery Practice Standards for the Practice of Midwifery	American Midwifery Certification Board (AMCB)	American College of Nurse-Midwives (ACNM) Accreditation Commission for Midwifery Education (ACME)
Midwifery CPM	Midwives Alliance of North America MANA Core Competencies for Basic Midwifery Practice MANA Standards and Qualifications for the Art and Practice of Midwifery	North American Registry of Midwives (NARM)	Midwifery Education Accreditation Council (MEAC)*

*Accredited midwifery program not required for certification examination.

Medical education

Allopathic medical schools are required to incorporate the fundamental principles of medicine through current concepts of basic and clinical science. The Liaison Committee on Medical Education (LCME) emphasizes the need for medical students to be concerned with the total needs of their patients and allows discretion by medical schools in providing a logical sequence of learning and the duration of exposure to core disciplines, of which obstetrics and gynecology is one [11]. Obstetrical education in medical school is generally conducted according to educational objectives prescribed by the Association of Professors of Gynecology and Obstetrics [12]. Obstetrics and maternity care education for medical students focuses on the physiologic changes of pregnancy, common obstetric problems, intrapartum care, postpartum care, and family planning. The medical student clerkship is a 6- to 10-week period of exposure to a combination of obstetrics, gynecology, and other related women's health educational objectives. Medical schools are required to maintain comparability of education across all clinical sites and comply with national standards set by LCME [12].

Osteopathic medical education includes preparation in family medicine, obstetrics and gynecology, and prevention medicine and public health in addition to other specialty areas [13]. "Osteopathic Core Competencies for Medical Students" [14] includes seven competencies for osteopathic medical education and seven additional concepts developed by an interdisciplinary group related to clinical prevention and population health. Osteopathic principles and practices include collaboration with other health professionals to maximize patient outcomes. Competency 14 is interprofessional collaboration and includes statements related to articulating one's own role and responsibilities, knowing roles and responsibilities of other health professionals, and participating in team-based care [14, p. 24].

Residency education

The Accreditation Council for Graduate Medical Education (ACGME) encourages innovation in residency education including emphasis on teamwork among disciplines.

Family medicine

The Family Medicine Residency Review Committee outlines the requirements for completion of the 3-year family medicine residency program. Primary care physicians are prepared to provide comprehensive care to the entire family with an emphasis on continuity of care. At the completion of their training, family medicine residents should be competent in a number of areas of patient care including pediatrics, adult medicine, women's health, and geriatrics with specific requirements within each of these areas [15].

The maternity care curriculum in family medicine residency training programs requires a minimum of 2 months of training that includes prenatal care, management of labor and birth, and postpartum care. Residents are expected to participate in a minimum of forty births by the end of residency, with ten of these as continuity births, where the resident has provided prenatal care, labor management, and postpartum care to the woman.

A portion of maternity care training involves continuity within the residency clinic with residency faculty but may also occur in an outside setting with appropriate supervision. Competence is determined by subjective assessment by residency faculty and others involved in the maternity care training of the residents.

A significant number of family medicine residency programs have residents work with obstetricians on the labor and delivery unit; some programs have midwives involved in their training. According to Residency Review Committee guidelines, "physicians in the other specialties must devote sufficient time to teaching and supervising, and to providing consultation to the family medicine residents in order to ensure that the program's goals for their specialty areas are accomplished" and "non-physician faculty must have appropriate qualifications in their field and hold appropriate institutional appointments" [15]. Although requirements for family medicine maternity care training allow for supervision of residents by professionals other than family medicine faculty, there are no specific guidelines or requirements for interprofessional education or training of obstetric and family medicine residents and midwifery students together, utilizing a shared curriculum.

Interprofessional education is not a new concept in family medicine, given the breadth of education and clinical practice of most family physicians. Residents often work on interprofessional teams that include residents and attending physicians from other specialties, nurses, social workers and pharmacists during their internal medicine, surgery, and other subspecialty rotations. Formalizing the partnerships that have been a foundation in the maternity care training of family medicine residents for decades into a truly interprofessional curriculum should not represent a radical change.

Obstetrics and gynecology

Obstetrics and gynecology resident education must be focused on "reproductive health care and ambulatory primary care for women, including health maintenance, disease prevention, diagnosis, treatment, consultation, and referral" [16]. Resident education in obstetrics and gynecology is a 4-year program conducted within a scholarly environment, with competency-based goals and objectives where residents become competent in the full range of obstetrics including medical and surgical complications, the full range of medical and surgical gynecology for all age groups, and primary and preventive care for women. Resident physicians demonstrate progressive acquisition of medical knowledge, practice-based learning, communication skills, professionalism, systems-based practice, and scholarly activities. Residents participate in structured evaluation and testing throughout the program [16], and graduates are eligible to take American Board of Obstetrics and Gynecology certification examinations, including scrutiny of the individual physician's patient case lists, written examination, and oral examination. Board certification is time limited and requires participation in ongoing maintenance of certification [17].

Obstetrics and gynecology residency training programs offer a favorable setting for development of interprofessional training models. Many Ob/Gyn residency programs have co-existing institutional educational programs for other disciplines including nurse-midwifery, physician assistants, nurse practitioners, and others. Along with the initiation of the ACGME requirement limiting resident physicians to an 80-hour workweek, there has been a significantly increased role for other health professionals in providing direct care to patients in teaching hospitals. Nurse practitioners, midwives, physician assistants, and other professionals are sharing responsibility for patient care traditionally provided primarily by resident physicians. Further development of interdisciplinary educational models in coordination with existing programs in obstetrics and gynecology is an opportunity to create quality and effective teams to meet women's health care needs.

Nonphysician faculty in obstetrics and gynecology training programs must have appropriate qualifications in their field and hold appropriate institutional appointments [16]. Participation of other faculty members in medical student and resident education varies significantly by institution and regions of the United States. However, these variations are not limitations of ACGME requirements. Nurse-midwives have been involved in the didactic and clinical teaching of medical students and residents within the Department of Obstetrics and Gynecology at the University of New Mexico since 1986 [18]. Brown University in Providence, Rhode Island [19], and the University of Vermont [20] are other examples of programs where nurse-midwives have effectively participated in the education of Ob/Gyn residents and medical students over an extended period of time. More than half of medical schools in the United States have certified nurse-midwives as educators for both graduate and undergraduate physician education [21]. The number of midwives involved in medical student and resident education has more than tripled since that reported in 1998 [22]. Medical educators will inevitably need to continue developing interprofessional models consistent with the evolution of the health care delivery system.

Midwifery education

Midwifery care in the United States is regulated under two sets of education and certification standards. Certified nurse-midwives (CNMs) practice and prescribe in all fifty states; certified midwives (CMs) are licensed to practice in three states—New York, New Jersey, and Rhode Island—and authorized to practice in Delaware and Missouri [23]. The practice of certified professional midwives (CPMs) is regulated in twenty-six states. The education process for CPMs may include formal education in a typical educational institution and an accreditation process. A table clarifying commonalities and differences among the midwife categories is available. (See Table 14.2.)

Midwifery education for CNMs and CMs is primarily framed by *Core Competencies for Basic Midwifery Education* and *Standards for the Practice of Midwifery* [24,25] and is at the graduate level [26]. Midwifery programs are directed by a CNM or CM certified by the American College of Nurse-Midwives (ACNM) or the American Midwifery Certification Board (AMCB). The majority of midwifery instruction, clinical supervision, and evaluation is provided by midwives. However, other qualified health professionals may participate in midwifery education and must be qualified and competent in the area of teaching responsibility, have a minimum of a master's degree, meet the institution's requirements for faculty, and be credentialed by appropriate national bodies for their profession [27].

Table 14.2

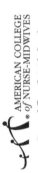
AMERICAN COLLEGE
of NURSE-MIDWIVES

Comparison of Certified Nurse-Midwives, Certified Midwives, and Certified Professional Midwives

Clarifying the distinctions among professional midwifery credentials in the U.S.

	CERTIFIED NURSE-MIDWIFE (CNM)®	CERTIFIED MIDWIFE (CM)®	CERTIFIED PROFESSIONAL MIDWIFE (CPM)®
PROFESSIONAL ASSOCIATION			
	American College of Nurse-Midwives (ACNM)		Midwives Alliance of North America (MANA) and National Association of Certified Professional Midwives (NACPM)
CERTIFICATION			
Certifying Organization	American Midwifery Certification Board (AMCB)**		North American Registry of Midwives (NARM)**
Certification Requirements (minimum degree and other requirements prior to taking national certifying exam)	Graduate degree required		No degree required
	1. Graduation from a nurse-midwifery education program accredited by ACNM Accreditation Commission for Midwifery Education (ACME); AND 2. Verification by program director of completion of education program; AND 3. Active registered nurse (RN) license	1. Graduation from a midwifery education program accredited by ACNM Accreditation Commission for Midwifery Education (ACME); AND 2. Verification by program director of completion of education program	1. Completion of NARM's Portfolio Evaluation Process (PEP) pathway; OR 2. Graduate of a midwifery education program accredited by Midwifery Education Accreditation Council (MEAC); OR 3. AMCB-certified CNM or CM; OR 4. Completion of state licensure program.
Recertification Requirement	Every five years		Every three years
EDUCATION			
Minimum Education Requirements for Admission to Midwifery Education Program	Bachelor's degree from accredited college/ university 1. Some programs require RN license. If the applicant has a bachelor's degree, but not an RN license, some programs will require attainment of an RN license prior to entry into the midwifery program; others will allow the student to attain an RN license prior to graduate study; OR 2. If the applicant is an RN but does not have a bachelor's degree, some programs provide a bridge program to a bachelor's degree prior to the midwifery portion of the program; other programs require a bachelor's degree before entry into the midwifery program.	Bachelor's degree from accredited college/ university and successful completion of specific science courses	There are two primary pathways for CPM education, with differing admission requirements: 1. Portfolio Evaluation Process (PEP) pathway: an apprenticeship program; no degree or diploma required. Student must find a midwife preceptor who is nationally certified or state licensed, has practiced for at least 3 years, and attended at least 50 out-of-hospital births; OR 2. Accredited formal education pathway: For this pathway, a high school diploma from an accredited state or private school is required for admission.
	Note: Currently, the majority of AMCB-certified midwives enter midwifery through nursing.		*Note: Currently, the majority of CPMs have completed the apprenticeship-only (PEP) pathway to the CPM credential.*

Continued...

Table 14.2   (Cont'd)

Comparison of Certified Nurse-Midwives, Certified Midwives, and Certified Professional Midwives

*Clarifying the distinctions among professional midwifery credentials in the U.S.**

	CERTIFIED NURSE-MIDWIFE (CNM®)	CERTIFIED MIDWIFE (CM®)	CERTIFIED PROFESSIONAL MIDWIFE (CPM)®
EDUCATION (continued)			
Clinical Experience Requirement	Attainment of clinical skills must meet Core Competencies for Basic Midwifery Education (ACNM 2008). Clinical education must occur under the supervision of an AMCB-certified CNM/CM or Advanced Practice RN (APRN) who holds a graduate degree and has clinical expertise and didactic knowledge commensurate with the content taught. Clinical skills include management of primary care for women throughout the lifespan, including reproductive health care, pregnancy, and birth; care of the normal newborn; and management of sexually transmitted infections in male partners.		Attainment of clinical skills must meet the Core Competencies developed by the Midwives Alliance of North America. Clinical education must occur under the supervision of a midwife who must be nationally certified, legally recognized and who has practiced for at least three years and attended 50 out-of-hospital births. Clinical skills include management of prenatal, birth and postpartum care for women and newborns.
Degree Granted	Master's or doctoral degree; a master's degree is the minimum requirement for the AMCB certification exam	Master's degree; a master's degree is the minimum requirement for the AMCB certification exam	No degree is granted through the PEP pathway. MEAC-accredited programs vary and may grant a certificate or an associate's, bachelor's, master's, or doctoral degree. Most graduates attain a certificate or associate degree; there is no minimum degree requirement for the CPM certification exam.
ACCREDITING ORGANIZATION			
	The Accreditation Commission for Midwifery Education (ACME) is authorized by the US Department of Education to accredit midwifery education programs and institutions.		The PEP pathway is not eligible for accreditation. The Midwifery Education Accreditation Council (MEAC) is authorized by the US Department of Education to accredit midwifery education programs and institutions.
LICENSURE			
Legal Status	Licensed in all 50 states plus the District of Columbia and US territories	Licensed in New Jersey, New York, and Rhode Island. Authorized by permit to practice in Delaware. Authorized to practice in Missouri.	Regulated in 26 states (variously by licensure, certification, registration, voluntary licensure, or permit)
Licensure Agency	Boards of Nursing, Boards of Medicine, Boards of Midwifery/Nurse-Midwifery, Departments of Health	Board of Midwifery, Board of Medicine, Department of Health	Departments of Health, Boards of Medicine, Boards of Midwifery

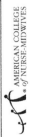

AMERICAN COLLEGE
of NURSE-MIDWIVES

Comparison of Certified Nurse-Midwives, Certified Midwives, and Certified Professional Midwives

Clarifying the distinctions among professional midwifery credentials in the U.S. * (Continued)

	CERTIFIED NURSE-MIDWIFE (CNM*)	CERTIFIED MIDWIFE (CM*)	CERTIFIED PROFESSIONAL MIDWIFE (CPMI)*
SCOPE OF PRACTICE			
Range of Care Provided	Independent management of women's health care throughout the lifespan, from adolescence through menopause. Comprehensive scope of practice including primary care and gynecologic care, family planning, annual exams (including breast and PAP screening), pregnancy, birth in all settings, and postpartum care. Care of the normal newborn. Management of sexually transmitted infections in male partners.		Independent management of care for women and newborns during pregnancy, birth, and postpartum. Birth in homes and birth centers. Care of the normal newborn.
Prescriptive Authority	All US jurisdictions	New York	None. However, may obtain and administer certain medications in some states.
Practice Settings	All settings — hospitals, birth centers, homes, and offices. The majority of CNMs and CMs attend births in hospitals.		Homes, birth centers, and offices. The majority of CPMs attend out-of-hospital births.
THIRD-PARTY REIMBURSEMENT			
	Most private insurances; Medicaid coverage mandated in all states; Medicare; Champus	New York, New Jersey, Rhode Island — most private insurance; Medicaid	Private insurance in some states; Medicaid in 10 states for home birth, additional states if birth occurs in birth center.

* This document does not address individuals who are not certified and who may practice midwifery with or without legal recognition.

** AMCB and NARM are accredited by the National Commission for Certifying Agencies, which "was created in 1987 ... to help ensure the health, welfare, and safety of the public through the accreditation of a variety of certification programs/organizations...Certification organizations ... are evaluated based on the process and products, not the content, and are therefore applicable to all professions and industries." (http://www.credentialingexcellence.org/ProgramsandEvents/NCCAAccreditation/tabid/82/Default.aspx)

Reviewed ACNM-MANA Liaison Committee February, 2011

Approved by ACNM Board of Directors March, 2011

Last updated August, 2011

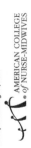

AMERICAN COLLEGE
of NURSE-MIDWIVES

ACNM's core competencies support interprofessional practice in the following ways: (1) a specific hallmark of midwifery practice is collaboration with other health team members; (2) the midwifery management process includes evaluating the need for consultation or collaboration with other health team members; and (3) specific care competencies include utilizing consultation, collaboration, and/or referral as indicated by the woman's health needs.

Midwifery education for CNMs and CMs is competency-based rather than requiring specific hour or experience numbers. Midwife graduates are expected to have competence as beginning practitioners in all areas defined by the core competencies. These areas include basic primary care, well-woman gynecology, and care of the childbearing woman and newborn.

There is no specific requirement that other health professionals participate in midwifery education, although the requirement to participate in interprofessional consultation and collaboration is clear. Interprofessional education is not specifically included in the key ACNM documents; however, a recent statement by three U.S. midwifery organizations, ACNM, the Midwives Alliance of North America (MANA), and the National Association of Certified Professional Midwives (NACPM), called for "competency-based, interdisciplinary programming for maternity health care clinicians and students" related to care promoting normal physiologic birth [28].

Barriers to interprofessional education

Improving collaboration among health care providers is a clear goal of government and other funding sources of health services. Policy-makers and leaders in health professions education have the ability to promote integrative interprofessional collaborative practice, but significant barriers exist [29]. Overcoming barriers to creating collaborative health care teams begins with an understanding of the nature of those barriers and why they exist.

Team model acceptance

The history of medical practice in the United States has cultivated a strong bond of individual provider/individual patient relationships. This mode of health care delivery has worked well in the past, at least in part, because of the previous simplicity of health science. There has been a massive expansion of scientific knowledge of human health and disease along with technologic advances in diagnosis and treatment that were unimaginable in the last century. It is no longer possible for a physician to deliver the entire scope of primary care to a patient, much less the variety of specialty care that might be required. The scope of nursing care has expanded and subspecialized. Other health care professions also have expanding roles and now provide significant contributions to the health of our population. Although patients still desire to have "their own doctor" or "their own nurse," there is a reality that every health care provider is a member of a highly interdependent team. The concept of the physician being the "captain of the ship" with sole responsibility and accountability for the patient's well-being is no longer valid. Yes, there is still the abiding human need for a personal relationship with the individual to whom a person entrusts their health. What has changed is that trusted person can be any member of a competent, well-coordinated team. The team can be quite capable of meeting the person's needs in a comprehensive and efficient manner. Despite the apparent advantages, some patients and providers may be reluctant to accept the team model of health care delivery.

Hierarchal conflicts

Hierarchal conflicts can be disruptive to interprofessional teams. The advantage of an interprofessional team is the combination of knowledge and skills of team members, with each member being empowered to bring her or his own unique contributions to the collective resources of the team. A disparity of power and authority is inherent in the health care setting. Teachers have power over students, practitioners have power over patients [30]. There are perceptions of power of one discipline over another, with physicians often acquiring an ambiguity of rank based upon the differences in education, knowledge, or skills. Effective collaboration requires an equal and mutual respect among team members for their individual contributions. Team members have a professional responsibility to clarify the role of teachers and students to patients whose care provides educational opportunities [30, p. 358]. Leadership of a collaborative team requires the skills of a team member who can best coordinate the resources of the team. The choice of team leadership should not be dependent on a hierarchy of tradition but rather on the pragmatism of choosing the best leader in each situation.

Scope-of-practice issues

Despite the rather idealistic analysis of team care and what it can offer, the lack of understanding of scope of practice, individual skills, and respect for differences in disciplinary values can be a significant barrier in both the educational and practice settings [31]. Our universities have conventionally been designed to function in "silos" of health disciplines [4]. Schools within a health science center are accustomed to structuring and executing their own curricula without significant interaction from other schools. In the clinical setting, faculty and students from various disciplines often do not effectively communicate, and consequently do not understand contributions of the other disciplines. For an interprofessional educational process to work, open communications among collaborators is essential, and any misunderstanding of the roles and capabilities of health care team members must be clarified. Mutual respect among disciplines requires an understanding of each discipline's scope of practice.

Ethical and legal constraints

Collaborative education must occur within the framework of both ethical and legal constraints of the health care system. Because the team approach necessarily involves multiple individuals, there is an increased risk for one or more persons on the team to inadvertently cross ethical or legal lines. Compliance with the Health Insurance Portability and Accountability Act of 1996, better known has HIPAA, is an example of potential increased vulnerability of interprofessional educational models. HIPAA has established national standards for patient privacy and electronic health care transactions [32]. Obviously, the more persons who have access to individual patient records, the higher the likelihood that information may be inappropriately shared. There is both a collective and individual responsibility associated with the health care team to protect patient privacy. Because there are financial implications and significant penalties for HIPAA violations, most hospitals and teaching institutions have compliance officers who have responsibility for monitoring institutional adherence to HIPAA regulations. Students and faculty frequently rotate in and out of interprofessional educational settings with knowledge of patients' health status. There is an ethical obligation for the interprofessional team to inform their patients of who might have access to health information and to assure them that their privacy will be protected. The legal obligation for privacy protection is similar, with the exception of having the defined penalties associated with violations. Compliance officers are understandably concerned about maintaining the integrity of medical information within the dynamics of interprofessional teams. Interprofessional educational team members are all interested in learning new skills and technologies while at the same time providing quality care to patients.

Teachers have an ethical obligation to maximize the learning experience of students while protecting the patient from harm [33]. Because different disciplines have valid alternatives for patient care, the team must collectively decide on the best approach to care for the individual patient and be consistent in delivery of that plan. Conflicting opinions and messages to patients from team members of different disciplines can leave patients confused and upset. An effective collaborative team values the differences among the disciplines represented and develops mutual respect for what each has to offer the patient. It can be easier to fulfill ethical obligations to patients within the confines of a single provider/single patient relationship than through a team approach. To compensate, interprofessional teams must abide by common understanding of the ethical boundaries of health care.

Resource limitations

Resource allocation is required for developing and sustaining interprofessional educational models, particularly at the undergraduate (basic nursing and medical education) level. Although much discussion has occurred related to the importance of collaborative education within health professions, funding resources have been limited. Most of the funding for program development has come from institutional reallocation rather than external sources [34]. Budgets in most health science centers are structured within the individual schools and their departments with minimal sharing of funds among schools. The first priority of deans of schools is to provide funding for their own faculty and programs. Our health education systems have not traditionally been designed to accommodate a collaborative educational model. Large-scale changes in philosophy with the intent of encouraging interactive education among students of different disciplines are best implemented at the level of an entire health sciences center [35]. Without a firm collective commitment of an institution to interprofessional education, internal reallocation of funds to support collaborative education will likely be difficult. Support from academic institutions, government, and accreditation bodies is important in the implementation of interprofessional education and the evolution into a truly collaborative system of health care delivery [4–6].

Call for interprofessional education in maternity care

Childbirth Connection is a nonprofit organization with roots dating back to 1918. First known as Maternity Center Association (MCA), the organization was initiated as nonprofit by individuals who worked to reduce maternal and infant mortality in New York City. MCA began the first nurse-midwifery education program in the United States in 1931 and the first free-standing birth center in 1975. The name change in 2005 highlighted a more contemporary focus on improving maternity care. The mission of the organization includes improving the quality and value of maternity care in the United States, engaging consumers and health care providers in transforming the health care system to provide safe, effective and evidence-based maternity care [36].

In April 2009, Childbirth Connection gathered multiple stakeholders in maternity care, including childbirth educators, consumer advocates, academics in health economics and health policy, administrators, employers, nurses, obstetricians, midwives, family medicine physicians, maternal fetal medicine specialists, and doulas. Together these representatives developed two key documents, *2020 Vision for a High-Quality, High-Value Maternity Care System* [37] and *Blueprint for Action: Steps toward a High-Quality, High-Value Maternity Care System* [38]. These documents outlined both the vision and a blueprint to help create the changes that need to occur within the U.S. maternity care system to meet the needs of women and their families and provide safe, effective, evidence-based care at a reasonable cost. The *Vision* document was more theoretical, with broad ideas and values. The *Blueprint* laid out a more detailed plan as to how to accomplish the goals of the *Vision*.

The *Blueprint* identified eleven critical areas for change including health professions education. The report addressed the scope, content, and availability of health professions education. It accurately pointed out the weaknesses of our current education of maternity care professionals with overemphasis on disease and intervention, separate and disparate education without content about working effectively in interdisciplinary teams, lack of adoption of evidence-based care, and continuing education programming that is not well focused. The stakeholders that created the *Blueprint* believed that a shift toward prevention, wellness, and physiologic childbirth is warranted and that interprofessional maternity care education is a way to accomplish the shift from overuse of some interventions toward a physiologic approach to pregnancy and birth. Proposed actions include creating a common core curriculum in maternity care for health professionals from different disciplines including clinical opportunities to learn with interprofessional teams [38].

Interprofessional education within collaborative practice models

In the fall of 2010, the American Congress of Obstetricians and Gynecologists (ACOG) and ACNM issued a call for papers describing effective models of collaborative practice between midwives and obstetricians. Sixty papers were submitted from across the United States describing how the collaborative practices developed and continue to function effectively in a variety of settings. Of four papers selected to receive awards from the two organizations, two presented models in which the synchrony of collaborative education and practice sustain the goal of high-quality patient-centered care [39,40]. An additional series of collaborative practice models papers was published in 2012, including a qualitative analysis of the published papers from the ACOG-ACNM project [41].

Certified nurse-midwives in the department of obstetrics and gynecology at Baystate Medical Center in Springfield, Massachusetts, serve a diverse population at a hospital-based clinic, neighborhood clinics, and a correctional facility. The practice also includes a collaborative hospital-based triage setting where nurse-midwives, resident physicians, and faculty physicians have significantly reduced patient waiting times and increased patient satisfaction. The certified nurse-midwives assume primary responsibility for teaching normal obstetrics to first-year residents and medical students. Effective communication, acceptance of differing philosophies of care, and maintaining trust among team members are keys to the success of this collaborative practice with interprofessional education [39].

San Francisco General Hospital has a 30-year history of collaborative maternity care and delivering high-quality care to women and their families. This model has been built on common financial management of the midwifery and obstetric services and a balance of independence and interdependence between the two disciplines of obstetrics and midwifery. This longstanding partnership includes mechanisms for conflict resolution and problem solving, and consequently has been an innovative success. The practice has had a model of interdisciplinary learning for many years, where medical students, midwifery students, and residents in obstetrics, pediatrics, family medicine, and anesthesia learn in an interprofessional practice environment and participate in learning activities together such as journal club and the Centering model of group prenatal care [40].

Boston Medical Center is an inner-city teaching hospital in the educational mecca of Boston, Massachusetts. In 2005, the leadership of the obstetrics and gynecology and family medicine departments developed an interdisciplinary collaborative practice on the labor and delivery and postpartum units utilizing the principle of teamwork. The team included an obstetrician, a family medicine physician, and a nurse-midwife, all attending and managing care of women on the labor unit. Obstetrical and family medicine residents work side by side and are taught by all three attending professionals. Educational rounds each morning include physicians and residents from OB and family medicine, midwives, and medical students. Care providers and nursing staff review the status of all laboring women twice daily and develop a care plan for the women based on input from all clinicians involved in the care. A similar structure is present on the postpartum unit. There are three rounding teams, one lead by a midwife working in conjunction with the pediatric team, one lead by a family physician, and one smaller team that is covered by the chief obstetrical resident and junior residents. Daily morning care rounds include the rounding team, care coordinator, social worker, lactation consultant, and head nurse together in conference rooms. Staff nurses present the individual women's cases and care plans, including discharge plans, are discussed as a team [42].

A key theme identified in an analysis of collaborative practice models was health professions education within the collaborative care environment. Interdisciplinary clinicians that practiced together also often educated health professionals from multiple disciplines, including nursing, medicine, midwifery, residents in family medicine and obstetrics and gynecology, and occasionally other specialties. The value of interprofessional education was discussed, and some authors described having become preferred clinical sites because of the interprofessional collaborative learning opportunities [41].

Interprofessional education models

Interprofessional education can occur at multiple levels. The core competencies [6] focus on basic health professions education including nursing, pharmacy, medicine, dentistry, and public health. Introduction of the basic competencies are important at the professional entry level and must also be included at advanced or graduate education levels such as medical specialty residencies, advanced practice nursing specialties (including midwifery), and other advanced education. Because the core competencies may not yet be included in all basic curricula, their inclusion and expansion is needed at all levels of health professions education.

A 2009 Cochrane review of research examining outcomes of interprofessional education found mixed results. Only six studies met the review criteria for inclusion. Four studies demonstrated some positive outcomes and two showed mixed outcomes, resulting in the authors' inability to draw general conclusion about the effectiveness of IPE. Continued research with more rigorous designs is needed to provide evidence of the benefits of IPE [43]. The initiation of new IPE projects in response to national calls is hopeful and may eventually provide data to support resulting changes in professional practice and in patient outcomes.

In fall 2010, the University of Minnesota introduced ONE Health, a new interdisciplinary curriculum that would cross the entire academic health center, involving the Medical School, the School of Dentistry, the School of Nursing, the College of Pharmacy, the College of Veterinary Medicine, and the School of Public Health. Although most students are located on the main campus in the Twin Cities, some students are based in programs on the Duluth and Rochester campuses. Starting in the first year of the basic health profession program, this curriculum brings together small groups of interprofessional students who meet with faculty facilitators from one of the schools and discuss ideas about collaborative health practice and learn more about other areas of health care. The program continues for 3 years and includes students working together in clinical settings [44].

A series of interprofessional opportunities have been offered at the University of British Columbia for medical, nursing, and midwifery students. These have included a 5-hour didactic and clinical simulation workshop on normal labor and birth and a "hands-on night" that included the opportunity to practice specific skills in a simulated setting, such as vaginal examinations, conduct of a vaginal birth, labor support, and admission of a woman in labor. Finally, students from these three disciplines partnered in a doula program where students from the three disciplines learned to provide labor support and then offer services to a specific group of underserved women. Student responses to these opportunities were positive [31].

Faculty from multiple health professions schools at Duke University partnered to develop a core women's health curriculum by examining core competencies from each discipline and then identifying universal competencies for all disciplines. Faculty for medical, nurse-midwifery, family nurse practitioner, and physician assistant students and residents in family medicine and obstetrics and gynecology participated in a content mapping exercise and then developed online self-directed content and clinical cases that could be used by each discipline. The content included both obstetric and nonobstetric aspects of women's health care. Universal concepts related to cultural competence, patient-centered care, communication, and collaborative practice were incorporated, along with health promotion, disease prevention, physical examination, laboratory test interpretation, differential diagnosis, and management plans. Content and cases developed are available to learners in a virtual online classroom [45].

The Colleges of Nursing and Medicine at Drexel University in Philadelphia have used simulation to create interdisciplinary learning opportunities in women's health. Faculty from medicine (ob/gyn), nursing, and the physician assistant (PA) programs worked with medical and undergraduate nursing students, women's health and family nurse practitioner students, nurse anesthetist students, and PA students. The program consisted of presimulation education utilizing online learning and live presentations of didactic material and online and live case discussions, as well as basic science and current literature related to women's health. Students then participated in interprofessional simulations of women's health emergency scenarios using low- and high-fidelity simulation over the course of an 8-hour day. Students collaborated in providing care and practiced respectful communication and principles of safety. Evaluation of the simulation experience was positive [46].

Interprofessional education for maternity care professionals

Maternity care is an ideal clinical practice area in which to continue to develop models of interprofessional education and practice. Multiple professionals provide care to women during pregnancy, labor, and birth, with overlapping scopes of practice and skill sets as well as distinct practice areas. Educating students and residents in this interprofessional setting utilizing evidence-based approaches [4,5] has the potential to improve care and reduce costs. Focusing on core IPE competencies at the graduate level among midwifery students and family medicine and ob/gyn residents would enrich their specialty education and prepare these professionals for collaborative practice postgraduation. Ideally, nursing and medical students would also be included in maternity care IPE activities. Discussion of the larger set of practitioners involved in maternity care is beyond the scope of this chapter.

We suggest that the Association of Women's Health, Obstetric and Neonatal Nurses (AWHONN), ACNM, ACOG, and the American Academy of Family Physicians (AAFP) partner in the development of a common curriculum in maternity care that would meet the needs of each profession's programmatic, accreditation, and scope-of-practice requirements. In addition, a set of measurable competencies specific to maternity care providers could be developed and adopted by each profession and related organizations, building on and further developing the work of others to date. Utilizing simulation and online education has been recommended as a way to reduce the barriers to IPE learning activities [8]. Specific components of the curriculum could include both broader interprofessional topics such as the IPE competencies and those specific to maternity care. Some practical suggestions are provided that build on the resources provided herein plus our own experience as educators and clinicians. (See Boxes 14.1–14.3.)

Box 14.1   Interprofessional collaborative practice concepts for maternity care

- Woman-centered care, shared decision making.
- Professionals working together collaboratively as a core value including effective communication.
- Mutual trust and respect, understand and respect each profession's roles and responsibilities for decision making.
- Consistent with a new approach to values/ethics professionalism, care focused on interprofessional practice vs. uniprofessional practice in a specific discipline.
- Common language such as SBAR (situation – background – assessment – recommendation).
- Environment where all practitioners are able to speak up, especially related to concerns about quality and safety.
- Cooperation among caregivers, recipients of care, others who support the care.
- Communicating difficult or complex information with families, communities.
- Coordinating care utilizing a team approach, accountability for care, manage overlapping skills, participation as both team leader and as member.
- Legal issues related to team care.
- Provide education for clinical preceptors and teachers of didactic courses about teaching in a multidisciplinary setting.

Box 14.2   Specific topics for a woman-centered physiologic approach to maternity care curriculum

- Normal physiology of pregnancy and birth.
- Psychobiological influences on pregnancy and birth.
- Screening and treatment of perinatal mental health conditions.
- Evidence-based care to promote normal pregnancy and birth.
- Labor support practices and techniques.
- Use of the birth plan by providers and women as a tool to promote woman-centered care.
- Intermittent auscultation and NICHD fetal monitoring guidelines.
- Techniques to promote birth over an intact perineum.
- Physiologic/expectant and active third stage labor management.
- Delayed cord clamping and immediate skin-to-skin contact.
- Breastfeeding support in the immediate postpartum period and first year.
- Recognition and management of complications and women with medically high-risk conditions, supporting normal processes where possible.

Box 14.3   Examples of clinical learning experiences in maternity care

- Online and/or face-to-face discussion of normal birth scenarios.
- Simulations of normal birth and methods to facilitate using high-fidelity simulation and standardized patients with task trainers.
- Simulation of high-risk birth scenarios and birth emergencies requiring interprofessional collaboration.
- "A day in the life" where students/residents spend a day with a clinician from a different profession.
- Interprofessional rounds on the labor unit, presentation of low-intervention and high-risk techniques for support and management.
- Participation with interprofessional facilitators of group model prenatal care.

The use of online learning paired with simulation or other common laboratory experiences avoids some of the difficulties associated with academic calendars and student schedules that are complex to organize among health professions education programs. The Drexel University and University of British Columbia programs provide examples of multiple professionals learning in simulated clinical scenarios with online preparation [31,46]. High-risk, emergency, and other scenarios requiring multiple professions collaboration are ideal for simulations. Other specific approaches to multilearner clinical learning activities provide some initial ideas [31,45]. Additional options could include interprofessional projects focused on research, community-based collaboration, clinical care innovation, and quality improvement implementation activities.

In addition to interprofessional education for basic learners in maternity care, the practice setting could be improved by clinicians participating in interprofessional continuing education opportunities [37]. Approvers and accreditors of these postlicensure and certification educational experiences for health professionals could easily and immediately begin planning interprofessional continuing education programs. Imagine if instead of each professional association developing programs for its respective members, organizations partnered in the development of programming for interprofessional teams that included opportunities for demonstrating achievement and maintenance of critical skills. Professional associations involved in maternity care could hold a joint professional meeting for maternity care clinicians, annually or every 3–5 years, similar to the American Public Health Association meeting.

Summary

We must transform the education of students/residents working in maternity care so that family medicine and obstetrical residents and midwifery students, as well as medical and nursing students, all learn and have clinical opportunities together. It is no longer an option to continue to educate our students/residents in silos. Clinical teachers in institutions providing clinical learning opportunities can and should demand to work with students in multiple health professions. Development of a common maternity care core curriculum is a first step in preparing clinicians to support a physiologic approach to pregnancy and birth in an interprofessional environment. The imperative is to partner in a team-based approach together with women and their families to provide high-quality, high-value care. Together, building on the examples that exist, we can reform our education programs and prepare maternity care clinicians for the future.

References

1. Wertz RW & Wertz DC. (1977). *Lying-in: A history of childbirth in America*. New York: Schocken Books.
2. Institute of Medicine of the National Academies. (1972). *Educating for the health team*. Washington, DC: National Academies Press.

3. O'Neil EH & the Pew Health Professions Commission. (1998). Recreating health professional practice for a new century: The fourth report of the Pew Health Professions Commission. San Francisco: Pew Health Professions Commission. December 1998.

4. Institute of Medicine of the National Academies. (2001). *Crossing the quality chasm: A new health system for the 21st century*. Washington, DC: National Academies Press.

5. Institute of Medicine of the National Academies. (2003). *Health professions education: A bridge to quality*. Washington, DC: National Academies Press.

6. Interprofessional Education Collaborative Expert Panel. (2011). *Core competencies for interprofessional collaborative practice: Report of an expert panel*. Washington, DC: Interprofessional Education Collaborative.

7. Cerra F & Brandt BF. (2011). Renewed focus in the United States links interprofessional education with redesigning health care. *Journal of Interprofessional Care*, *25*(6), 394–396.

8. Institute of Medicine of the National Academies. (2010). *The future of nursing: Leading change, advancing health*. Washington, DC: National Academies Press.

9. American Association of Colleges of Nursing. (2008). The essentials of baccalaureate education for professional nursing practice. Retrieved from: http://www.aacn.nche.edu/education-resources/baccessentials08.pdf. Accessed October 20, 2012.

10. National League for Nursing Accrediting Commission, Inc. (2008). NLNAC standards and criteria—baccalaureate. Retrieved from: http://www.nlnac.org/manuals/SC2008_Baccalaureate.pdf. Accessed October 20, 2012.

11. Liaison Committee on Medical Education Accreditation Standards. (2012). Functions and structure of a medical school. Washington, DC, May.

12. Peska ED, ed. (2009). *APGO medical student educational objectives*, 9th ed. Crofton, MD: Association of Professors of Gynecology and Obstetrics.

13. American Osteopathic Association Commission on Osteopathic College Accreditation. (2012). Accreditation of osteopathic colleges of medicine: COM accreditation standards and procedures. Chicago: American Osteopathic Association Commission on Osteopathic College Accreditation.

14. American Association of Colleges of Osteopathic Medicine. (2012). Osteopathic core competencies for medical students. Retrieved from: http://www.aacom.org/InfoFor/educators/mec/cc/Documents/CoreCompetencyReport2012.pdf.

15. Accreditation Council for Graduate Medical Education. (2007). Family medicine program requirements. Retrieved from: http://www.acgme.org/acWebsite/RRC_120/120_prIndex.asp.

16. Accreditation Council for Graduate Medical Education. (2008). Program requirements for graduate medical education in Obstetrics and Gynecology. Chicago: Accreditation Council for Graduate Medical Education.

17. American Board of Obstetrics and Gynecology. (2011). Bulletin for basic certification in obstetrics and gynecology. Dallas: American Board of Obstetrics and Gynecology.

18. Sedler KD, Lyndon-Rochelle M, Castillo YM, Craig EC, & Albers L. (1993). Nurse-midwifery service model in an academic environment. *Journal of Nurse-Midwifery*, *38*, 241–245.

19. Afriat CI. (1993). Nurse-midwives as faculty preceptors in medical education. *Journal of Nurse-Midwifery*, *38*, 349–352.

20. Blake KD & Magrane DM. (1995). Reorganization of postpartum rounds. *Academic Medicine*, *70*(5), 432.

21. Harman PJ, Summers L, King T, & Harman TF. (1998). Interdisciplinary teaching: A survey of CNM participation in medical education in the United States. *Journal of Nurse-Midwifery*, *43*, 27–35.

22. McConaughey E & Howard E. (2009). Midwives as educators of medical students and residents: Results of a national survey. *Journal of Midwifery & Women's Health*, *54*, 268–274.

23. American College of Nurse-Midwives. (2011). Comparison of certified nurse-midwives, certified midwives, and certified professional midwives. Silver Spring, MD: American College of Nurse-Midwives.

24. American College of Nurse-Midwives. (2011). *Standards for the practice of midwifery.* Silver Spring, MD: American College of Nurse-Midwives.

25. American College of Nurse-Midwives. (2012). *Core competencies for basic midwifery education.* Silver Spring, MD: American College of Nurse-Midwives.

26. American Midwifery Certification Board. (2011). Information for candidates of the National Certification Examination in Nurse-Midwifery and Midwifery. Linthicum, MD: American Midwifery Certification Board.

27. Accreditation Commission for Midwifery Education. (2012). Criteria for programmatic accreditation of midwifery education programs with instructions for elaboration and documentation. Retrieved from: http://www.midwife.org/ACNM/files/ccLibraryFiles/Filename/000000002761/ ACME% 20Programmatic%20Criteria%2012%202009%20%2810%202012%20%20%20IV% 2012%202012%29.pdf. Accessed October 20, 2012.

28. American College of Nurse-Midwives. (2012). Supporting healthy and normal physiologic childbirth: A consensus statement by the American College of Nurse-Midwives, the Midwives Alliance of North America the Midwives Alliance of North America, and the National Association of Certified Professional Midwives.

29. Angelini DJ. (2011). Interdisciplinary and interprofessional education. *Journal of Perinatal Medicine, 25,* 175–179.

30. American Congress of Obstetricians and Gynecologists. (2007). Professional responsibilities in obstetric-gynecologic education. ACOG Committee Opinion no. 358. Washington, DC: American Congress of Obstetricians and Gynecologists.

31. Saxell L, Harris S, & Elarar L. (2009). The collaboration of maternal and newborn health: Interprofessional maternity care education for medical, midwifery, and nursing students. *Journal of Midwifery & Women's Health, 54,* 314–320.

32. Health Insurance Portability and Accountability Act of 1996. (1996). PUB.L. 104–191, 110 STAT. 1936, enacted August 21, 1996.

33. American College of Obstetricians and Gynecologists. (2002). Ethical issues in obstetric-gynecologic education. In *Ethics in obstetrics and gynecology,* pp. 35–37. Washington, DC: American College of Obstetricians and Gynecologists.

34. Barker KK, Bosco C, & Oandasan IF. (2005). Factors in implementing interprofessional education and collaborative practice initiatives: Findings from key informant interviews. *Journal of Interprofessional Care, Supplement 1,* 166–176.

35. Zwarenstein M, Reeves S, & Perrier L. (2005). Effectiveness of pre-licensure interprofessional education and post-licensure collaborative interventions. *Journal of Interprofessional Care, Supplement 1,* 148–165.

36. Childbirth Connection. (2012). History. Retrieved from: http://www.childbirthconnection.org/ article.asp?ck=10076. Accessed September 29, 2012.

37. Transforming Maternity Care Vision Team. (2010). 2020 vision for a high-quality, high-value maternity care system. *Women's Health Issues, 20,* S7–17.

38. Transforming Maternity Care Symposium Steering Committee. (2010). Blueprint for action: Steps toward a high-quality, high-value maternity care system. *Women's Health Issues, 20,* S18–49.

39. Dejoy S, Burkman RT, Graves BW, Grow D, Sankey HZ, Delk C, & Hallisey A. (2011). Making it work: Successful collaborative practice. *Obstetrics & Gynecology, 118*(3), 683–686.

40. Hutchinson MS, Ennis L, Shaw-Battista J, Myers K, Cragin L, & Jackson RA. (2011). Great minds don't think alike: Collaborative maternity care at San Francisco General Hospital. *Obstetrics & Gynecology, 118*(3), 678–682.

41. Avery MD, Montgomery O, & Brandl-Salutz E. (2012). Essential components of successful collaborative maternity care models: The ACOG-ACNM Project. *Obstetrics & Gynecology Clinics of North America, 39,* 423–434.

42. Pecci CC, Mottl-Santiago J, Culpepper L, Heffner L, McMahan T, & Lee-Parritz A. (2012). The birth of a collaborative model: Obstetricians, midwives, and family physicians. *Obstetrics & Gynecology Clinics of North America, 39,* 323–334.

43. Reeves S, Zwarenstein M, Goldman J, Barr H, Freeth D, Hammick M, & Koppel L. (2009). Interprofessional education: Effects on professional practice and health care outcomes. *Cochrane Library*, DOI: 10.1002/14651858.CD002213.pub2.

44. University of Minnesota, Academic Health Center, Office of Education. (2012). ONE health. Retrieved from: http://www.ach.umn.edu/1health. Accessed February 10, 2012.

45. Taleff J, Salstrom J, & Newton ER. (2009). Pioneering a universal curriculum: A look at six disciplines involved in women's health care. *Journal of Midwifery & Women's Health, 54,* 306–313.

46. Montgomery K, Morse C, Smith-Glasgow ME, et al. (2012). Promoting quality and safety in women's health through the use of transdisciplinary clinical simulation educational modules: Methodology and a pilot trial. *Gender Medicine, 9,* S48–54.

Chapter 15

Women's health and maternity care policies: Current status and recommendations for change

Heather M. Bradford

Key points

- Government agencies, health care systems, third-party payers, and health professions associations have multiple incentives to create policies that support women's health and normal birth.
- Continue to foster interprofessional relationships and collaborative models of care in order to expand the maternity care workforce, increase access to quality health care, and improve patient outcomes.
- State legislatures should adopt the "Consensus Model for APRN Regulation" recommendations, with Boards of Midwifery as the ultimate goal when feasible.
- All third-party payers should be required to credential and equitably reimburse all licensed health professionals.
- Reform payment methods for maternity care including the National Priorities Partnership 2011 and 2012 recommendations.
- Maintain Affordable Care Act provisions that support expanded health care access for women.
- Joint Commission should incorporate all components of the Baby-Friendly Hospital Initiative into the requirements for accreditation of all maternity services.

Improved insurance coverage and access to affordable, appropriate health care is an essential first step to help address the nation's disparities in maternal and child health.

Adam Sonfield, Guttmacher Institute

Introduction

Government agencies, health care systems, third-party payers, and health professions associations have multiple incentives to create policies that support normal birth given the current cesarean section rate of 32.8% in 2010 and increasing U.S. maternity mortality and severe maternal complications [1,2]. Of all births in the United States, one-third involve

Supporting a Physiologic Approach to Pregnancy and Birth: A Practical Guide, First Edition.
Edited by Melissa D. Avery.
© 2013 John Wiley & Sons, Inc. Published 2013 by John Wiley & Sons, Inc.

complications, such as a 12% preterm birth rate and an 8% low-birth weight rate [1]. With obstetric care accounting for 25% of all hospital stays, the increase in cesarean births also places a financial burden on both public and commercial insurers, as the facility charges for cesarean deliveries are nearly double that of vaginal births [3,4]. In 2008, 8.5% of total U.S. hospital charges were pregnancy-related, with mother's pregnancy and delivery and newborn hospital stays representing two of the top five most costly conditions in aggregate [5].

This chapter will provide an overview of existing and needed policies that support a woman's ability to have a normal birth, as well as those that improve her health status prior to pregnancy. Policies written and implemented by professional associations, hospital systems, third-party payers, and state and federal governments all have the potential to improve outcomes and control costs. Breastfeeding policies at the state and federal level, as well as within the hospital and workplace setting, will also be examined. When appropriate policies exist within the health care system, maternity and women's health care providers can practice to their broadest scope and provide unencumbered care in a collaborative environment, thereby offering women full access to affordable well-woman and maternity care, improving maternal and infant outcomes, and reducing health care costs.

Policies for women's health and maternity care providers

Although there are other women's health and maternity care providers, this chapter focuses primarily on policies pertaining to physicians and American Midwifery Certification Board (AMCB)-certified midwives, who together attend 94% of all U.S. births and provide well-woman care [6]. Specifically, maternity care providers are guided by health professions association statements with respect to collaboration, scope-of-practice regulations, and third-party payers' rules on credentialing and reimbursement for health care providers.

Collaboration among health care providers

Collaborative practice has been defined as "the provision of health care by an interdisciplinary team of professionals who collaborate to accomplish a common goal" and is associated with increased efficiency, improved clinical outcomes, and enhanced provider satisfaction [7]. From the 1950s throughout the 1980s, nurse-midwifery care was seen as a solution for quality, low-cost health care for the poor. Some physicians felt threatened when nurse-midwives sought independent practice, and physicians were more welcoming of those who were salaried employees of hospitals or physician-owned practices [6]. Over the past 30 years, relationships between the physician and midwifery communities, as well as the health professions organizations that represent them, has evolved. Relationships among the American Congress of Obstetricians and Gynecologists (ACOG), the American Academy of Family Physicians (AAFP), and the American College of Nurse-Midwives (ACNM) can impede or contribute to patient care, ultimately affecting patient satisfaction and clinical outcomes [8].

ACOG and ACNM: Finding new opportunities for collaboration

The relationship between ACOG and ACNM, as reflected in the ACOG/ACNM joint statement, has improved dramatically in the last 10 years. As early as 2002, ACOG recognized the equivalency of the certified midwife (CM) and certified nurse-midwife (CNM) credentials in the ACOG/ACNM joint statement of practice relations [9]. This 2002 joint statement was revised in 2011 to assert that "Ob-gyns and CNMs/CMs are experts in their respective fields of practice and are . . . independent providers who may collaborate with each other based on the needs of their patients" [10]. The statement also asserts that "to provide high quality and seamless care, ob/gyns and CNMs/CMs should have access to a system of care that fosters collaboration among licensed, independent providers" [7]. This new statement positions obstetrics and midwifery as separate fields of expertise and provides opportunities to develop and implement interprofessional interventions to improve collaborative practice.

Some physician resistance to midwifery practice remains at the local level, especially as midwives expand their scope of practice and attend more births. However, in 2011, the leadership of ACNM and ACOG requested articles written jointly by midwives and obstetricians describing successful collaborative models of care in community and academic settings. Selected papers were published in *Obstetrics & Gynecology* [7]. Additional papers have been published in the *Journal of Midwifery & Women's Health* and *Obstetrics and Gynecology Clinics of North America* [11,12]. Further collaborative discussions to address the maternity care shortage have also occurred, asking obstetricians and midwives to join together at local and global levels to share in policy development, continuing education, research, and preparation of the future maternity care workforce [11]. With this knowledge sharing, relationships and cooperation between ob/gyn physicians and midwives will be enhanced, with the ultimate goal of improved access to quality health care and clinical outcomes [13].

> *Recommendation*: Continue to foster interprofessional relationships and collaborative models of care in order to expand the maternity care workforce, increase access to quality health care, and improve patient outcomes.

AAFP and ACNM: A gap remains

Ten percent of nurse-midwives work directly with family physicians and 18% of AAFP members attended births in a hospital setting [14]. Midwives and family practice physicians have a shared philosophy of family and woman-centered maternity care, and both have lower intervention rates (as compared to obstetricians) including episiotomy, use of Pitocin, and cesarean section [15]. Despite these commonalities, formal collaboration between the two disciplines has been limited, although several successful collaborative models have been reported [15–18].

In 1993, AAFP issued a statement "opposing nurse-midwifery licensure" and asserting that "the use of nurse-midwives is not in the best interest of quality patient care . . . the AAFP does not believe that the midwife can adequately substitute for the physician in obstetrics" and "has recommended the abolishment of midwifery for many years" [19]. In 2004, AAFP revised its opinion to allow for practice of certified nurse-midwives only "in an integrated practice arrangement under the direction and responsible supervision of a practicing, licensed physician qualified in maternity care" [20]. AAFP proposed legislation in 2010 inferring that nurse practitioners are misleading the public with their credentials and training, specifically related to the doctorate of nursing practice, and in 2012 published a document describing health care teams as a licensed physician supervising one or more nonphysician providers such as nurse practitioners or CNMs [21,22].

A 2010 editorial in the *Journal of Family Practice* called for a fundamental change, encouraging family practice physicians to embrace a full partnership with advanced practice nurses, citing: (1) the recent Institute of Medicine Future of Nursing recommendations, which argues for the removal of all scope-of-practice barriers (such as physician supervision), (2) the belief that nursing professionals do indeed practice within their experience and training boundaries, (3) interprofessional fighting reduces family practice's effectiveness with legislative, business, and consumer advocates, and (4) joined forces will create innovative models of care and lead to better health outcomes [23,24].

> *Recommendation*: ACNM and AAFP can build on collaboration between ACNM and ACOG with an updated practice statement highlighting examples of CNM/CM and family practice physician shared philosophy and successful collaborative practice models.

Regulation and scope of practice

There are many entities involved with defining a provider's scope of practice, including professional associations, educational institutions, credentialing and accrediting organizations, and regulatory agencies. Definition of women's health and maternity care providers' scope and standards of practice begins with core competency documents written by the medical, professional, nursing, and specialty organizations [25]. For example, the ACNM publishes the *Core Competencies for Basic Midwifery Practice* [26]. These essential documents, specific to each profession, serve as the foundation for legislation and regulatory policy making among each state, which, through a licensing and regulatory body, regulates scope of practice [25].

Variations in state regulations for nonphysician providers

Each state has strong influence over scope of practice and is critical in a health care professional's ability to provide care, including prescribing medication, assessing patient conditions, and ordering and evaluating tests. Historically, most states base their licensure frameworks on the underlying principle that physicians are able to treat all human conditions, with corresponding provisions making it illegal for nonphysicians to perform these services. Thus, any nonphysician provider groups are required to "carve out" their scope of practice through legislative exception making, resulting in a very circumscribed practice authority that is or may be much less than their education and training [24]. In order to practice to their full scope as defined by their professional standards, education, and certification, nonphysician providers must request a legislative revision in state laws and/or regulations, which is usually a costly and challenging undertaking, often requiring a lobbyist and grassroots legislative advocacy [27,28].

In addition, state regulatory boards are not required to accept the professions' approved educational routes, certification process, and defined scope of practice. Therefore states can limit the scope of practice for any health care professional, often based on the political climate of the state and not on principles of safe care [6]. It was likely not a coincidence that Illinois, headquarters of the American Medical Association, was one of the last states where CNMs were granted prescriptive authority [29]. In some states, statutory language includes vague provisions open to interpretation and varied enforcement, where in others, language is very detailed. Most states require collaboration with physicians, but the definition of collaboration may range from direct supervision to unclear requirements for written protocols [30]. For example, while CNMs/CMs are educated and certified as independent practitioners, twenty-eight states require a written practice agreement between physician and midwife or physician supervision for some aspect of practice. CNMs practice without the requirement for supervision or contractual agreements in twenty-three jurisdictions (twenty-two states plus D.C.) [31]. Other legal practice barriers include onsite physician oversight and chart review requirements, as well as maximum ratios for physicians who collaborate with more than one CNM/CM [24]. These restrictions limit midwives' ability to practice when physicians are unwilling to enter into these relationships [6,32].

Variations in licensing boards

In addition to variations in scope-of-practice laws, licensing boards that regulate health care providers also vary. Physicians are regulated by Boards of Medicine and CNMs are primarily licensed by Boards of Nursing, although some states license CNMs under other boards. CMs are statutorily recognized with licensure to practice in three states and are licensed under other boards, including the Board of Regents-State Education Department, the Board of Medical Examiners, and the Department of Health (Table 15.1) [33].

Recent efforts have been made by the National Council of State Boards of Nursing (NCSBN) to develop more uniform standards for licensing, accreditation, certification, and education of advanced practice nurses, including CNMs. Specifically, the "Consensus Model for APRN Regulation" requirements call for state Boards of Nursing to be the regulatory body that issues licenses and provides oversight of advanced practice registered nurses (APRNs) [34]. However, ACNM supports the development of Boards of Midwifery as the ultimate decision makers regarding the licensure and practice of CNM/CMs [35]. Currently, only one state has a Board of Midwifery regulating midwifery prescriptive authority, licensing, and practice. Expansion of this model has been proposed and would alleviate potential problems when state Boards of Nursing are not well acquainted with issues specific to midwifery [9,32]. However, feasibility may be difficult given the time and cost involved. An additional benefit to the adoption of the "Consensus Model for APRN Regulation" could be greater autonomy for APRNs in all states, including CNMs, given the model's ability to help eliminate variations in scope-of-practice regulations [36].

> *Policy Recommendation*: All state legislatures adopt the "Consensus Model for APRN Regulation" recommendations to have common regulations under nursing for full scope independent midwifery practice, with Boards of Midwifery as the ultimate goal when feasible.

Table 15.1 Agencies/boards that regulate CNMs and CMs. *Journal of Midwifery & Women's Health, 56*(6), November/December 2011, p. 544.

Regulatory agency/board	States regulated	Title(s) used
Board of Nursing	Alaska, Arizona, Arkansas, California, Colorado, Delaware, District of Columbia, Florida, Georgia, Hawaii, Idaho, Indiana, Iowa	ANP/APN/APNP/ APON/APPN/ APRN/ARNP/CNM/ NMNP/RNP
	Kansas, Kentucky, Louisiana, Maine, Maryland, Massachusetts, Michigan, Minnesota, Mississippi, Missouri, Montana, Nevada	
	New Hampshire, North Dakota, Ohio, Oklahoma, Oregon, South Carolina, Tennessee, Texas, Vermont, West Virginia, Wisconsin, Wyoming	
Department of Financial and Professional Regulation	Illinois	APN
Department of Health and Human Services–Division of Public Health	Nebraska	APRN-CNM
Board of Regents–State Education Department	New York	LM
Board of Medical Examiners	New Jersey	CNM/CM
Board of Medicine	Pennsylvania	CNM
Department of Commerce–Division of Occupational and Professional Licensing	Utah	CNM
Nursing Care Quality Assurance Commission	Washington	ARNP
Department of Health	New Mexico, Rhode Island	CNM/CM/Midwife
Department of Public Health	Connecticut	CNM/Licensed nurse-midwife
Joint Regulation: Board of Nursing and Board of Medicine	Alabama, North Carolina, South Dakota, Virginia	APN/Midwife/CNM

A tipping point for nonphysician providers: The IOM report

Movement to amend the state regulations appears to be at a tipping point, primarily following a 2010 report by the Institute of Medicine (IOM) and the Robert Wood Johnson Foundation. *The Future of Nursing: Leading Change, Advancing Health* calls for the removal of scope-of-practice barriers for APRNs, and urges that APRNs practice to the full extent of their education and training. These recommendations have also been supported by the American Association of Retired Persons and the Federal Trade Commission [37, 38]. Noted scope-of-practice expert Barbara Safriet, JD, LLM, has called upon the federal government to intervene via the regulatory process in order to facilitate the use of APRNs to their full scope, given "organized medicine's continued opposition to expanding the authority of other providers to practice [39]."

Policy Recommendations:
For maternity care providers: Partner to support full scope and safe practice for all appropriately educated, certified, and licensed providers.

For Congress: (1) Expand the Medicare program to include coverage of services by APRNs and CMs that are within their scope of practice as defined by their professional standards, education, and certification. (2) Amend Medicare regulations so APRNs and CMs are authorized to perform admission assessments as well as certification of patients for home health services and for admission to hospice and skilled nursing facilities.

For the Federal Trade Commission and the Antitrust Division of the Department of Justice: Review current and proposed state laws regarding APRNs and CMs that might be anticompetitive in nature. Amend all state restrictive regulations to allow APRNs and CMs to practice according to their qualifications [24].

In conjunction with the IOM report, other signs of progress indicate growing opportunities for expansion of scope of practice for nonphysician providers. These include:

- After passage of the Patient Protection and Affordable Care Act (ACA) in 2010, twenty-eight states began examining their laws regarding scope of practice for APRNs [24].
- A 2010 *New England Journal of Medicine* paper argued for expanded scope of practice for nurse practitioners to their fullest knowledge and competence in order to meet expanding needs for primary care services and to improve quality of care [40].
- In a 2011, Health and Human Services Secretary Kathleen Sebelius and Dr. Bill Frist, former U.S. Senate majority leader, urged examination of state laws that restrict the practice of APRNs, supporting expansion of scope of practice [41].
- The National Institute for Health Care Reform 2011 report proposes the expansion of APRNs scope of practice to respond to the growing need for primary care providers under the ACA [42].
- In 2012, *Womens Health Issues* published a review of twenty-one studies over 18 years finding that CNMs have outcomes at least comparable to care managed exclusively by physicians, including lower rates of cesarean delivery, episiotomy, and severe perineal

trauma. The authors concluded that care by CNMs is safe and effective. In addition, women cared for by CNMs were more likely to choose nonpharmacologic approaches to manage pain and have higher breastfeeding rates [43].

Credentialing and reimbursement by third-party payers

The ability of a health care professional to be paid for her/his services is essential to professional viability. State and federal governments (through Medicaid and Medicare), as well as third-party private entities, pay for most health care in the United States. Medicare has universal reimbursement rates for all health care providers, and as of January 1, 2011, under the ACA reimburses CNMs the same as physicians for the same services [2]. While physician and nurse-midwife services under Medicaid are mandated by federal law, the decision as to whether a specific service is covered, and the reimbursement rate, is determined by the state [24] (Table 15.2).

Credentialing and reimbursement by third-party payers is also complex and regulated by the state, although much more loosely [6]. Third-party payers often refuse to credential and/or recognize nonphysician providers on their provider panel, typically because of state requirements for physician supervision in prescribing medications [44,45]. A National Nursing Centers Consortium study found that almost half of all managed-care organizations do not credential or contract with nurse practitioners as primary care providers [44].

Policy Recommendations:
For Congress: Expand equitable reimbursement under Medicare to all APRNs and CMs.
   For state legislatures: Increase Medicaid reimbursement for APRNs and CMs to 100% of physician payments.
   For state legislatures: Require all third-party payers to credential and equitably reimburse all health professionals licensed in that state.

Payment reform leads to improved clinical outcomes?

A major limitation of the current health care system is the fee-for-service payment structure, which rewards increasing volume of services, regardless of whether use of more services leads to improved clinical outcomes [46]. With pregnancy and birth, which require a limited number of routine tests and unlimited hands-on care, the payment system provides little or no reimbursement for non-procedure-based interventions that have been shown to improve outcomes [47]. An upward trend in payment reform favors reimbursement based on meeting or exceeding certain quality standards and/or clinical outcomes [48]. For example, third-party payers should provide equal compensation for vaginal and cesarean births, with successful vaginal birth following a history of previous cesarean compensated at a higher rate than a normal vaginal birth [49]. A 2011 article highlighting a gold standard CNM/obstetrician collaborative model attributed their 18.5% primary cesarean rate for all women (including high risk) and their 31% vaginal birth after cesarean

Table 15.2 ACNM medicaid table.

State	Rate
Alabama	80%
Alaska	85%
Arkansas	80%
Arizona	90%
California	100%
Colorado	100%
Connecticut	90%
Delaware: CNMs and CMs	100%
District of Columbia	100%
Florida	80%
Georgia	100%
Hawaii	75%
Idaho	85%
Illinois	100%
Indiana	75%
Iowa	85%
Kansas	75%
Kentucky	75%
Louisiana	80%
Maine	100%
Maryland	100%
Massachusetts	100% for independent practitioners; 85% for dependent practitioners
Michigan	100%
Minnesota	90%
Mississippi	90%
Missouri: CNMs	100%
Missouri: CMs	Not Eligible
Montana	90%
Nebraska	100%
Nevada	88%
New Hampshire	100%
New Jersey: CNMs	70%
New Jersey: CMs	Not Eligible
New Mexico	100%
New York: CNMs and CMs	85%
North Carolina	97%
North Dakota	75%
Ohio	100%
Oklahoma	100%
Oregon	100%
Pennsylvania	100%
Rhode Island: CNMs and CMs	100%
South Carolina	100%
South Dakota	100%
Tennessee	90%
Texas	92%
Utah	100%
Vermont	100%
Virginia	100%
Washington	100%
West Virginia	100%
Wisconsin	90% if non-master's prepared, or 100% with master's degree
Wyoming	100%

(VBAC) rate (superior to national trends) to the lack of compensation for health care providers based on the number and type of procedures completed [50]. Removing economic incentive for intervention (i.e., cesarean section) allows the team to focus on research evidence and safety concerns in order to improve patient satisfaction, alleviate unnecessary costs, and improve clinical outcomes.

The National Priorities Partnership (NPP), a multistakeholder group of forty-eight public and private sector national organizations that offers consultative support to the U.S. Department of Health and Human Services, recently called for ongoing payment and delivery system reform "that rewards value over volume; promotes patient-centered outcomes, efficiency, and appropriate care; and seeks to improve quality while reducing or eliminating waste from the system" [51]. Specifically, NPP noted inappropriate care and overuse of maternity care interventions, specifically related to cesarean sections. Their 2011 recommendations include:

1 Implement new payment programs and care delivery models emphasizing shared learning and public and private stakeholder collaboration.
2 Address underlying cost drivers that affect payment and delivery models.
3 Ensure transparency to allow for informed decision making as an integral component of all payment and delivery models.
4 Address underlying workforce and technology constraints that impede progress.

In January 2012, the NPP formed the Maternity Action Team to address inappropriate maternity care. Specifically, the goals of the group are to reduce elective inductions and cesarean sections prior to 39 weeks and reduce the cesarean section rate for low-risk women [52].

Policy Recommendation to Maternity Care Stakeholders: Reform payment methods for maternity care including the NPP 2011 and 2012 recommendations.

Hospital policies

Many hospital policies directly impact a maternity care provider's ability to support normal birth. These include hospital bylaws that dictate credentialing, scope of practice, and admitting/discharge privileges, as well as safe staffing policies, clinical improvement initiatives, and policies related to transfers of women from home and birth center settings onto the hospital labor unit.

Hospital bylaws and hospital privileging legislation

Despite potential state restrictions of health professions scope of practice, hospital policies also may restrict a care provider's ability to practice independently in caring for women. Medical staff, composed primarily of physicians, are often responsible for writing hospital bylaws, as well as making decisions about credentialing and admitting privileges, which can pose a barrier for nonphysicians. For example, one hospital may allow independent admissions by a midwife, and a different hospital in the same community may not allow midwives to have admitting privileges [6]. Examples of high-quality collaborative practices without restrictions have been outlined elsewhere [50,53,54].

The IOM 2010 report highlighted the need to reduce barriers and improve access to services provided by APRNs. The report called for ensuring that APRNs are eligible for hospital clinical privileges (including admitting privileges) and medical staff membership [55]. Existence of these barriers was confirmed by a 2011 ACNM member survey, which found that:

- 14.8% of respondents had been told that they could not apply for clinical privileges because the hospital would not consider a midwife application.
- 66.2% of respondents stated that they or a midwife they know had been denied access to clinical privileges, thus reducing access to services for women in their community.
- 65.4% of respondents stated they had been granted practice privileges, but limitations were applied such as supervision or co-signature requirements that are not required of other clinicians on medical staff, or restricted scope of practice.
- 70.3% of respondents did not have full medical staff privileges.
- 79.3% of respondents did not have full voting privileges within the medical staff [56].

A coalition of eight nursing-related organizations, including the American Nurses Association (ANA) and ACNM, are supporting reforms to the Medicare Hospital Conditions of Participation to ensure that APRNs are eligible for clinical privileges, admitting privileges, and membership on medical staff. The coalition aims to correct the processes for clinical privileges and appointments to full medical staff to ensure decisions are based on an objective evaluation of an applicant's credentials, free of anticompetitive intent or purpose [55].

> *Policy Recommendation for U.S. Congress*: Passage of federal legislation regarding the requirements for hospital participation in the Medicare program to ensure that: (1) APRNs are eligible for clinical privileges, admitting privileges, and membership on medical staff, and (2) APRNs are accorded all categories of medical staff privileges, including voting rights [57].

Safe staffing

Higher RN staffing levels are associated with improved patient outcomes, fewer deaths and complications, and fewer prolonged hospital stays [58,59]. Research correlates continuous nursing support during labor with improved outcomes, including shorter labor, decreased use of analgesia/anesthesia, decreased operative vaginal births or cesarean births, decreased need for oxytocin/uterotonics, increased likelihood of breastfeeding, and increased satisfaction with the childbirth experience [60–62].

The Association of Women's Health, Obstetric and Neonatal Nurses' (AWHONN) "Guidelines for Professional Registered Nurse Staffing for Perinatal Units" can assist hospital executives and nurse leaders in planning adequate registered nurse staffing in order to provide safe and effective perinatal nursing care. Specifically, AWHONN recommends a one-to-one RN-to-patient ratio for women in labor with medical or obstetric complications, who are receiving oxytocin, who choose minimal intervention (e.g., decline analgesia or anesthesia, opt for intermittent fetal heart monitoring), or who are in second stage labor [63].

> *Policy Recommendation*: Adopt AWHONN guidelines in order to attain improved patient outcomes.

Clinical improvement initiatives

With the increasing focus on pay for performance, specific clinical improvement initiatives can be used to decrease rates of cesarean section and improve maternal and infant outcomes. These initiatives can be implemented by both hospitals and/or maternity care providers.

First, hospital quality improvement programs can be implemented to assist maternity care providers in their decision making to support normal birth, including VBAC. In 2011, the California Maternal Quality Care Collaborative found growing evidence that provider-dependent indications (i.e., those that rely on provider judgment) combined with provider discretion play a large role in the upward trend of cesarean births. Suggested hospital quality improvement programs include:

1 Achieve a maternity care department commitment to lowering cesarean rates with a stated goal.
2 Implement a self-evaluation and strong peer review program among the maternity care team and clinical staff, including a review of current VBAC and induction policies and cases of primary cesarean deliveries. Consider a required second opinion for all cesarean sections, especially when indicated for dystocia prior to the active phase of labor [49].
3 Incentives can be used to motivate maternity care providers and hospital administration, along with nursing staff, to engage together in changing the culture on labor and delivery units [4].
4 Engage in external sharing and benchmarking of quality outcomes measures, such as with the National Perinatal Information Center, the Leapfrog Group, and other subgroups, including academic perinatal centers, nonacademic perinatal centers, or the Council of Women's and Infant Specialty Hospitals [49].
5 Eliminate nonmedically indicated (elective) deliveries before 39 weeks gestation. For example, the Florida Perinatal Quality Collaborative, funded through the March of Dimes, is engaging six Florida hospitals to develop successful quality improvement programs on this topic in a year-long pilot test [64].
6 Reestablish the teaching and training of physicians for breech and operative vaginal births [49].
7 Seek assistance regarding VBAC programs through ACOG's Voluntary Review of Quality Program, which provides an on-site evaluation and a customized and confidential report [65].

Home and birth center transfers

While 99% of births occur in a hospital setting, some women choose to give birth outside the hospital. If these women require a higher level of care, the transfer process to a hospital setting can be a frightening experience, affecting a woman's ability to labor effectively. Therefore, a family centered and collaborative approach among all care providers is of utmost importance.

In 2011, a task force of Washington state licensed midwives, obstetrician-gynecologists, and those with expertise in public health and policy published a document that addressed this important transfer process. The MAWS "Planned Out-of-Hospital Birth Transport

Guideline" was reviewed and approved by members of the Statewide Perinatal Advisory Committee (PAC), the Midwives' Association of Washington State (MAWS), and the Physician-Licensed Midwife Work Group. The document aims to improve maternal and neonatal outcomes and patient satisfaction by creating unobstructed hospital admittance, good communication, and continuity of care, as well as appropriate and timely medical attention. Highlights of the document include a concise list of expectations for both the out-of-hospital birth attendant and the hospital staff. This Washington state project is ongoing; the next phase will include adoption of these guidelines by hospitals and the formation of more intentional relationships between out-of-hospital birth attendants and physicians [66]. See additional recommendations in Chapter 13.

> *Policy Recommendation*: Implement out-of-hospital transport guidelines in each hospital in order to improve communication and maternal and neonatal outcomes.

Federal and state policies affecting women's health and maternity care

Many federal and state laws and programs exist that impact a woman's ability to have a normal birth. This section will first address the current medico-legal environment and how professional liability laws may affect a maternity care provider's clinical decision making. The federal and state health insurance programs, Medicare and Medicaid, and the federal and state interplay with private insurance mandates and coverage will be reviewed with respect to women's health. Finally, state and federal legislative progress with respect to reproductive health care policy from 1990 to the present will be highlighted, with a special focus on the ACA.

Medico-legal liability and its effect on clinical decision making

Many experts believe that the current medico-legal climate and fear of malpractice litigation in particular leads health care providers to practice "defensive" medicine [4]. In obstetrics, this is likely one reason for the rising cesarean rate. Has anyone been sued over an unnecessary cesarean section? Fear of litigation is especially strong in clinical decision making for a trial of labor after cesarean section [67]. A recent ACOG survey revealed that 25.9% of obstetricians stopped offering or performing VBAC births because of the risk or fear of professional liability claims or litigation [68].

Organized medicine's recommendation for professional liability reform at the state and federal level has been made for decades. Many argue that limiting frivolous lawsuits would make it possible for obstetric care providers to recommend cesarean delivery less often when an element of risk presents, such as nonreassuring fetal heart tones [49]. Researchers have attempted to model the impact of caps on noneconomic damages on rates of primary and repeat cesarean deliveries, demonstrating that new laws would be associated with a reduction in cesarean sections [69].

While the trial lawyers who represent injured patients argue against reform, many health care experts have recommended other less controversial options, such as "no fault" compensation models (alternative dispute resolution, early offers, and birth injury compensation funds) and health courts [70]. In addition, thirty-six states have passed immunity for apology laws, which allow health care providers to apologize and offer expressions of grief (not fault) without their words being used against them in court [71]. Five states have passed mandatory written disclosure laws that require the health care provider to document the adverse event to patients and their families [72,73]. The state of Colorado is exceptional in that it also makes "admissions of fault" inadmissible in a court of law [73].

Policy Recommendations: (1) Passage of "I'm sorry" legislation in all fifty states. (2) Passage of "no fault" compensation models and health courts.

Federal and state health insurance programs

Federal and state governments have many policies that determine women's scope of health insurance coverage, affordability, and ultimately access to health care. The federal government has primary jurisdiction over two major health programs: Medicare (for seniors and women with disabilities) and Medicaid (for low-income women), which insures 10% of all women. Medicaid is the largest payer of maternity services, funding 40–50% of all care, primarily because an uninsured woman is more likely to qualify for Medicaid when she is pregnant. States typically set their income-eligibility levels for pregnant women at or near 200% of the federal poverty level (FPL), which is $44,700 for a family of four [2]. Medicaid typically covers prenatal care and screenings, labor and birth services, as well as postpartum care for 60 days. However, a recent Kaiser Family Foundation survey found that some services are excluded under Medicaid, such as genetic screenings, breastfeeding support services, and access to birth centers or doulas [2].

Women need access to care outside of the maternity cycle, which can improve their health status at the time of conception, thereby increasing their opportunity to have a normal birth. In fact, the most important way to improve birth outcomes is to improve preconception and interconceptional care [74]. It is important for providers to work with women to assure care extending beyond pregnancy when covered by Medicaid. Several federal and state programs include family planning services, well-women exams, and sexually transmitted infection testing. Title X provided funding that served 4.7 million women in 2008 and helped avoid 973,000 unintended pregnancies. Without these services, unintended pregnancy and abortion in the United States would be one-third higher [75]. Twenty-seven states extend Medicaid eligibility for family planning services to low-income women who do not qualify for full Medicaid benefits [76]. Many state, city, and/or county agencies oversee additional programs for women who are underinsured or uninsured, such as prescription drug assistance, breast and cervical cancer screenings, and public education and outreach [77].

State and federal government's role with private insurance

Having health insurance does not necessarily equate to access to care. State governments play an important role in regulating private insurance plans, making decisions about which provider services and benefits, such as maternity care, are mandatory [77]. Mandatory services vary greatly by state and by health plan and can have significant influence on birth outcomes. For example, while all fifty states require cancer screening, only five states require private insurance to cover the human papillomavirus (HPV) vaccine. If all states reimbursed for the costs associated with this vaccination, the rate of cervical cancer would decline, decreasing the risk of cervical incompetence and preterm birth [78,79].

In order to increase health insurance coverage of maternity services, Congress passed the Pregnancy Discrimination Act in 1978, an amendment to the Title VII sex discrimination section of the Civil Rights Act of 1964. This act, which only applies to employers with fifteen or more employees, states that discrimination on the basis of pregnancy, childbirth, or related medical conditions is unlawful, and women who are pregnant or affected by pregnancy-related conditions must be treated in the same manner as other employees with similar abilities or limitations. Employer-sponsored health insurance must cover expenses for employees and their spouses for pregnancy-related conditions, including prenatal care, birth, and postpartum care, on the same basis as costs for other medical conditions [80]. Despite this landmark law, legal gaps still exist, such as businesses with less than fifteen employees, or health insurance plans that exclude "nonspouse dependents" such as daughters of employees and their infants [2].

Another legal gap related to this act is with private insurers. Although most women of childbearing age have health insurance through Medicaid or an employer, 6% of women purchase individual insurance directly from private insurers, who in this scenario are not required under the act to cover maternity care and delivery services, prescription benefits, or contraception, leaving many women needing to purchase costly supplemental insurance. Women with a history of certain health conditions may not qualify for private insurance, thus making them uninsurable [77]. Historically, women have been denied coverage or payment for conditions such as an existing pregnancy, a prior cesarean section, or a history of domestic violence [81]. Payment for prenatal care and hospital delivery can be cost-prohibitive, deterring women from seeking care until later in pregnancy, thus increasing their risk for pregnancy complications [82].

Government agencies are not able to regulate affordability with employer-sponsored private insurance. Health insurance premiums increased 80% between 2000 and 2007, with employee contributions more than doubling during that period, exceeding the rate of inflation and employee compensation. Costs of co-payments and deductibles have also increased substantially. A 2004 Kaiser Family Foundation survey of women with health insurance during the previous 12 months showed that women delayed or went without care they thought they needed. Reasons cited were difficulty finding the time for an appointment or taking time off work, or difficulty securing childcare or transportation [77].

Legislative progress in women's health policy: The ACA

Despite these public and private insurance options for women, 20% of U.S women (ages 19–64) were uninsured in 2010, and an additional almost 18% were underinsured; that is, they had insurance but were at risk of high out-of-pocket costs relative to their income [83]. The majority of uninsured women fall into the category of "the working poor," as two-thirds live in households with at least one full-time worker [77]. Recent research indicates that women without health insurance lack access to care and have poorer health outcomes [24].

Many state and federal laws have addressed women's health services and prevention to ameliorate these shortfalls over the past 25 years. In 1990, the Breast and Cervical Cancer Mortality Prevention Act provided funding for pap smears and mammograms for underserved women [6]. In 1992, the Infertility Prevention Act authorized the screening, treatment, and necessary follow-up for sexually transmitted diseases (STDs) that can lead to infertility. Violence against women was categorized as a federal crime in 1994 and penalties were increased for the offender under the Violence Against Women Act. The Newborns' and Mothers' Health Protection Act (NMHPA) of 1996 requires all health insurance plans to cover a postpartum hospital stay of at least 48 hours for a vaginal birth and 96 hours for an uncomplicated cesarean section [84]. In 2000, breast and cervical cancer screenings were funded for women eligible for Medicaid through the Breast and Cervical Cancer Prevention and Treatment Act [6]. Between 1994 and 2001, forty-two states and the District of Columbia passed laws requiring health plans and provider networks to permit direct access to women's health care services without a prior "gatekeeper" referral, including ob/gyn physicians and CNMs [85]. The exclusions included Alaska, Arizona, Hawaii, Iowa, North Dakota, Oklahoma, South Dakota, and Wyoming [86].

Despite these policy improvements, many gaps still existed in women's health coverage. In 2010, President Barack Obama signed the Patient Protection and Affordable Care Act (ACA) into law, creating substantial changes for all health care providers and women with its provision of health insurance by 2014 for an estimated 32 million Americans who were previously uninsured [87]. Three key elements of the ACA that may improve a woman's health status prior to pregnancy, thereby optimizing her chance for a normal birth are (1) expanding coverage and access to care, (2) mandatory essential benefits and preventive services, and (3) reimbursement.

The ACA: Expanding coverage and access to women's health care

While most of the ACA changes take effect in 2014, some insurance market reforms directly impacting a woman's access to care were implemented in 2010:

- For women uninsurable because of pre-existing conditions such as a prior cesarean section or history of domestic violence, a temporary high-risk pool was developed.
- For new plans offered, dependent coverage was extended to age 26 from age 18 (adults with one of the highest uninsured rates of all age groups) [88]. This drastically increased women's access to well-woman care, including breast and cervical cancer screenings and contraception.
- Insurers can no longer rescind coverage due to illness, particularly important for women with mental health diagnoses or chronic health conditions [89].

When the law takes full effect in 2014, 54% of uninsured women will most likely qualify for Medicaid, and 37% will be required to purchase private coverage but will receive federal assistance to help cover the cost (Figure 15.1) [76,89]. Medicaid coverage

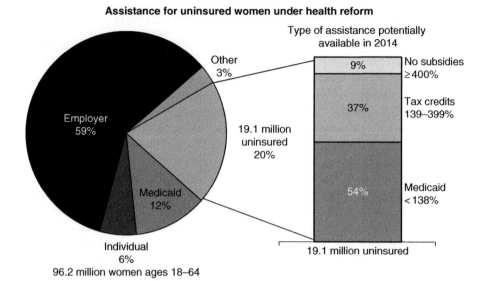

Figure 15.1   The Kaiser Family Foundation, KaiserEDU.org. Health Reform: Impact on Women's Health Coverage and Access to Care, November 2010, available at http://www. kaiseredu.org/Tutorials-and-Presentations/Women-and-Health-Reform.aspx. "Other" includes programs such as Medicare and military-related coverage. The federal poverty level for a family of four in 2009 was $22,500. The original source for the data is KFF/Urban Institute analysis of 2010 ASEC Supplement to the Current Population Survey, U.S. Census Bureau.

has been expanded because of a new mandatory Medicaid eligibility category created for all individuals with income at or below 133% of the FPL. Thirty-five percent of uninsured women with income between 133% and 399% of the FPL will qualify to purchase health insurance through the American Health Benefits Exchanges, or "exchanges" that will serve as a marketplace where consumers can compare and buy health insurance. Both individuals and small businesses will be able to buy insurance through this mechanism [90]. Exchanges should end anticompetitive practices by third-party payers that have limited women's access to their choice of providers [91].

Access will be further improved under a provision prohibiting new plans from denying coverage based on pre-existing conditions. Also, health plans will no longer be able to set premiums based on gender; they may use only two criteria—smoking status and age. Finally, plans will be required to offer renewable coverage, regardless of whether a woman becomes sick [89].

With this expanded coverage, more women will have access to a regular health care provider, and fewer women will have to pay for pregnancy and newborn care. In addition, more women will be able to plan their pregnancies having access to contraception, ensure they are healthy prior to pregnancy, access early prenatal care, and achieve overall better health outcomes [2]. Only one in ten uninsured women will not qualify for health insurance because their income is above 400% of the FPL ($90,000 for a family of four). New immigrants or undocumented immigrants will not qualify for Medicaid coverage [89].

The ACA: Mandatory preventive services and essential benefits

In 2010, new health plans were required to provide minimum coverage without cost sharing for certain preventive services (rated by the U.S. Preventive Services Task Force), many of which pertain to women (Table 15.3) [89]. As of 2012, new plans must require certain women's preventive health and maternity services, with no co-payments or deductibles (see Box 15.1) [90,92].

Many other specific programs have received funding aimed at maternity care and women's health. For example, the U.S. Department of Health and Human Services allocated $40 million in grants for Strong Start, focused on two key maternity care initiatives. First, the Center for Medicare and Medicaid Innovation awarded funding to health care providers and coalitions to improve prenatal care to women covered by Medicaid. The grants support enhanced prenatal care through group prenatal care, birth centers providing case management, and maternity care homes where pregnant women have expanded access to better coordinated, enhanced prenatal care. The second initiative aims to reduce the rate of early elective deliveries (less than 39 weeks). The existing infrastructure of the Partnership for Patients, including the participating Hospital Engagement Networks, is leveraged by implementing a quality improvement platform to share best practices, providing technical assistance to hospitals, and creating support for change with a broad-based campaign to engage providers, patients, and the public. Finally, Strong Start supports efforts to collect performance data, measure success, and promote transparency and continuous improvement [93].

Table 15.3   ACA covered preventive screening services identified by the U.S. Preventive Services Task Force.

U.S. Preventive Services Taskforce: A and B level recommendations				
Lifestyle/Healthy Behaviors	Cancer	STI/STDs	Chronic Conditions	Pregnancy
Alcohol screening	Colorectal screening	HIV testing	Hypertension	Tobacco interventions
Depression screening	Breast screening	Gonorrhea screening	Diabetes	Rh incompatibility screening
Healthy diet counseling	Breast chemoprevention	Chlamydia screening	Obesity screening	Hepatitis B screening
Tobacco interventions	Breast/ovarian High risk/BRCA	Syphilis screening	Osteoporosis	Iron deficiency anemia screening
Immunizations	Cervical cancer	STI counseling	Lipid disorders	Bacteriurea screening

In addition to these benefits individuals in these exchange plans and other qualifying plans will be covered for all the services that are recommended by the USPSTF without cost-sharing. This will apply to Medicare as well, where beneficiaries have had to make co-payments or co-insurance for these benefits in the past. Cost has been documented as one of the many barriers to appropriate use of preventive services and the intent was to reduce the barriers to care for these effective services.

This is a broad list, but it should be noted that not all preventive services that are important to women are included in the TF recommendations.

> **Box 15.1   Required women's preventive health and maternity services under the ACA**
>
> • Well-woman visits.
> • All FDA-approved contraception methods and counseling.
> • Mammograms.
> • Colonoscopies.
> • Blood pressure tests.
> • Sexually transmitted infections.
> • Domestic violence screenings and counseling.
> • HIV screening and counseling.
> • Breastfeeding support, counseling, and equipment, including breast pumps.
> • Gestational diabetes screening.
> • HPV testing as part of cervical cancer screening for women 30 years and older.
>
> References [90,92].

Forty-nine states also received funding to create a maternal, infant, and early childhood home-visiting program to reduce infant and maternal mortality by improving prenatal, maternal, and newborn health, child health and development, parenting skills, school readiness; reducing juvenile delinquency; and enhancing family economic self-sufficiency [92]. The new Personal Responsibility Education Program (PREP) allocates funding to states to educate adolescents about evidenced-based sex education and contraception to decrease teen pregnancy and sexually transmitted infections [81,89]. Title V funding has also been restored for the Abstinence Education Grant Program [89]. Finally, funds have been allocated to states to provide services to individuals and their families with, or at risk, of postpartum depression [92].

ACA exchanges will require a more uniform, fifty-state standard coverage of "essential benefits" in 2014. For the first time, maternity and newborn care are now considered an essential benefit under qualified health plans, prohibiting private insurers from adding charging for this benefit [2]. Other essential benefits that may impact women's health care coverage prior to or during pregnancy include mental health and substance use disorder services, including behavioral health treatment, and prescription drugs (Box 15.2) [90].

Comprehensive tobacco cessation services for pregnant women in Medicaid without cost sharing are also required under ACA. Specific recommendations for pregnant women include person-to-person psychosocial interventions that exceed minimal advice to quit, as well as tobacco-dependence interventions to pregnant smokers at the first prenatal visit and throughout the pregnancy [89,92].

Family planning services are not an essential benefit, but the ACA supports states who wish to establish family planning programs without a federal waiver to prenatal eligibility levels, thus making it easier for states to provide this service [89].

The ACA and reimbursement

With the expansion and improvement of insurance coverage, Congress also addressed limited access to health care providers. First, Congress designated family planning clinics and community health clinics as "essential community providers," thus requiring insurance

---

Box 15.2 Essential health benefits package

Essential health benefits, as defined in Section 1302(b) of the Patient Protection and Affordable Care Act, will include at least the following general categories:

- Ambulatory patient services.
- Emergency services.
- Hospitalization.
- Maternity and newborn care.
- Mental health and substance use disorder services, including behavioral health treatment.
- Prescription drugs.
- Rehabilitative and habilitative services and devices.
- Laboratory services.
- Preventive and wellness and chronic disease management.
- Pediatric services, including oral and vision care.

Adapted from National Conference of State Legislatures, Understanding Mandated Health Insurance Benefits. http://www.ncsl.org/issues-research/health/state-ins-mandates-and-aca-essential-benefits. aspx#Understanding Accessed October 5, 2012.

---

plans in the new exchanges to contract with these health centers and other safety-net providers [2,89]. The ACA also funds the establishment of interdisciplinary "community health teams" to support primary care, ob/gyn, and midwife-owned practices to serve as central coordinators of care [2,94].

Two other major changes specific to pregnant women were made under the ACA. First, free-standing birth centers are covered under Medicaid, including the licensed caregiver professional fee and the facility fee [81,89]. Second, as of January 2011, CNMs are now reimbursed by Medicare at the same rate as physicians, which should influence the reimbursement rates of Medicaid and private plans [2]. Currently, CNMs are reimbursed under Medicaid at less than 100% as compared to physicians in twenty-two states (Table 15.2). ACNM and ANA are working to correct this inequity using Medicare as the gold standard [91,95]. Altogether, these ACA reimbursement improvements should make it more financially viable for women to choose birth centers and midwives for care, thus mitigating the current shortage of maternity care providers [2].

Policies supporting breastfeeding

Breastfeeding is associated with many health benefits. Short- and long-term benefits to mothers include decreased risks of breast and ovarian cancers, diabetes, rheumatoid arthritis, and cardiovascular disease. For infants, breastfeeding decreases the incidence and severity of many infectious diseases, reduces infant mortality, and optimally supports neuro-development. Breastfeeding also decreases their risk of obesity later in childhood [96].

Multiple recommendations are available for families, health care providers, and for breastfeeding initiation and duration. The American Academy of Pediatrics recommends exclusive breastfeeding (no solids or other liquids) for the first 6 months of life, and then continued breastfeeding, with the introduction of iron-rich foods, for at least the first year of an infant's life [97]. The U.S. Department of Health and Human Services Healthy People 2020, the latest science-based, 10-year national objective plan, includes four

Table 15.4 Healthy people 2020 breastfeeding objectives.

Objectives	Baseline	Target
MICH-21: Increase the proportion of infants who are breastfed.		
MICH-21.1 Ever	74.0% of infants born in 2006 were ever breastfed as reported in 2007–2009	81.9%
MICH-21.2 At 6 months	43.5% of infants born in 2006 were breastfed at 6 months as reported in 2007–2009	60.6%
MICH-21.3 At 1 year	22.7% of infants born in 2006 were breastfed at 1 year as reported in 2007–2009	34.1%
MICH-21.4 Exclusively through 3 months	33.6% of infants born in 2006 were breastfed exclusively through 3 months as reported in 2007–2009	46.2%
MICH-21.5 Exclusively through 6 months	14.1% of infants born in 2006 were breastfed exclusively through 6 months as reported in 2007–2009	25.5%
MICH-22: Increase the proportion of employers that have worksite lactation support programs.	25% of employers reported providing an on-site lactation/mother's room in 2009	38%
MICH-23: Reduce the proportion of breastfed newborns who receive formula supplementation within the first 2 days of life.	24.2% of breastfed newborns born in 2006 received formula supplementation within the first 2 days of life as reported in 2007–2009	14.2%
MICH-24: Increase the proportion of live births that occur in facilities that provide recommended care for lactating mothers and their babies.	2.9% of 2007 live births occurred in facilities that provide recommended care for lactating mothers and their babies as reported in 2009	8.1%

U.S. Department of Health and Human Services. Healthy People 2020, Maternal, Child and Infant Health, MICH 21. December 2010. Available at http://www.cdc.gov/breastfeeding/policy/hp2010.htm.

major objectives related to breastfeeding (Table 15.4) [98]. AWHONN's position statement supports an even higher exclusive breastfeeding initiation rate of 90%, a 75% 6-month breastfeeding rate, and a 50% 1-year breastfeeding goal by 2025 [99].

State laws regarding breastfeeding

Many state laws have been enacted to achieve these goals and support a woman's choice to breastfeed. Forty-five states plus the District of Columbia specifically allow women to breastfeed in any public or private location. Twenty-eight states and the District of Columbia articulate that the act of breastfeeding is not indecent exposure. Twenty-four states and the District of Columbia have various laws related to breastfeeding in the workplace. For example, in Washington state, an employer may use the designation "infant friendly" on its promotional materials if the employer has an approved workplace breastfeeding policy. Twelve states exempt breastfeeding mothers from jury duty, and five states have encouraged development or have implemented a breastfeeding awareness education campaign. Several states have more unique laws such as California, which requires health departments to assist hospital staff in developing policies aimed at those patients ranked in the lowest 25% for exclusive breastfeeding rates. New York passed a law that allows a breastfed child under 1 year of age to accompany the mother to a correctional facility [100]. In 2011, Rhode Island became the first state to pass legislation prohibiting hospitals from providing free infant formula to mothers upon discharge [101]. Despite these improvements, many laws, states, and employers fail to support a woman's ability to breastfeed in all locations and to provide the necessary education and support.

Policy Recommendation: States should enact legislation that supports breastfeeding including laws that: (1) Allow women to breastfeed in any public or private location. (2) Encourage employers to implement an infant-friendly work environment through tax incentives. (3) Allocate funding to support breastfeeding education campaigns and training of local hospital staff. (4) Require local hospitals to prohibit distributing free infant formula.

Hospital breastfeeding policies fall short

Maternity practices and policies in hospitals and birth centers can also help achieve these aforementioned goals and increase initiation and duration of breastfeeding. The World Health Organization (WHO) and United Nations Children's Fund (UNICEF) Baby-Friendly Hospital Initiative outlined "Ten Steps to Successful Breastfeeding" in 1989 (Box 15.3), delineating evidence-based hospital practices to improve breastfeeding initiation, duration, and exclusivity [102]. To be designated as baby-friendly by WHO/UNICEF, a hospital must implement the "Ten Steps to Successful Breastfeeding" and comply with the International Code of Marketing of Breastmilk Substitutes, which requires that hospitals pay fair market value for infant formula and not promote items detrimental to breastfeeding, including discharge bags containing infant formula [103]. In 2011, only 4.5% of babies were born in U.S. hospitals with this designation [104].

Box 15.3   Ten steps to successful breastfeeding

Every facility providing maternity services and care for newborn infants should:

1. Have a written breastfeeding policy that is routinely communicated to all health care staff.
2. Train all health care staff in skills necessary to implement this policy.
3. Inform all pregnant women about the benefits and management of breastfeeding.
4. Help mothers initiate breastfeeding within half an hour of birth.
5. Show mothers how to breastfeed and how to maintain lactation even if they should be separated from their infants.
6. Give newborn infants no food or drink other than breast milk, unless medically indicated.
7. Practice rooming-in—that is, allow mothers and infants to remain together—24 hours a day.
8. Encourage breastfeeding on demand.
9. Give no artificial teats or pacifiers to breastfeeding infants.
10. Foster the establishment of breastfeeding support groups and refer mothers to them on discharge from the hospital or clinic.

Source: Protecting, Promoting and Supporting Breastfeeding: The Special Role of Maternity Services, a joint WHO/UNICEF statement published by the World Health Organization.

In 2007 and 2009, the Centers for Disease Control and Prevention invited all U.S. hospitals and birth centers that provide maternity care to participate in the first national Maternity Practices in Infant Nutrition and Care (mPINC) survey to determine the prevalence of facilities using maternity care practices consistent with the "Ten Steps to Successful Breastfeeding." The 2009 results were that most U.S. hospitals fall short. Although staff members at most hospitals provide prenatal breastfeeding education (93%) and teach mothers breastfeeding techniques (89%) and feeding cues (82%), few hospitals have model breastfeeding policies (14%), limit breastfeeding supplement use (22%), or support mothers after discharge (27%). The Joint Commission, which accredits and certifies U.S. hospitals, added exclusive breastfeeding in the hospital as a new quality of care measure in 2010 [105].

Beginning in 2012, the National Initiative for Children's Healthcare Quality (NICHQ), with support from the CDC, recruited and enrolled ninety hospitals in a 22-month learning collaborative with other participating hospitals to make system-level changes in order to become baby-friendly. Teams will work together and with national breastfeeding and quality improvement experts; regional collaboratives will be established to help participating teams work together and connect to local resources.

Policy Recommendations: (1) Hospitals aim to become baby-friendly under the WHO/ UNICEF designation by adopting evidence-based practices and apply to participate in this NICHQ project or similar programs as they become available. (2) Public health agencies review their individual CDC mPINC benchmark report and incorporate the breastfeeding measures into their quality standards. (3) The Joint Commission should incorporate all components of the Baby-Friendly Hospital Initiative into the requirements of accreditation of all maternity services.

New ACA breastfeeding policies in the workplace

Women comprise half of the U.S. workforce, therefore government and employer policies that support breastfeeding in the workplace are needed. Under the ACA in 2012, new health insurance plans must provide breastfeeding support, counseling, and equipment, including breast pumps, with no co-payments or deductibles [90,92]. In addition, a new law called the "Break Time for Nursing Mothers" amends the Fair Labor Standards Act of 1938 and requires employers with more than fifty employees to provide a reasonable break time for a nursing mother to express breast milk and provide adequate space other than a bathroom where the employee can pump her breast milk until the child is 1 year old [92]. AWHONN also recommends tax credits or other incentives for employers to facilitate lactation in the workplace, as well as enhanced family medical leave policies that provide opportunities for women to have extended maternity leave in order to fully establish breastfeeding [106].

Policy Recommendations: (1) Expand ACA requirements for breastfeeding support to all third-party payers. (2) Expand ACA law regarding reasonable break times for breastfeeding to all employers. (3) Adopt AWHONN breastfeeding in the workplace policies through state and federal legislation.

Summary

In this new era of the Affordable Care Act and its inherent political environment, it is important to remain focused on moving policy development forward. We need policy improvements in maternity care in order to respond to the national call to meet the triple aim—better care, better health outcomes, and lower cost. To achieve those goals, women need access to regular, affordable, and high-quality care, so they are healthy preconceptionally and prenatally and can optimize their chances for a normal birth. When appropriate policies exist within the health care system, maternity and other health care providers can practice to their broadest scope and provide unencumbered care in a collaborative and noncompetitive environment.

References

1. Hamilton B, Martin J, & Ventura S. (2010). Births: Preliminary data for 2009. U.S. Department of Health and Human Services. Contract No.: 3.
2. Sonfield A. (2010). The potential of health care reform to improve pregnancy-related services and outcomes. *Guttmacher Policy Review, 13*. Retrieved from: http://www.guttmacher.org/pubs/gpr/13/3/gpr130313.html.
3. Ranji U. (2011). Reproductive health care policy for women. Tutorials and presentations, Henry J. Kaiser Family Foundation.
4. Main E, Morton C, Hopkins D, Giuliani G, Melsop K, & Gould J. (2011). Cesarean deliveries, outcomes, and opportunities for change in California: Toward a public agenda for maternity care safety and quality. Retrieved from: http://www.cmqcc.org.
5. Wier L & Andrew R. (2011). The national hospital bill: The most expensive conditions by payer, 2008. Healthcare Cost and Utilization Project. Retrieved from: http://www.hcup-us.ahrq.gov/reports/statbriefs/sb107.pdf.
6. Ament LA. (2007). *Professional issues in midwifery*. Sudbury, MA: Jones and Bartlett.
7. Waldman R & Powell Kennedy H. (2011). Collaborative practice between obstetricians and midwives. *Obstetrics & Gynecology*, 118(3), 503–504.
8. Mann S. (2011). New reports announce competencies, action strategies for interprofessional collaboration. Washington, D.C.: Association of American Medical Colleges.
9. American College of Nurse-Midwives, Accreditation Commission for Midwifery Education, & American Midwifery Certification Board. (2011). Midwifery in the United States and the consensus model for APRN regulation.
10. American College of Nurse-Midwives & American College of Obstetricians and Gynecologists. (2011). Joint statement of practice relations between obstetrician-gynecologists and certified nurse-midwives/certified midwives. College statement of policy. Retrieved from: http://www.midwife.org/ACNM/files/ccLibraryFiles/Filename/000000000751/CollegeACNMPolicyStatementFeb2011_2.pdf.
11. Waldman R & Powell Kennedy H. (2012). The long and winding road to effective collaboration. *Obstetrics and Gynecology Clinics of North America*, 39(3), xix–xxii. Retrieved from: http://www.obgyn.theclinics.com/article/S0889-8545%2812%2900057-5/fulltext.
12. Anand Nijagal M & Wice M. (2012). Expanding access to midwifery care: Using one practice's success to create community change. *Journal of Midwifery & Women's Health*, 57(4), 376–380.

13. Kaplan LK. (2011). ACOG and ACNM publish shared principles to improve inter-professional cooperation in serving the needs of women. *Quickening*, 15.
14. Miller S, King T, Lurie P, & Choitz P. (1997). Certified nurse-midwife and physician collaborative practice piloting a survey on the internet. *Journal of Nurse-Midwifery*, *42*, 308–315.
15. Payne P & King V. (1998). A model of nurse-midwife and family physician collaborative care in a combined academic and community setting. *Journal of Nurse-Midwifery*, *43*(1), 19–26.
16. Wingeier R, Bloch S, & Kvale J. (1988). A description of a CNM-family physician joint practice in a rural setting. *Journal of Nurse-Midwifery*, *33*(2), 86–82.
17. Hueston W & Murray M. (1998). A three-tier model for the delivery of rural obstetrical care using a nurse-midwife and family physician copractice. *Journal of Rural Health*, *3*, 283–290.
18. Mengel M & Phillips W. (1987). The quality of obstetric care in family practice: Are family physicians as safe as obstetricians? *Journal of Family Practice*, *24*, 159–164.
19. American Academy of Family Physicians. (1994). 1993–1994 compendium of AAFP positions on selected health issues. Kansas City: American Academy of Family Physicians.
20. American Academy of Family Physicians. (2011). Nurse-midwife, certified 2012. Retrieved from: http://www.aafp.org/online/en/home/policy/policies/n/nursemidwivescertified.html. Accessed November 1, 2011.
21. American Society of Anesthesiologists. (2010). ASA supports new health care provider transparency legislation. Retrieved from: http://www.asahq.org/news/asanews051310.htm.
22. American Academy of Family Physicians. (2012). Primary care for the 21st century: Ensuring a quality, physician-led team for every patient.
23. Susman J. (2010). It's time to collaborate—not compete—with NPs. *Journal of Family Practice*, *59*(12), 672.
24. Institute of Medicine. (2011). The future of nursing: Leading change, advancing health. Washington, DC: The National Academies Press.
25. American Nurses Association. (2012). Standards and scope of practice. Retrieved from: http://www.nursingworld.org/scopeandstandardsofpractice. Accessed October 5, 2012.
26. American College of Nurse-Midwives. (2012). *Core competencies for basic midwifery practice*.
27. American College of Nurse-Midwives. (2006). After years of hard work, victory on EMTALA. Contract No.: 6.
28. Rostant D & Cady R. (1999). *AWHONN liability issues in perinatal Nursing*, 2nd ed. Philadelphia: Lippincott Williams & Wilkins.
29. American College of Nurse-Midwives. (2008). Certified nurse-midwives in Illinois. Retrieved from: http://www.midwife.org/index.asp?bid=59&cat=11&button=Search&rec=186. Accessed June 27, 2012.
30. Cunningham R. (2010). Tapping the potential of the health care workforce: Scope-of-practice and payment policies for advanced practice nurses and physician assistants. Retrieved from: http://www.nhpf.org/library/background-papers/BP76_SOP_07-06-2010.pdf.
31. King J, Director of Government Relations, ACNM. E-mail correspondence, 2012.
32. Collins MK. (2005). Midwifery Model Practice Act.
33. Federation of State Medical Boards. (2006). Trends in physician regulation. 2006.
34. APRN Consensus Work Group & the National Council of State Boards of Nursing APRN Advisory Committee. (2008). Consensus model for APRN regulation: Licensure, accreditation, certification, & education.
35. American College of Nurse-Midwives. (2009). Principles for licensing and regulating midwives.
36. Kline Kaplan L. (2002). Join the action. *Quickening*, 2.
37. American Association of Retired Persons. (2010). AARP policy supplement: Scope of practice for advance practice registered nurses. Retrieved from: http://championnursing.org/sites/default/files/2010 AARPPolicySupplementScopeAvailable from: ofPractice.pdf.

38. Federal Trade Commission. (2012). FTC staff: West Virginia should consider expanding advanced practice registered nurses' role in patient care. Retrieved from: http://www.ftc.gov/opa/2012/09/wva.shtm. Accessed September 29, 2012.

39. Safriet B. (2010). Federal options for maximizing the value of advanced practice nurses in providing quality, cost-effective health care. Institute of Medicine.

40. Fairman J, Rowe J, Hassmiller S, & Shalala D. (2011). Broadening the scope of nursing practice. *New England Journal of Medicine, 364*, 193–196.

41. Iglehart J. (2011). The uncertain future of Medicare and graduate medical education. *New England Journal of Medicine, 365*(14), 1340–1345.

42. Carrier E, Yee T, & Stark L. (2011). Matching supply to demand: Addressing the U.S. primary care workforce shortage. Policy analysis. Retrieved from: http://www.nihcr.org/PCP_Workforce.pdf.

43. Johantgen M, Fountain L, Zangaro G, Newhouse R, Stanik-Hutt J, & White K. (2012). Comparison of labor and delivery care provided by certified nurse-midwives and physicians: A systematic review, 1990 to 2008. *Womens Health Issues, 22*(1), e73–81.

44. Hansen-Turton T. (2009). NNCC research shows insurer contracting policies threaten success of health care reform. Retrieved from: http://www.phmc.org/site/index.php?option=com_content&view=article&id=372:nncc-research-shows-insurer-contracting-policies-threaten-success-of-health-care-reform&catid=29&Itemid=1465.

45. Craven G & Ober S. (2009). Massachusetts nurse practitioners step up as one solution to the primary care access problem: A political success story. *Policy, Politics, & Nursing Practice, 10*(2), 94–100.

46. MedPAC. (2006). Report to the Congress: Medicare payment policy.

47. Cragin L & Kennedy H. (2006). Linking obstetric and midwifery practice with optimal outcomes. *JOGNN, 35*(6), 779–785.

48. Institute of Medicine Committee on Quality of Health Care in America. (2001). *Crossing the quality chasm: A new health system for the 21st century.* Washington, DC: National Academies Press. Retrieved from: http://www.nap.edu/openbook.php?isbn=0309072808.

49. Queenan J. (2011). How to stop the relentless rise in cesarean deliveries. *Obstetrics & Gynecology, 118*(2, Part 1), 199–200.

50. Darlington A, McBroom K, & Warwick S. (2011). A northwest collaborative practice model. *Obstetrics & Gynecology, 118*(3), 673–677.

51. National Priorities Partnership. (2011). Input to the Secretary of Health and Human Services on priorities for the national quality strategies. Retrieved from: http://www.qualityforum.org/Setting_Priorities/National_Priorities_Partnership_Input_to_HHS_on_the_National_Quality_Strategy.aspx.

52. National Quality Forum. (2012). NPP action teams. Retrieved from: http://www.qualityforum.org/Setting_Priorities/NPP/NPP_Action_Teams.aspx.

53. Hutchison M, Ennis L, Shaw-Battista J, Delgado A, Myers K, Cragin L, et al. (2011). Great minds don't think alike: Collaborative maternity care at San Francisco General Hospital. *Obstetrics & Gynecology, 118*(3), 678–682.

54. Shaw-Battista J, Fineberg A, Boehler B, Skubic B, Woolley D, & Tilton Z. (2011). Obstetrician and nurse-midwife collaboration: Successful public health and private practice partnership. *Obstetrics & Gynecology, 118*(3), 663–672.

55. American Nurses Association. (2012). Conditions of participation. Retrieved from: http://www.nursingworld.org/conditionsofparticipation. Accessed October 5, 2012.

56. Schuiling K. (2011). ACNM credentialing and hospital privileging survey.

57. Weston M. (2011). Medicare and Medicaid programs: Reform of hospital and critical access hospital conditions of participation.

58. Aiken L, Clarke S, Sloane D, Sochalski J, & Silber J. (2002). Hospital nurse staffing and patient mortality, nurse burnout and job satisfaction. *Journal of the American Medical Association, 288*(16), 1987–1993.

59. Aiken L, Sloane D, Cimiotti J, Clarke S, Flynn L, & Seago J. (2010). Implications of the California nurse staffing mandate for other states. Health Services Research. *45*(4), 904–921.

60. Hodnett E, Gates S, Hofmeyr G, & Sakala C. (2003). Continuous support for women during childbirth. *Cochrane Database of Systematic Reviews, 3*. Art. No.: CD003766.

61. Kennell J & Klaus M. (2002). Continuous nursing support during labor. *Journal of the American Medical Association, 288*(11), 1373–1381.

62. Hofmeyr G, Nikodem V, Wolman W, Chalmers B, & Kramer T. (1991). Companionship to modify the clinical birth environment: Effects on progress and perceptions of labour and breastfeeding. *British Journal of Obstetrics and Gynecology, 98*(8), 756–764.

63. Association of Womens' Health Obstetric and Neonatal Nurses. (2011). Guidelines for professional registered nurse staffing for perinatal units. Retrieved from: http://www.awhonn. org/awhonn/store/productDetail.do?productCode=SG-910.

64. Detman L. (2012). Florida perinatal quality collaborative. Retrieved from: http://health.usf. edu/publichealth/chilescenter/services.html-Florida%20Perinatal%20Quality%20 Collaborative. Accessed May 5, 2012.

65. Scott J. (2011). VBAC: A common sense approach. *Obstetrics & Gynecology, 118*, 342–350.

66. Midwives of WA State Transport Guideline Committee with the Ad Hoc Physician-Licensed Midwife Workgroup of the WA State Perinatal Advisory Committee. (2011). Planned out-of-hospital birth transport guideline. Retrieved from: http://www.washingtonmidwives.org/docu-ments/MAWS-OOH-transport-policy0211.pdf.

67. Socol M. (2010). Trial of labor versus elective repeat cesarean: An administrator's perspective. *Seminars in Perinatology, 34*(5), 311–313.

68. Klagholz B & Strunk A. (2009). Overview of the 2009 ACOG survey on professional liability. *ACOG Clinical Review, 14*, 1–16.

69. Yang T, Mello M, Subramanian S, & Studdert D. (2009). Relationship between malpractice litigation pressure and rates of Cesarian section and vaginal birth after Cesarian section. *Medical Care, 47*, 234–242.

70. Positioning Midwifery in Health System Reform: A Policy Review. (2010).

71. Page L. (2011). Ohio's "I'm sorry" law doesn't protect against admitted errors. Retrieved from: http://www.outpatientsurgery.net/news/2011/11/28-Ohio-s-I-m-Sorry-Law-Doesn-t-Protect-Against-Admitted-Errors. Accessed January 22, 2012.

72. Sorry Works Coalition. (2011). States with apology laws. Retrieved from: http://www.sorry-works.net/laws.phtml. Accessed January 22, 2012.

73. The Doctors Company. (2006). "I'm sorry" law differs in each state. Retrieved from: http://www.thedoctors.com/KnowledgeCenter/PatientSafety/Alerts/CON_ID_000167. Accessed January 22, 2012.

74. Johnson K, Atrash H, & Johnson A. (2008). Policy and finance for preconception care: Opportunities for today and the future. *Women's Health Issues, 188*, S2–S9.

75. Guttmacher Institute. (2011). Title X–supported family planning services nationally and in each state. News in Context. Retrieved from: http://www.guttmacher.org/media/inthe-news/2011/02/16/index.html. Accessed December 1, 2011.

76. Ranji U. (2011). Reproductive health care policy for women: Henry J. Kaiser Family Foundation. Retrieved from: http://www.kaiseredu.org/Tutorials-and-Presentations/Reproductive-Health-Care-Policy-for-Women-in-the-United-States.aspx. Accessed December 1, 2011.

77. Salganicoff A. (2008). Women's health policy: Coverage and access to care: Henry J. Kaiser Family Foundation. Retrieved from: http://www.kaiseredu.org/Tutorials-and-Presentations/Womens-Health-Policy-Coverage-and-Access.aspx. Accessed December 15, 2011.

78. Sjoborg K & Eskild A. (2009). Vaccination against human papillomavirus—an impact on pre-term delivery? Estimations based on literature review. *Acta Obstetricia et Gynecologica Scandinavica, 88*(3), 255–260.

79. Lu B, Kumar A, Castellsagué X, & Giuliano AR. (2011). Efficacy and safety of prophylactic vaccines against cervical HPV infection and diseases among women: A systematic review & meta-analysis. *BMC Infectious Diseases, 11:13.*

80. The U.S. Equal Employment Opportunity Commission. (2008). Facts about pregnancy discrimination 2008. Retrieved from: http://www.eeoc.gov/facts/fs-preg.html. Accessed December 1, 2011.

81. Corry M, Childbirth Connection. E-mail regarding benefits of health care reform for the patients we serve, 2011.

82. Abu-Ghanem S, Sheiner E, Sherf M, Wiznitzer A, Sergienko R, & Shoham-Vardi I. (2011). Lack of prenatal care in a traditional community: Trends and perinatal outcomes. *Archives of Gynecology and Obstetrics.* Epub November 29, 2011.

83. Robertson R, Squires D, Garber T, Collins S, & Doty M. (2012). Realizing health reform's potential. Retrieved from: http://www.commonwealthfund.org/~/media/Files/Publications/Issue Brief/2012/Jul/1606_Robertson_oceans_apart_reform_brief.pdf.

84. Department of Health and Human Services. (1999). The Newborns' and Mothers' Health Protection Act of 1996. Retrieved from: http://library.findlaw.com/1999/Jan/6/127039.html. Accessed January 13, 2012.

85. Baker L & Chan J. (2007). Laws requiring health plans to provide direct access to obstetricians and gynecologists, and use of cancer screening by women. *Health Services Research, 42*(3, Part 1), 990–1007.

86. Cauchi R. (2010). Managed care state laws and regulations, including consumer and provider protections. Retrieved from: http://www.ncsl.org/default.aspx?tabid=14320.

87. U.S. Department of Health and Human Services. (2012). Understanding the Affordable Care Act. Washington, D.C.

88. National Conference of State Legislatures. (2012). Covering young adults through their parents' or guardians' health policy. Retrieved from: http://www.ncsl.org/default.aspx?tabid=14497. Accessed January 13, 2012.

89. Salganicoff A. (2010). Health care reform: Impact on women's health coverage and access to care. Tutorials and presentations, Henry J. Kaiser Family Foundation.

90. Cauchi R. (2011). State health insurance mandates and the ACA essential benefits provision. Denver, CO: National Conference of State Legislatures.

91. Summers L, American Nurses Association. E-mail, 2011.

92. Ewig B. (2011). The Patient Protection and Affordable Care Act: Summary of key maternal and child health related highlights with updates on status of implementation. Washington, D.C.: Association of Maternal & Child Health Programs.

93. Centers for Medicaid and Medicare Services. (2012). Strong start initiative improving maternal and infant health. In: CMS Office of Public Affairs, editor. Baltimore, MD.

94. H.R. 3590 Patient Protection and Affordable Care Act. Sect. 3602 (2009).

95. King J, Director of Government Relations, ACNM.

96. National Initiative for Childrens' Healthcare Quality. (2012). Best Fed Beginnings Project summary. Retrieved from: http://www.nichq.org/our_projects/BFB One-Pager March 2012 FINAL.pdf. Accessed May 4, 2012.

97. American Academy of Pediatrics. (2005). Breastfeeding and the use of human milk. *Pediatrics, 115*(2), 496–506.

98. Centers for Disease Control and Prevention. (2011). Healthy People 2020 objectives for the nation. Retrieved from: http://www.cdc.gov/breastfeeding/policy/hp2010.htm. Accessed January 20, 2012.

99. Association of Women's Health, Obstetric and Neonatal Nurses. (2007). Breastfeeding position statement. Retrieved from: http://www.awhonn.org/awhonn/content.do?name=05_HealthPolicyLegislation/5H_PositionStatements.htm. Accessed January 20, 2012.

100. National Conference of State Legislatures. (2011). Breastfeeding laws. Retrieved from: http://www.ncsl.org/issues-research/health/breastfeeding-state-laws.aspx. Accessed January 20, 2012.
101. Go Local Prov Health Team. (2011). RI eliminates free infant formula giveaways at hospitals in move to boost breastfeeding. Go Local Prov Retrieved from: http://www.golocalprov.com/health/new-ri-first-state-in-us-to-eliminate-free-infant-formula/.
102. World Health Organization. (2012). Exclusive breastfeeding. Retrieved from: http://www.who.int/nutrition/topics/exclusive_breastfeeding/en/. Accessed January 20, 2012.
103. World Health Organization. (1981). International code of marketing of breast-milk substitutes. Geneva, Switzerland.
104. Centers for Disease Control and Prevention. (2012). Breastfeeding report card—United States. Retrieved from: http://www.cdc.gov/breastfeeding/data/reportcard.html. Accessed January 20, 2012.
105. Joint Commission. (2011). Specifications manual for Joint Commission—national quality care measures: perinatal care. Retrieved from: http://manual.jointcommission.org/releases/TJ2011A/PerinatalCare.html. Accessed January 20, 2012.
106. Association of Women's Health Obstetrics and Neonatal Nurses. (2008). Breastfeeding and lactation in the workplace position statement. Retrieved from: http://www.awhonn.org/awhonn/content.do?name=05_HealthPolicyLegislation/5H_PositionStatements.htm. Accessed January 20, 2012.

Resources for physiologic pregnancy and childbirth

Maternity Care Health Professions Associations

American Academy of Family Physicians, www.aafp.org.
American College of Nurse-Midwives, www.midwife.org.
American Congress of Obstetricians and Gynecologists, www.acog.org.
Association of Women's Health, Obstetric and Neonatal Nurses, www.awhonn.org.
Midwives Alliance of North America, http://mana.org/.
National Association of Certified Professional Midwives, www.nacpm.org.

Advocacy, Consumer, and Related Organizations

Centering Healthcare, https://www.centeringhealthcare.org/pages/centering-model/pregnancy-over
    view.php.
Childbirth Connection, www.childbirthconnection.org.
Coalition for Improving Maternity Services, http://www.motherfriendly.org/.
Lamaze International, http://www.lamazeinternational.org/.
March of Dimes, http://www.marchofdimes.com/.

Quality Organizations and Maternity Care Measures

American Medical Association and the National Committee for Quality Assurance, Maternity Care
    Performance Measurement Set, http://www.ama-assn.org/resources/doc/cqi/no-index/maternity-
    care-measures.pdf.
California Maternal Quality Care Collaborative, http://www.cmqcc.org/.
Joint Commission, Perinatal Care Measures, http://manual.jointcommission.org/releases/
    TJC2011A/PerinatalCare.html.
National Quality Forum, Endorsement Summary: Perinatal and Reproductive Health Measures,
    http://www.qualityforum.org/Projects/n-r/Perinatal_Care_Endorsement_Maintenance_2011/
    Perinatal_and_Reproductive_Healthcare_Endorsement_Maintenance_2011.aspx.
World Health Organization, Care in Normal Birth: A Practical Guide, Safe Motherhood, http://
    www.who.int/maternal_child_adolescent/documents/who_frh_msm_9624/en/.

Supporting a Physiologic Approach to Pregnancy and Birth: A Practical Guide, First Edition.
Edited by Melissa D. Avery.
© 2013 John Wiley & Sons, Inc. Published 2013 by John Wiley & Sons, Inc.

Maternity care data, guides, and tools

BMI calculator, http://nhlbisupport.com/bmi/.

California Department of Public Health, Model Hospital Policy Recommendations On-Line Toolkit, http://www.cdph.ca.gov/healthinfo/healthyliving/childfamily/Pages/MainPageofBreast feedingToolkit.aspx.

Centers for Disease Control and Prevention, National Vital Statistics System, http://www.cdc.gov/nchs/nvss.htm.

Childbirth Connection, Rights of Childbearing Women, http://www.childbirthconnection.org/pdfs/rights_childbearing_women.pdf.

Childbirth Connection, Transforming Maternity Care, http://transform.childbirthconnection.org/.

Holistic Pregnancy & Childbirth, Center for Spirituality and Healing, http://www.takingcharge.csh.umn.edu/explore-healing-practices/holistic-pregnancy-childbirth.

Lamaze International, Introduction to the Six Lamaze Healthy Birth Practices, http://www.lamaze international.org/HealthyBirthPractices.

March of Dimes Less than 39 Weeks Toolkit, http://www.marchofdimes.com/professionals/medicalresources_39weeks.html.

National Center for Complementary and Alternative Medicine, http://nccam.nih.gov/.

NHS Institute for Innovation and Improvement, Maternity Improvement: Optimizing Opportunities for Normal Birth and Reducing Intervention Rates, 2013, http://www.institute.nhs.uk/quality_and_value/introduction/improving_maternity_care.html.

Northern New England Perinatal Quality Improvement Network, VBAC Resources, http://www.nnepqin.org/VBAC.asp.

Royal College of Midwives Campaign for Normal Birth, http://www.rcmnormalbirth.org.uk/.

U.S. Breastfeeding Committee Toolkit for Implementing Exclusive Breastfeeding Core Measure, http://www.usbreastfeeding.org/HealthCare/HospitalMaternityCenterPractices/Toolkit ImplementingTJCCoreMeasure/tabid/184/Default.aspx.

U.S. Department of Health and Human Services, Office of Disease Prevention and Health Promotion, Healthy People 2020, Maternal Infant and Child Health Objectives, http://www.healthy people.gov/2020/topicsobjectives2020/objectiveslist.aspx?topicId=26#93911.

Acupuncture and acupressure

Websites, associations, and organizations

Acupoint Locator, http://www.acupuncture.com/.

American Association of Acupuncture and Oriental Medicine, http://www.aaaom.edu/.

American Organization for Bodywork Therapies of Asia, http://www.aobta.org/.

Associated Bodywork & Massage Professionals, http://www.abmp.com.

Debra Betts website, http://acupuncture.rhizome.net.nz/.

Federation of Acupuncture and Oriental Medicine Regulatory Agencies, http://www.faomra.org/.

National Acupuncture and Oriental Medicine Alliance, http://www.acuall.org/.

National Certification Commission for Acupuncture and Oriental Medicine, http://www.nccaom.org/.

National Institutes of Health's MedlinePlus, http://www.nlm.nih.gov/medlineplus/.

Webinars, http://medigogy.com/archives.

World Federation of Acupuncture-Moxibustion Societies, http://www.wfas.org.cn/en/.

Books

Baur, Cathryn. (1987). *Acupressure for Women*. Langhorne, PA: Crossing Press.
Betts, Debra. (2006). *The Essential Guide to Acupuncture in Pregnancy and Childbirth*. East Sussex, UK: Journal of Chinese Medicine.
Maciocia, Giovanni. (2011). *Obstetrics and Gynecology in Chinese Medicine*. Beijing: Elsevier.
Roemer, A.T. (2005). *Medical Acupuncture in Pregnancy—a Textbook*. New York: Thieme.
West, Zita. (2008). *Acupuncture in Pregnancy and Childbirth*, 2nd ed. New York: Elsevier.
Yates, S. (2003). *Shiatsu for Midwives*. London: BFM.

Aromatherapy

Alliance for International Aromatherapists, http://www.alliance-aromatherapists.org.
National Cancer Institutes at the National Institutes of Health, Aromatherapy and Essential Oils, http://www.cancer.gov/cancertopic/pdq/cam/aromatherapy/HealthProfessionals/page2.
Tiran, D. (2000). Massage and Aromatherapy. In D. Tiran & S. Mack, eds., *Complementary Therapies for Pregnancy and Childbirth*, 2nd ed. (pp. 129–167). Edinburgh: Ballière Tindall.

Touch therapies

Center for Reiki Research, www.centerforreikiresearch.org/.
Healing Touch, www.healingtouch.net.
Healing Touch International, Inc., www.healingtouchinternational.org.
Healing Touch online module, Taking Charge of Your Health, Center for Spirituality and Healing, http://www.takingcharge.csh.umn.edu/explore-healing-practices/healing-touch.
International Center for Reiki Training, www.reiki.org.
Reiki online module, Taking Charge of Your Health, Center for Spirituality and Healing, http://www.takingcharge.csh.umn.edu/explore-healing-practices/reiki.
Therapeutic Touch online module, Taking Charge of Your Health, Center for Spirituality and Healing, http://www.takingcharge.csh.umn.edu/explore-healing-practices/therapeutic-touch.
Touchstone Process, http://www.centerforreikiresearch.org/RRTouchstone.aspx.

Water immersion

Garland D. (2010). *Revisiting Waterbirth: An Attitude to Care*, 3rd ed. New York: Palgrave Macmillan.
Waterbirth International, http://www.waterbirth.org/.

Out-of-hospital birth

American Association of Birth Centers, www.birthcenters.org/.
Home Birth Consensus Summit, http://www.homebirthsummit.org/summit-outcomes.html.

Additional books, monographs, and reports for care providers and clients

Boston Women's Health Book Collective. (2008). *Our Bodies, Ourselves: Pregnancy and Birth*. New York: Simon & Schuster.

Childbirth Connection. (2008). *Evidence-Based Maternity Care: What It Is and What It Can Achieve.* New York: Childbirth Connection, the Reforming States Group, and the Milbank Memorial Fund.

England, P., & Horowitz R. (1998). *Birthing from Within.* Albuquerque, NM: Partera Press.

Gabriel, Cynthia. (2011). *Natural Hospital Birth: The Best of Both Worlds.* Boston: Harvard Common Press.

Goer, H., & Romano, A. (2012). *Optimal Care in Childbirth: The Case for a Physiologic Approach.* Seattle: Classic Day Publishing.

Hale, M.F., & Chalmers, L. (1994). *The Childbirth Kit: Ideas and Images to Help You Through Labor.* Spring, TX: Swanstone Press.

Institute of Medicine of the National Academies. (2001). *Crossing the Quality Chasm: A New Health System for the 21st Century.* Washington, DC: National Academies Press.

Interprofessional Education Collaborative Expert Panel. (2011). *Core Competencies for Interprofessional Collaborative Practice: Report of an Expert Panel.* Washington, DC: Interprofessional Education Collaborative.

Simkin, P. (2008). *The Birth Partner: A Complete Guide to Childbirth for Dads, Doulas, and All Other Labor Companions*, 3rd ed. Boston: Harvard Common Press.

Simkin, P., & Ancheta, R. (2011). *The Labor Progress Handbook: Early Interventions to Prevent and Treat Dystocia*, 3rd ed. Oxford: Wiley-Blackwell.

Wagner, Marsden, with Stephanie Gunning. (2006). *Creating Your Birth Plan: The Definitive Guide to a Safe and Empowering Birth.* New York: Penguin Group.

Index

action potentials 19, 22
acupuncture/acupressure 8, 9, 25, 38, 56,
    58, 97, 138, 140, 141, 183,
    197–226, 332
  definition 198
  Eastern theories 199–203
  history 199
  meridians 202
  pregnancy and postpartum 209
    breech presentation 214–15
      moxibustion 214–15
    carpel tunnel 211, 212
    common uses table 209
    contraindicated acupoints 209
    emotional health (anxiety,
      depression) 219–21
    Yintang point 219–21
    labor encouragement 215–16
      spleen 6 point 216–18
    labor pain 218
      spleen 6 point 218
    low back pain 213
    nausea and vomiting 210
      P6 acupressure and
        acupuncture 210–212
  safety 207
  training, licensure
    acupressure 222
    acupuncture 221
      other regulated providers 222

Western theories 203–7
  acupoints 204
  acupuncture stimulation 206
  cupping 203, 205
  mechanism of action 207
adrenocorticoptroic hormone
    (ACTH) 15, 17
Affordable Care Act (ACA) 5, 301, 307,
    316–20, 324
American Academy of Family
    Physicians 5, 231, 294, 302, 331
American Academy of
    Pediatrics 5, 231
American Association of Birth
    Centers 254, 264, 333
American College of Nurse-Midwives 5,
    34, 58, 64, 92, 231, 251, 281,
    284, 302, 331
  ACNM Home Birth Practice
    Handbook 254, 264
  Appropriate Use of Technology in
    Childbirth 121, 254
  Consensus Statement Supporting
    Healthy and Normal Physiologic
    Childbirth 5, 49, 251
  philosophy 34, 80, 121
American College (Congress) of
    Obstetricians and Gynecologists
    5, 6, 57, 58, 167, 231, 269, 270,
    291, 292, 294, 302–4, 313, 331

Supporting a Physiologic Approach to Pregnancy and Birth: A Practical Guide, First Edition.
Edited by Melissa D. Avery.
© 2013 John Wiley & Sons, Inc. Published 2013 by John Wiley & Sons, Inc.

American College (Congress)
    of Obstetricians and
    Gynecologists (*cont'd*)
  Joint statement of practice relations
    between obstetrician-
    gynecologists and certified
    nurse-midwives/certified
    midwives 302
  obstetric analgesia and anesthesia 30
American College of Osteopathic
    Obstetricians and
    Gynecologists 5, 281
American Medical Association (AMA)
    6, 34, 305, 331
  Physician Consortium for Performance
    Improvement 6
anticipatory guidance 29, 33, 34, 43, 51, 136
aromatherapy 58, 97, 98, 125, 138, 141,
    166, 173–95, 333
  application 179–80
    cautions 184
  botanical medicines 175–6
  within botanical medicines 175
    continuum of plant medicines 176
  chemical constituents 179
  credentialing 191
  definition 174
  evidence for therapeutic effects 184–6
    in labor and birth 186
    perineal healing 187
    postpartum 187
  history 174
  incorporating into practice 188–91
  physiological effects 178
  processing of essential oils 177–8
  safe in pregnancy 183
  safety 182–3
    skin sensitivity 182
    toxicity 180–182
art of doing 'nothing' well 8, 101, 251
Association of Women's Health
    Obstetrical, and Neonatal
    Nurses (AWHONN) 5, 58, 64,
    91, 93, 94, 167, 242, 294, 311,
    321, 323, 331
Autonomic nervous system 128

birth centers *see* out-of-hospital births
Birth plan *see* birth preferences
birth preferences 40, 42, 44, 252
breastfeeding 31, 36, 38, 39, 41, 53,
    57, 69, 142, 232, 244–6, 263,
    265, 295, 308, 311, 314,
    319–23, 332
  increased initiation in midwife
    lead care 31
  support for mothers 5
Business of Being Born 254, 266

California Maternal Quality Care
    Collaboration 4, 312, 331
Centering Pregnancy 36–7, 41
Centers for Medicare and Medicaid
    Services (CMS) Center for
    Medicare and Medicaid
    Innovation 6
  Strong Start for Mothers and
    Newborns 6
cervical cancer screening 5, 314,
    316, 319
cesarean section
  breech presentation and 214, 215
  cesarean delivery 4, 5
  EFM contributions to 59
  liability and 33
  nurse-patient ratio contributions to 93
  overused interventions 41, 93, 310
  in overweight 32
  percent of births 229
  post partum stay 316
  preexisting condition 315, 316
  previous cesarean 4
  quality measurement 234, 312
  rate 3, 4, 6, 29, 31, 37, 59, 92,
    231, 301
    reduced with continuous labor
    support 92, 101
  relaxation techniques and 123
  touch therapies and 123, 139
  waterbirth and 160
Chakra system
  Healing touch 135
  Seven chakras 134

change on maternity units 229–49
  adapting the electronic health
    record 238
  barriers to change 236–7
  case study 240, 243, 245
  change process 233–9
    FOCUS 234
    Plan, Do, Check, and Act
      (PDCA) 234, 235
  environment 232–3
  leadership 234
  staff education 237
  transformed labor unit 239
Childbirth Connection 39, 84, 92, 271,
  331, 332, 334
  Blueprint for Action: Steps toward a
    High-Quality, High-Value
    Maternity Care System 6,
    232, 291
  Maternity Care Shared Decision
    Making Initiative 41
  Transforming Maternity Care 254
  2020 Vision for High-Quality, High
    Value Maternity Care
    System 291
Childbirth education 36, 38, 39,
  43, 44, 105, 107, 120,
  125, 261
Coalition for Improving Maternity
  Services 137, 331
  Mother-Friendly Childbirth
    Initiative 232
Collaborative practice 9, 275–99,
  302–4
comfort 8, 39–44, 51, 52, 55–8, 63,
  65–8, 70
  nonpharmacologic measures 58, 125
  physical support 96, 231–2
  promoting 57, 58, 79–87, 97
comfort, conceptual 80–89
  art of nursing 80–81
  definition 82
  Kolcaba's theory 81–3, 87
  labor pain and 83–5
  measures 39, 43, 83, 85, 125
  midwifery and 85–7

comfort line 83
common discomforts of pregnancy 37–8,
  124, 127, 158
  constipation 37, 38, 127, 139, 142,
    183, 209
  low back pain 37, 38, 44, 95, 123, 127,
    138, 139, 142, 213
  nausea and vomiting 37, 38, 41, 138,
    141, 183, 202, 209–12
Complementary and Alternative Medicine
  (CAM) *see* Integrative
  Therapies
Complementary and Alternative
  Medicine Survey of
  Hospitals 125
confidence xi, 7, 8, 25, 38, 39, 57, 92,
  101, 236, 242, 262, 266
  care providers 7
  climate/culture of 29, 39–40, 43, 261
    birth setting 40, 261
    meet and greet appointments 39
  labor nurses 237, 238
  out-of-hospital practitioners 261
Consensus Statement Supporting Healthy
  and Normal Physiologic
  Childbirth 5, 49, 251
continuous labor support 41, 91–103,
  137, 231, 232, 237
  barriers to 94–5
  benefits 92
  components of 94–9
  labor support providers 92–3
    nurses 93–4
  reassurance 25, 38, 96, 98–9, 101, 136,
    138, 242, 265
control (women in pregnancy and
  birth) 7, 31, 34, 35, 39, 41, 42,
  82–5, 96, 101, 138, 159, 232,
  252, 258, 259, 262
Coping with Labor Algorithm 49,
  55–7, 96
corpus luteum 15, 22
corticotropin-relasing hormone
  (CRH) 14, 16, 17, 22
cortisol 17, 20, 24, 82, 124, 138,
  184, 206

Creating Your Birth Plan: The Definitive
        Guide to a Safe and
        Empowering Birth 42
culture change 101, 231
cytokines 15, 17, 22

dehydroepiandrosterone sulfate
        (DHEAS) 16, 17
delayed cord cutting 41, 44, 49,
        69, 295
Dick-Read, Grantly 95, 106, 253
directed (Valsalva) pushing 63, 64
doula 36, 40, 42–4, 51, 56, 57, 70, 83,
        92–5, 120, 136, 166, 291,
        293, 314

emotions in pregnancy and labor 92
endocrine adaptations in
        pregnancy 15–16
    growth factors 15
    maternal-placental-fetal unit 15
endorphins 84, 206, 219
epidural analgesia 84, 161, 186, 232
    adverse effects of 84
    in birth centers and home birth 257
    in delayed pushing 244
    with second stage labor 243
epidural rate 229, 230, 242
estrogen 15, 16, 18, 21, 23, 24, 214, 215
    cervical remodeling 17
    estriol 16
    estrogen dominance 13, 21
    labor initiation 19
ethics
    in acupuncture 222
    in aromatherapy 191
    in interprofessional practice 278, 295
    in providing touch therapy 135–6
Evidence Based Maternity Care 6, 291
    Milbank Report 41, 92
evidenced-based care/practice 36, 40, 41,
        43, 50–52, 67, 69, 92, 94, 121,
        277, 291, 295, 323

fear-tension-pain cycle 39, 95, 106, 253
fetal growth 13, 19

fetal heart monitoring
    continuous 58, 59, 97, 99, 157, 166, 167
    intermittent auscultation 49, 54, 58, 59,
        70, 167, 235, 241, 259, 265,
        295, 311

gap junctions 16, 19–22
Gate Control Theory of Pain 124, 160
Gross Domestic Product (GDP) % for
        healthcare 4
group prenatal care 29, 36–7, 43, 318
    centering model 36–7, 41, 292, 331

Healing Touch 120–122, 126–30,
        139–41, 333
health policy *see* Women's health and
        maternity care health policy
health-seeking behaviors 81, 82, 87
Healthy People 2020 3, 321, 332
hospital charges 4, 302
    liveborn infant 4
    pregnancy and childbirth 4, 302
Hover-Kramer, Dorothea 156
    Creating Healing Relationships 135
human chorionic gonadotropin
        (hCG) 14, 15
human placental lactogen (hPL) 14, 15

immunization 318
    preconception 31
inclusivity of partners, families, and
        support persons 40
infant mortality
    African American infants 4, 30
    rate 30
    United States 4, 229
    White infants 4
Institute of Medicine (IOM) 277, 304, 307
    Summit on Integrative Medicine and
        the Health of the Public 121
integrative therapies 8, 9, 180, 183, 190
    acupuncture and acupressure 197–226
    aromatherapy 173–96
    ginger 38
    touch therapies 119–55
    water immersion/water birth 157–72

interdisciplinary education *see*
    interprofessional education
interprofessional education (IPE)
    275–99
  barriers 276, 288–90
  competencies, health professions
    education 279
    medical 282
    residency 282–4
    midwifery 284–8
    comparison among CNM, CM,
      CPM 285–7
    nursing 279–81
  competencies IPE 275, 278
  continuing education
    opportunities 296
  definition IPE, WHO 277
  documents recommending IPE
    Core Competencies for
      Interprofessional Collaborative
      Practice 277
    Health Profession Education:
      A Bridge to Quality 277
    Institute of Medicine Crossing the
      Quality Chasm 277
    Interprofessional Education
      Collaborative (IPEC) 277
    Pew Health Commission five
      recommendations 277
  Maternity care IPE 291–6
  maternity care models
    collaborative practice between
      midwives and
      obstetricians 291–3
    proposed maternity care IPE 294–6
    concepts 295
    examples 295
    topics 295
  models of IPE existing 293–4

Joint Commission 6, 234, 254, 301,
    323, 331

Kaiser Family Foundation 314, 315, 317
Krieger, Dolores 126, 129
Kunz, Dora 126, 128

labor admission 53–4, 239, 240
laboring down 243, 268
labor physiology 8, 19–23
  labor initiation 19
  uterine phases summary 24
labor support *see* physiological labor
    and support
Lamaze International 39, 92, 237, 331
  six care practices 52–3, 230–231,
    237, 246
Listening to Mothers II survey 84,
    92, 270
low birth weight 29, 30, 32, 33, 124, 302
  Black infants 29
  White infants 29

March of Dimes 4, 312, 331, 332
Maslow's hierarchy 134
Massage 24, 38, 39, 44, 56, 58, 85,
    97, 99, 114, 120, 121,
    124–7, 136–41, 180, 183,
    186–9, 203, 222, 232, 233,
    238–40, 262, 268
maternal-fetal circulation 13, 15
maternal mortality
  African American women 4
  rate 4
  United States 229, 301
  White women 4
maternal weight gain 18
Maternity Care Working Party 5
McGill Pain Questionnaire 55, 137
Medicaid 4, 6, 308, 309, 313–20
Medicare 6, 307, 308, 311, 313, 314, 317,
    318, 320
  American College of Nurse Midwives
    reimbursement table 309
midwifery model of care 30, 50, 80,
    85–7, 263
mind-body-spirit connection 119

National Center for Complementary and
    Alternative Medicine
    (NCCAM) 125, 175, 332
National Institute of Child Health and
    Human Development 6

National Quality Forum 6, 234, 331
Natural Hospital Birth: The Best of Both
        Worlds 42, 334
nitric oxide (NO) 14
normal birth *see* physiologic birth
nurses role in labor 94

Odent, Michel 158, 258
Optimality Index û US 6
optimized prenatal care setting 29, 36
oral hydration 49, 69
Organization for Economic
        Co-operation and
        Development (OECD) 4, 5
Our Bodies Ourselves: Pregnancy and
        Birth 40, 236, 333
out-of-hospital birth 6, 8, 42, 230,
        251–74, 312, 313, 333
    authority, centrality, privacy 251,
        258–9, 265
    barriers 269–71
    consultation networks 252, 263
    direct reimbursement 270
    evidence for 256–8
    Future of Home Birth in the United
        States: Addressing Shared
        Responsibility 254–6
    history 252–4
    home birth case study 260–261
    hospital response to patient
        preferences 270
    liability insurance 270
    Planned Out-of-Hospital Birth
        Transport Guidelines 312–13
    prenatal preparation for 264
    principles for safe 257
    quality improvement 266
    students 271
    transfer 264–6, 313, 314
        case study 266–9
        communication in 264
oxytocin 15, 16, 19–24, 27, 52, 94,
        160, 162, 206, 216, 242, 244,
        265, 311
    oxytocin receptor 16, 21
    oxytocin sensitivity 21

pain in labor 23–5, 83–5, 87, 106, 113,
        125, 137
    gate control theory 124, 160
partograph 59–61
perinatal paradox 5
physiologic changes in pregnancy
    cervical remodeling 17
    cervical ripening 16, 21, 22
    coagulation factors 17
    endocrine 15–16
    hematologic 17–18
    nutritional 18–19
    respiratory 18
    uterine adaptation 16
physiologic support during pregnancy
    anticipatory guidance 34
    centering pregnancy 36
    childbirth education 39
    definition 33
    family centered care 35
    group prenatal care 36
    listening to women 34
    mindfulness 115
    partners/family involved 35, 40
    prenatal care, supportive 33–43
    psychological support 35
    therapeutic alliance 34–5
    Yoga 25, 109, 115, 123
physiologic support in labor and
        birth 50–71
    admission process 53–4
    assessing coping 55–7
    assessing progress 59
    definition 50–51, 231
    disrupts physiologic processes 69, 70
    environment 94, 114, 232
        PLACE 233
    2nd stage
        care during birth 66–8
        heat and cold 112
        laboring down 243
        positioning 243, 268
        positive encouragement 65
        principles to encourage progress 65
        pushing
            final phases of 65, 66

promoting intact perineum 67–8
spontaneous 41, 49, 63, 111, 231, 237
supporting the woman 64–5
nonpharmacologic strategies 25, 56, 58, 79, 83, 136, 166, 185, 232, 261, 308
physical hygiene 114
promoting comfort 57–8
3rd stage
maternal/newborn bonding 245
physiological management of third stage 244
third stage case study 245
1st stage
breathing techniques 56, 58, 107, 111
epidural support 242
first stage labor case study 240
heat and cold 105, 112
imagery 82, 105, 111–12, 114, 139, 189
language use 57, 108, 128
movement (mobility) 44, 49, 51, 57, 61, 115, 137, 140, 160, 166, 231, 233, 237, 241, 259, 261
music 56, 82, 97, 98, 105, 108–9, 122, 137, 233, 238–40, 260
one-to-one nursing care 231, 241, 242, 265
positioning 113, 137
progressive relaxation 242
transition to the care environment 82
Pitocin 62, 93, 165–7, 268
placenta 13–16, 18–24, 95, 163, 170, 181, 184, 214, 215, 243, 245, 261
positions for birth 41, 64–5, 243
hands and knees 57, 58, 65, 67, 113, 168, 240, 242, 243, 260, 261
high Fowler's 70
side lying 64, 65, 67, 70, 113, 242, 243
squatting 65, 67, 113, 168, 238, 243, 244
supine 54, 65, 67, 68, 113, 231, 237, 244
posterior pituitary 16, 20, 21

preconception care 30–33, 38, 43, 141, 314
exercise 31, 32
folic acid 31, 32, 43
healthy weight 32, 43
immunizations 31, 318
nutrition 32, 43
previous risks/adverse outcomes 33
unhealthy practices 32–33
preferred birth experience 40
prenatal care
reduced visit schedule 30
risk-based approach 30
typical schedule 30
presence xi, 51, 57, 61, 65, 80, 91, 92, 96, 97, 99–101, 121, 122, 128, 136, 189, 253, 258, 261, 263, 265
preterm birth 5, 32, 33, 41, 124, 315
rate 4, 30, 37, 302
progesterone 13–21, 24
progesterone receptor Pr-A 21
progesterone receptor Pr-B 21
prolactin 21
prostacyclin 14, 16
prostaglandin (PG) 13, 15, 16, 19–22, 24, 163, 206, 214, 215
PG receptor 16, 20, 22
PG sensitivity 22
psychobiological responses to labor 23–5

quality measurement 5
triple aim 5, 6, 234, 279

racial disparities 4 *see also* infant mortality; maternal mortality
Reiki 119–28, 130–134, 136, 137, 139–42, 333
relaxation 105–18 *see also* Physiologic support in labor and birth
relaxin 14, 16, 22
reproductive life plan 31, 43
respiratory alkalosis 18
Rights of Childbearing Women 36
Royal College of Obstetricians and Gynecologists 5

Safriet, Barbara 307
Science and Sensibility blog 254
self-care (health clinicians) 130
shared decision making 5, 29, 33, 40–41,
        43, 57, 231, 254, 255, 295
Simkin, Penny 40, 95, 98, 125, 136, 334
    Birth Partner: A Complete Guide to
        Childbirth for Dads, Doulas,
        and All Other Labor
        Companions 40
skin-to-skin contact 41, 49, 69, 232, 245,
        246, 295
Society for Maternal-Fetal
        Medicine 5, 6, 231
Staffing guidelines 94
supportive direction 64
sympathetic nervous system 95, 123, 184

therapeutic touch 119–22, 124–9, 135,
        137, 139, 333
touch therapies 119–55 *see also* Healing
        touch; Massage; Therapeutic
        touch; Reiki
    case studies 140–141
    light touch sequence for laboring
        women 135
Traditional Chinese Medicine
        (TCM) 197
    typical TCM treatment 202, 203
transcutaneous electrical
        nerve stimulation
        (TENS) 84, 203
transition for the newborn 69

United Nations Children Fund
        (UNICEF) 232, 322, 323
uterine phases in pregnancy
    activation 14
    involution 14
    quiescence 14, 15, 19
    stimulation 14, 19, 22
    summary of changes 24

water immersion/water birth 157–72, 333
    candidate selection 165
    case study 170
    contraindications 165

developing water immersion
        guidelines 166–8
    history 158
    incorporating into clinical
        practice 164–9
    infant outcomes 159
    managing complications 168–9
    maternal outcomes 159–60
    positive physiological effects 160
        buoyancy 160
        hydrostatic pressures 161
        specific gravity 160
        specific heat 161
        thermal effect 161
    risks to baby 162–4
    theoretical risks to mother 161–2
woman-centered 5, 8, 29, 37, 38, 40, 66,
        71, 81, 86, 87, 100, 230, 231,
        275, 295, 303
women's health and maternity care health
        policy 301–29
    Affordable Care Act 301, 307, 316–20
        Breastfeeding policies in the
            workplace 323
        Covered preventive screening
            services 318
        Mandatory essential
            benefits 316–8, 320
    AWHONN-Guidelines for Professional
            Registered Nurse Staffing for
            Perinatal Units 311
    breastfeeding support 320
        AWHONN breastfeeding in the
            workplace policies 324
        Baby-friendly 322, 323
        facility support for successful
            breastfeeding 322
        Healthy People 2020 breastfeeding
            objectives 321
    collaboration among clinicians 302–4
    Department of Justice 307
    federal and state health insurance 314
    Federal Trade Commission 307
    Future of Nursing: Leading Change,
            Advancing Health 307
        scope of practice for nonphysician
            providers 307

government's role with private
      insurance 315
   Kaiser Family Foundation 315
home and birth center transfers 312
   Planned Out-of-Hospital Birth
         Transport Guidelines 313, 314
hospital policies
   American College of Nurse
         Midwives member survey 311
   bylaws 310
   Medicare Hospital Conditions of
         Participation 311
medico-legal climate 313
payment reform 308
   Maternity Action Team 310
   National Priorities Partnership 310

quality improvement
   California Maternal Quality Care
         Collaborative 312
   reimbursement by third-party
         payers 308
   scope of practice 304
      American Medical
            Association 305
      Board of Midwifery 305
      Consensus Model for APRN
            Regulation 301, 305
      variations in licensing
            boards 305
World Health Organization 50, 52,
      92, 222, 231, 232, 277, 322,
      323, 331

Printed and bound by CPI Group (UK) Ltd, Croydon, CR0 4YY

27/10/2024

14580244-0001